Spinal Injuries in the Athlete

Guest Editors

PIERRE A. D'HEMECOURT, MD
LYLE J. MICHELI, MD

CLINICS IN
SPORTS MEDICINE

www.sportsmed.theclinics.com

Consulting Editor
MARK D. MILLER, MD

July 2012 • Volume 31 • Number 3

SAUNDERS an imprint of ELSEVIER, Inc.

W.B. SAUNDERS COMPANY
A Division of Elsevier Inc.

1600 John F. Kennedy Blvd. • Suite 1800 • Philadelphia, Pennsylvania 19103

http://www.theclinics.com

CLINICS IN SPORTS MEDICINE Volume 31, Number 3
July 2012 ISSN 0278-5919, ISBN-13: 978-1-4557-4947-8

Editor: Jessica McCool

Clinics in Sports Medicine (ISSN 0278-5919) is published quarterly by Elsevier Inc., 360 Park Avenue South, New York, NY 10010-1710. Months of issue are January, April, July, and October. Business and Editorial Offices: 1600 John F. Kennedy Blvd., Ste. 1800, Philadelphia, PA 19103-2899. Customer Service Office: 3251 Riverport Lane, Maryland Heights, MO 63043. Periodicals postage paid at New York, NY and additional mailing offices. Subscription prices are $324.00 per year (US individuals), $503.00 per year (US institutions), $160.00 per year (US students), $367.00 per year (Canadian individuals), $608.00 per year (Canadian institutions), $223.00 (Canadian students), $446.00 per year (foreign individuals), $608.00 per year (foreign institutions), and $223.00 per year (foreign students). Foreign air speed delivery is included in all *Clinics* subscription prices. All prices are subject to change without notice. **POSTMASTER:** Send address changes to *Clinics in Sports Medicine,* Elsevier Health Sciences Division, Subscription Customer Service, 3251 Riverport Lane, Maryland Heights, MO 63043. Customer Service (orders, claims, online, change of address): Elsevier Health Sciences Division, Subscription Customer Service, 3251 Riverport Lane, Maryland Heights, MO 63043. Tel: 1-800-654-2452 (U.S. and Canada); 314-447-8871 (outside U.S. and Canada). Fax: 314-447-8029. E-mail: journalscustomerservice-usa@elsevier.com (for print support); journalsonlinesupport-usa@elsevier.com (for online support).

Reprints. For copies of 100 or more of articles in this publication, please contact the Commercial Reprints Department, Elsevier Inc., 360 Park Avenue South, New York, NY 10010-1710. Tel.: 212-633-3812; Fax: 212-462-1935; E-mail: reprints@elsevier.com.

Clinics in Sports Medicine is covered in *MEDLINE/PubMed (Index Medicus) Current Contents/Clinical Medicine, Excerpta Medica,* and *ISI/Biomed.*

Printed and bound by CPI Group (UK) Ltd, Croydon, CR0 4YY
Transferred to Digital Print 2012

Contributors

CONSULTING EDITOR

MARK D. MILLER, MD
S. Ward Casscells Professor of Orthopaedic Surgery, University of Virginia, Charlottesville, Virginia; Team Physician, James Madison University, Harrisonburg, Virginia

GUEST EDITORS

PIERRE A. D'HEMECOURT, MD, FACSM
Director, Primary Care Sports Medicine Fellowship, Children's Hospital Boston, Boston, Massachusetts

LYLE J. MICHELI, MD
O'Donnell Family Professor of Orthopaedic Sports Medicine; Director, Division of Sports Medicine, Children's Hospital Boston; Clinical Professor of Orthopaedic Surgery, Harvard Medical School, Boston, Massachusetts

AUTHORS

MEGAN E. ANDERSON, MD
Orthopaedic Surgeon, Children's Hospital Boston; Orthopaedic Surgeon, Beth Israel Deaconess Medical Center; Instructor, Harvard Medical School, Boston, Massachusetts

JOANNE BORG-STEIN, MD
Associate Professor of Physical Medicine and Rehabilitation, Harvard Medical School, Spaulding Rehabilitation Hospital; Director, Harvard/Spaulding Sports Medicine Fellowship, Boston; Medical Director, Spine Center and Chief of Physical Medicine and Rehabilitation, Newton Wellesley Hospital, Newton; Medical Director, Spaulding Wellesley Center, Wellesley, Massachusetts

ERIK BRAND, MD, MSc
Sports Medicine Fellow, Department of Physical Medicine and Rehabilitation, Harvard Medical School, Spaulding Rehabilitation Hospital, Boston, Massachusetts

DANIEL V. COLONNO, MD
Sports Medicine Fellow, Department of Rehabilitation Medicine, University of Washington, Seattle, Washington

PIERRE A. D'HEMECOURT, MD, FACSM
Director, Primary Care Sports Medicine Fellowship, Children's Hospital Boston, Boston, Massachusetts

DONN DIMOND, PT, OCS
Director of Clinical Development, The KOR Physical Therapy and Athletic Wellness, Beaverton, Oregon

ROBERT DONATELLI, PhD, PT
Physiotherapy Associates, Las Vegas, Nevada

LAUREN ELSON, MD
Instructor of Physical Medicine and Rehabilitation, Harvard Medical School, Spaulding Rehabilitation Hospital, Boston, Massachusetts

MARK A. HARRAST, MD
Medical Director, Seattle Marathon and Clinical Associate Professor of Rehabilitation Medicine, Orthopaedics and Sports Medicine, University of Washington, University of Washington Medicine Sports and Spine, Seattle, Washington

BRIAN M. HAUS, MD
Division of Sports Medicine, Department of Orthopaedic Surgery, Children's Hospital Boston, Boston, Massachusetts

STANLEY A. HERRING, MD
Director, Spine, Sports and Musculoskeletal Medicine, University of Washington Medicine Health System; Co-Medical Director, Seattle Sports Concussion Program; Clinical Professor of Rehabilitation Medicine, Orthopaedics and Sports Medicine, University of Washington, Seattle, Washington

MATT HOLLAND, PT, SCS, CSCS
Methodist Center for Sports Medicine, Houston, Texas

M. TIMOTHY HRESKO, MD
Associate Professor of Orthopaedic Surgery, Harvard Medical School, Children's Hospital Boston, Boston, Massachusetts

MANDY J. HUGGINS, MD
Staff Physician, Broward Health Sports Medicine, Weston, Florida

S. BABAK KALANTAR, MD
Assistant Professor in Orthopaedic Surgery, Division of Spine Surgery, Department of Orthopaedic Surgery, Georgetown University Hospital, Washington, DC

CHRISTOPHER K. KEPLER, MD, MBA
Thomas Jefferson University and Rothman Institute, Philadelphia, Pennsylvania

WILLIAM LAUERMAN, MD
Professor in Orthopaedic Surgery, Division of Spine Surgery, Department of Orthopaedic Surgery, Georgetown University Hospital, Washington, DC

YING LI, MD
Assistant Professor of Orthopaedic Surgery, Division of Pediatric Orthopaedic Surgery, University of Michigan, Ann Arbor, Michigan

ALBERTO F. LOVELL, BS
Research Assistant, Department of Orthopaedic Surgery, University of California, San Francisco, San Francisco, California

ANTHONY LUKE, MD
Associate Professor of Clinical Orthopaedic Surgery, University of California, San Francisco Medical Center, University of California, San Francisco; Director, Primary Care Sports Medicine and Director, University of California, San Francisco Human Performance Center, University of California, San Francisco Orthopedic Institute, San Francisco, California

KEN R. MAUTNER, MD
Assistant Professor of Medicine, Department of Physical Medicine and Rehabilitation, Department of Orthopedics, Emory University, Atlanta, Georgia

LIONEL N. METZ, MD
Orthopaedic Surgery Resident, Department of Orthopaedic Surgery, University of
California, San Francisco, San Francisco, California

LYLE J. MICHELI, MD
O'Donnell Family Professor of Orthopaedic Sports Medicine; Director, Division of Sports
Medicine, Children's Hospital Boston; Clinical Professor of Orthopaedic Surgery,
Harvard Medical School, Boston, Massachusetts

MARK R. PROCTOR, MD
Associate Professor of Neurosurgery, Department of Neurosurgery, Children's Hospital
Boston, Harvard Medical School, Boston, Massachusetts

AENOR J. SAWYER, MD, MSc
Assistant Clinical Professor, Department of Orthopaedic Surgery, University of
California, San Francisco, San Francisco, California

R. MICHAEL SCOTT, MD
Associate Professor of Surgery, Department of Neurosurgery, Children's Hospital
Boston, Harvard Medical School, Boston, Massachusetts

KONSTANTINOS M. TRIANTAFILLOU, MD
Resident Physician in Orthopaedic Surgery, Department of Orthopaedic Surgery,
Georgetown University Hospital, Washington, DC

ALEXANDER R. VACCARO, MD, PhD
Thomas Jefferson University and Rothman Institute, Philadelphia, Pennsylvania

ROSANNA WUSTRACK, MD
Orthopaedic Surgery Resident, Department of Orthopaedic Surgery, University of
California, San Francisco, San Francisco, California

Contents

> Athletes consistently recruit or transfer high levels of repetitive force through the spine and injuries to the cervical, thoracic and lumbar spine are relatively common. The paper's introduction includes a review of the functional anatomy of the spine as it relates to movements of the spine during sporting activities. Following the review of functional anatomy the paper will review special considerations and rehabilitation of spinal injuries in various sports. The specific sports reviewed in this paper will include the overhead throwing athlete in crewing, golf, football, soccer, baseball, and tennis.

> Aesthetic athletes are well recognized to suffer back pain. It is often overuse and growth related. Each aesthetic sport has biomechanical factors that are specific to the sport. These factors are crucial in understanding the injury patterns and prevention.

> Spinal pathology is relatively common among athletes. Spinal injections represent an appealing treatment option for athletes with spine conditions, as they have the potential to facilitate earlier return to play. This article reviews the utility of epidural, facet, and sacroiliac interventions in athletes with lumbar spine conditions. The existing literature regarding efficacy and potential complications of these interventions are discussed. General guidelines for the use of these procedures in athletes and for return to play are also presented.

Back pain is becoming more common in young athletes, due in part to injuries sustained during organized sports. The spectrum of clinical entities in young athletes is different from that in adults; back pain usually arises from either an acute traumatic event or chronic overuse. Acute injuries include thoracolumbar fractures, spinal cord injury without radiographic abnormality, acute disc herniation, apophyseal ring fractures, and muscular sprains. Problems associated with overuse include spondylolysis, spondylolisthesis, degenerative disc disease, hyperlordotic mechanical back pain, and atypical Scheurmann disease. It is important to remember that infection, neoplasm, or a rheumatologic condition may be mistaken for a sports injury.

Spinal deformity refers to abnormal or excessive curvature of the spine, which may occur during growth unrelated to sports but may be aggravated by sports. This article discusses these variances and their relationship to sports activities.

The prevalence of low back pain in young adult athletes is surprisingly high, with internal disc disruption being the most common etiology in this population. This article provides a brief review of the pertinent anatomy. It also addresses key findings in the clinical history, physical examination, and imaging for discogenic pain, radiculopathy, and pain from the sacroiliac joint. Nonoperative treatment recommendations are the focus, including medications, physical therapy, and interventional procedures.

As the baby boomers age, there are an increasing number of masters athletes aged 50 and beyond who remain active in sports and physically demanding recreational activities. This population is at risk for degenerative disorders of the lumbar spine, including degenerative disc disease, lumbar facet arthropathy, spinal stenosis, and osteoporosis with compression fracture, deformity, and kyphosis. The clinical presentations of spine pathology can include axial back pain, radiculopathy, neurogenic claudication, or acute/subacute fracture and deformity with resultant pain, impairment of alignment, and decreased balance. Comprehensive treatments may include medications, exercise, injec-

tion, activity modification and biomechanical correction, sports-specific
training, and surgery.

Athletes can return to their preinjury level of performance after discectomy for lumbar disc herniation. Athletes who undergo direct pars
repair for spondylolysis may be able to return to sports, but their
participation level may vary. Athletes and military personnel who
undergo lumbar total disc replacement can return to contact sports and
unrestricted full-service military duty. Distal fusion level may be a
significant negative predictor of successful return-to-play after fusion
for scoliosis. There is great variability in published return-to-play
criteria. Physicians must base their decision to release athletes back to
sport on each individual's condition and the sport.

Sporting injuries are a relatively common cause of spinal cord injury in
the United States, particularly among those younger than 30 years.
Many cervical injuries have characteristic mechanisms of injury, which
often helps to understand the nature of resulting neurologic injury.
Return-to-play guidelines are presented for cervical fractures, stingers,
transient neuropraxia, and other acquired and congenital forms of
cervical pathology. The role of the sideline physician in treating cervical
spine injury is reviewed. Literature that documents the rate of return to
play after cervical injury can help treating physicians counsel players
about the likelihood of return to play after their own cervical injury.

Cervical spine degeneration incidence appears higher in athletes with
long-term participation in competitive collision sports. However, the
clinical relevance of premature cervical degeneration in athletes is
unknown. Degenerative disease of the cervical spine is one cause of
cervical stenosis, which is thought to increase the severity of irreversible spinal cord injury and the frequency of reversible spinal cord injury.
Athletes with transient spinal cord injury should be screened for
functional cervical stenosis and counseled against return to play if
discovered. Treatment guidelines will continue to evolve as magnetic
resonance imaging and a focus on clinical outcomes are emphasized in
future studies.

CLINICS IN SPORTS MEDICINE

RELATED INTEREST

Orthopedic Clinics of North America, January 2012 (Volume 43, Issue 1)
Treatment of Complex Cervical Spine Disorders
Frank M. Phillips, MD, and Safdar N. Khan, MD, *Guest Editors*
Available at: http://www.orthopedic.theclinics.com/

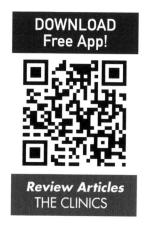

**DOWNLOAD
Free App!**

Review Articles
THE CLINICS

NOW AVAILABLE FOR YOUR iPhone and iPad

Foreword

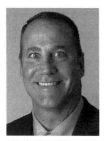

Mark D. Miller, MD
Consulting Editor

Congratulations to Drs d'Hemecourt and Micheli—they've got our back! The guest editors of this edition of *Clinics in Sports Medicine* have done a super job of recruiting an all-star lineup to produce a wonderful treatise on Spinal Injuries in the Athlete. The issue begins with two nice articles on spine biomechanics. An overview of spinal interventions is followed by a well-organized discussion of back problems in a chronologic fashion—from pediatric to aging patients. Both lumbar and cervical spine topics are covered, as well as articles on spinal cord abnormalities, metabolic diseases, and spinal tumors. This is a very well done issue and I encourage you to read it carefully and not put it on the back shelf!

Mark D. Miller, MD
S. Ward Casscells Professor of Orthopaedic Surgery
University of Virginia
Team Physician, James Madison University
400 Ray C. Hunt Drive, Suite 330
Charlottesville, VA 22908-0159, USA

E-mail address:
mdm3p@hscmail.mcc.virginia.edu

Clin Sports Med 31 (2012) xiii
http://dx.doi.org/10.1016/j.csm.2012.03.014   **sportsmed.theclinics.com**
0278-5919/12/$ – see front matter

Preface

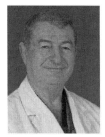 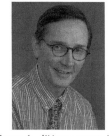

Lyle J. Micheli, MD   Pierre A. d'Hemecourt, MD
Guest Editors

The explosion in organized sports has resulted in a concomitant increase in sports injuries. While the incidence of acute injuries may actually be decreasing due to improvements in equipment and safety education, overuse injuries are on the rise—an inevitable consequence of intensive training programs that emphasize repetition of key maneuvers in the quest for performance success.

Sports injuries involving the spine are part of this trend. Here at the sports medicine division of Boston Children's Hospital we are seeing a steady increase in the number of young athletes presenting with overuse sports injuries of the spine, in particular, athletes engaged in endeavors whose training regimens involve repetitive flexion, extension, and rotation of the spine such as gymnasts, figure skaters, and dancers. Prior to the era of organized sports, it was uncommon to see an overuse spine injury in an athlete.

Adult athletes are becoming increasingly involved in recreational and competitive sports that have vigorous physical demands involving the spine—tennis and golf, for example—that may result in spinal conditions.

It is timely, then, that an issue of *Clinics in Sports Medicine* should be devoted to spinal injuries in the athletic population.

We are pleased to have secured contributions from some of the most eminent professionals in the field, who in turn have produced articles focusing on key issues in the area of sports medicine of the spine. In many cases the articles address topics that are controversial, and this makes for especially engaging reading. It stimulates the recognition of the need for continued research in the area of spine care. How exciting it is that these contributions should be gathered together in one issue!

Assembling these articles would not have possible without the assistance of several key people. Our thanks to Mark Jenkins, editorial manager at the Sports Medicine Division of Boston Children's Hospital, as well as the team of editors at *Clinics in Sports Medicine*—especially Jessica McCool, who was essential in keeping this project on schedule.

Clin Sports Med 31 (2012) xv–xvi
http://dx.doi.org/10.1016/j.csm.2012.03.012
0278-5919/12/$ – see front matter © 2012 Elsevier Inc. All rights reserved.

sportsmed.theclinics.com

Of course, none of this would have been possible were not so many respected professionals willing to give of their time, effort, and knowledge to contribute to this issue of the *Clinics in Sports Medicine*. It is a given that these men and women are all exceptionally busy, which makes us especially grateful for their involvement. It is a testament to the importance of this topic and their commitment to their field that they should set aside the time to share their expertise with us and our readers.

We hope you will appreciate and enjoy the fruits of our combined efforts.

Lyle J. Micheli, MD
Division of Sports Medicine, Children's Hospital Boston
Harvard Medical School
319 Longwood Avenue
Boston, MA 02115, USA

Pierre A. d'Hemecourt, MD
Primary Care Sports Medicine
Division of Sports Medicine
Children's Hospital Boston
300 Longwood Avenue
Boston, MA 02115, USA

E-mail addresses:
Lyle.micheli@childrens.harvard.edu (L.J. Micheli)
Pierre.dhemecourt@childrens.harvard.edu (Pierre A. d'Hemecourt)

Sport-Specific Biomechanics of Spinal Injuries in the Athlete (Throwing Athletes, Rotational Sports, and Contact-Collision Sports)

Robert Donatelli, PhD, PT[a], Donn Dimond, PT, OCS[b],*,
Matt Holland, PT, SCS, CSCS[c]

KEYWORDS

- Perturbation • Axial rotation • Cocontraction • Lumbopelvic • Spinal injuries
- Athletes • Synopsis

KEY POINTS

- Biomechanical etiology of spinal injuries in the athlete. The most common etiologies of spinal injuries in sporting activities are improper mechanics and overuse that adversely affect the stability of the spine. These forces may cause instability of the spine through disruption of the spinal support mechanisms.
- Neural control of the spinal segments. Joint mobility is complicated and involves movement in multiple planes, which is a result of the coordinated action of muscles and joints. The spine is a kinetic chain where movement at one joint is influenced by other joints in the chain.
- Dynamic stabilization. Dynamic stabilization is usually referred to as co-contraction of muscles. As previously noted, co-contraction of muscle will enhance stability and joint stiffness and serve to regulate the stress distributions during joint contact.

Athletic injuries to the cervical, thoracic, and lumbar spine are relatively common, depending upon the specific sport. In most sporting activities, injuries are secondary to overuse. With proper evaluation and treatment, it is possible to resolve the majority of injuries quickly and allow for rapid return to sport. One of the most common etiologies of spinal injuries in sporting activities is improper mechanics and overuse that adversely affect the stability of the spine. These forces may cause instability of

[a] 5920 Bella Citta Street, Las Vegas, NV 89178, USA; [b] The KOR Physical Therapy & Athletic Wellness, 735 SW 158th Avenue, Suite 160, Beaverton, OR, USA; [c] Methodist Center for Sports Medicine, 3100 Timmons Lane Suite 120, Houston, TX 77027, USA
* Corresponding author.
E-mail address: donn.dimond@gmail.com

Clin Sports Med 31 (2012) 381–396
doi:10.1016/j.csm.2012.03.003
0278-5919/12/$ – see front matter Published by Elsevier Inc.

sportsmed.theclinics.com

the spine through disruption of the spinal support mechanisms. White and Panjabi[1] have divided the spinal support mechanisms into the passive, active, and neurological. The spinal column provides intrinsic (passive) stability. It incorporates the osseous and articular structures and the spinal ligaments. The passive system is integral to the spinal stabilization by offering most of their restraint at the end of range of movement. The muscles that surround the spine provide dynamic (active) stability. Lastly, the neural control system modulates the muscle system. The muscle system changes spinal stiffness dependent on the demands of internal and external forces. During movements, the muscle activity is modulated by feedback from spindle and ligament afferents.[2] In other words, the neural system evaluates and determines the requirements for stability by coordinating the active muscular response, which we will refer to as *neuromuscular control*.

The development of an appropriate treatment plan depends on a thorough assessment of the musculoskeletal and neuromuscular systems that provide spinal stability followed by the proper prescription of therapeutic exercises to correct the identifiable deficits. A comprehensive rehabilitation program should include correction of muscle imbalances that are a result of flexibility, strength, endurance, and balance deficits.

The purpose of this article is to review current concepts regarding the functional anatomy and biomechanics of spinal movements related to spinal stability and rehabilitation in the athlete. The introduction includes a review of the functional anatomy of the spine to include spinal kinematics and muscle function as they relate to movements of the spine during sporting activities. After the review of functional anatomy, we review special considerations and rehabilitation of spinal injuries in various sports. The specific sports reviewed here include crewing, golf, football, soccer, baseball, and tennis.

SPINAL KINEMATICS
Neural Control

Joint mobility is complicated and involves movement in multiple planes, which is a result of the coordinated action of muscles and joints. The spine is a kinetic chain in which movement at one joint is influenced by other joints in the chain. In addition, the joints are interconnected by muscle and ligaments. An athlete must have greater-than-average full range of movement because often the movement exceeds the "normal" range. It is a biomechanical requirement to have excessive glenohumeral mobility for a baseball pitcher to throw a baseball at extremely high velocities. Why do some baseball pitchers have shoulder injuries and others never experience shoulder problems? Why do some athletes have a 1-time ankle sprain and others have ankle instabilities that may require surgical intervention? The answer to both questions is a combination of strength, endurance, and neuromuscular control. Depending on the situational demands of the sporting activity, the central nervous system derives or selects specific programs for the motor solution to the problem. The motor program then recruits the specific motor units to execute a coordinated motor response.[2] The muscle must be set on a higher state of readiness to prevent injury by protecting joints from perturbation forces and be able to execute exceptionally skilled activities performed at high velocities. This higher state of readiness of the neural control of the muscle system can be achieved through neuromuscular training.

Spinal Mobility

The principal motions of the spine are flexion, extension, lateral flexion, and rotation. Variations among individuals are considerable. Men were determined to have more mobility in flexion-extension and women had greater flexibility in lateral flexion.[3] McGill and coworkers[3] determined that there was a reduced range of motion in full flexion and lateral bending, but not in axial twist, when elderly were compared with younger subjects. Pearcy and colleagues[4] noted that during flexion and extension of the lumbar spine, each vertebra undergoes an arcuate motion in relation to the next lower vertebra, which is caused by a combination of rotation and translation in the sagittal plane. Bogduk[5] reported that for any arch of movement from a starting position to the end position of the moving vertebra, the center of movement is known as the *instantaneous axis of rotation*. In normal conditions, the instantaneous axis of rotation of flexion-extension and lateral flexion lies within the disc and generally in the posterior part of the disc.[6,7]

Pearcy and Bogduk[8] determined that the relative movement of any vertebrae follows a pattern, a spinal rhythm, referred to as a *coupled motion,* that is a result of the elasticity and tensile strength of the passive tissues and the coordinated action of spinal muscles. The above studies show the interdependence of movement in the spine.

Ochia and colleagues[9] studied the complex coupling motion of the spinal segments using computed tomography scanning. The results of this study showed that the segmental movements were small, with the greatest motion in axial rotation, lateral bending range, and frontal translations; all of the above movements are important to many complex athlete movement patterns. The greatest amount of movement was at the L1–2 and L3–4 segments. The amount of movement was dependent on facet orientation; L1–2 facet orientation is more sagittal and L5–S1 is a more coronal position.

Chronic low back pain has been associated with spinal instabilities. In sports such as baseball, tennis, and golf, rotational movement patterns are essential to performance; however, repetitive rotational movement patterns can cause microtrauma. If dynamic stabilization is not present, the repetitive aggressive rotational movements can be destructive to the spinal segments, causing instability and pain.

Kong and coworkers[10] found that the range of motion, intradiscal pressure, forces in ligaments, and load across facets increased nonlinearly with the increases in trunk flexion and with a load held in hands. At greater loads carried in the hands or at larger flexion postures, muscles were found to play a more crucial role in stabilizing the spine compared with the passive structures. Muscle "dysfunction" destabilizes the spine, reduces the role of facet joints in transmitting load, and shifts loads to the discs and ligaments. Potvin and O'Brien[11] found that prolonged, submaximal, isometric, lateral bend contractions were sufficient to fatigue the agonist trunk muscles. The test participants then responded to this fatigue by increasing the activation levels of the agonist and antagonist trunk muscles such that cocontraction forces were estimated to increase. Based on the above findings, the fatigue of the agonist trunk muscles response was assumed to cause an increase in spine compression, resulting in increased trunk stiffness and a subsequent enhancement of spine stability. Although initially, this type of finding seems to be contradictory, there seems to be a neural adaptation that takes place that increases activation of the muscle to augment the increased fatigability of the actual muscle fibers. This type of response can then be considered a protective mechanism. In addition to augmenting stability and joint stiffness, cocontraction also can serve to regulate the stress distributions during joint contact.[12,13]

One of the areas that we have observed in athletes with thoracic spine facet strains is pain with palpation of the costovertebral joints and limited rib mobility. Watkins and colleagues[14] showed the biomechanical role of the costovertebral joints and rib cage in stabilizing the thoracic spine is significant, especially in lateral bending and axial rotation. The costovertebral joints are important stabilizers of the thoracic spine motion segments, and the state of the costovertebral joints should be assessed in evaluating the stability of the thoracic spine.[14]

The above studies have significant implications for athletes because the majority of athletic movement patterns are focused around axial rotations such as twisting and lateral bending in a swing or throwing an object, lateral bending in pulling and pushing activities, and frontal translations in a lunge or squat/lift. In addition, all of the above activities need to be performed while maintaining balance and agility during a dynamic gait. McGill[15] describes all movement as broken down into 6 functional patterns: (1) squat/lift, (2) push/pull, (3) twist, (4) maintaining balance, (5) lunge, and (6) gait.

Furthermore, the above spinal movements must be an arch motion of the vertebra above and the next lower vertebra, which is caused by a combination of rotation and translation in the sagittal plane with an instantaneous axis of rotation. This movement follows a spinal rhythm, referred to as a *coupled motion*, that is a result of the elasticity and tensile strength of the passive tissues and the coordinated action of spinal muscles. The above studies show the interdependence of movement in the spine.[6–9]

Spinal Dynamic Stabilization

Bergmark[16] categorized the trunk muscles into global and local muscle systems. The local muscles included deep muscles and the deep portions of other muscles that had their insertions on the vertebrae. These muscles control the stiffness and the intervertebral relationship of the spinal segments and the posture of the segments. The global muscle system encompasses the large, superficial muscles of the trunk that do not have direct attachment to the vertebrae. These muscles are the torque generators and control spinal posture, balance the external loads applied to the trunk, and transfer loads from the thorax to the pelvis.[16] Muscle dysfunction may reduce the stability of the spinal system and shift loads to the intervertebral discs, ligaments, and facet joints.[9]

Dynamic stabilization is usually referred to as *cocontraction of muscles*. As previously noted, cocontraction of muscle will enhance stability and joint stiffness and serve to regulate the stress distributions during joint contact.[12,13] However, strength deficits of back muscles do not seem to be related to low back pain. Biering-Sorensen[17] found that isometric back strength did not predict the appearance of low back pain in previously healthy subjects over a 1-year follow-up period. However, Luoto[18] and Biering-Sorensen[17] suggested that poor static back endurance scores are related to the onset of back pain. Muscle endurance appears to be linked with better back health. A recent study by McGill and coworkers[19] observed that low back trouble is associated with poor endurance of the back extensors when compared with the flexor endurance.

The athlete is fixated on the development of power as a means to improving performance. Power equals the velocity of movement times the force. McGill[15] indicates that power generated in the spine is specific to angular motion of the vertebrae, which results in greater force to the spine, creating an increased risk of injury and decreased performance. Therefore, generating rapid spinal movements is much safer when the spine is not bending, thus, creating lower forces.[15] Marras and colleagues[20] also determined that spine velocity is associated with greater risks of back problems. In most athletic activities, the power is generated by the hips with a stable trunk. Often we hear the hitting coach talk about the power in a baseball swing is in the core.

We have observed and tested hundreds of athletes with low back pain and lower extremity injuries that demonstrate tightness of the hip flexors and weakness of the gluteal maximus, posterior fibers of gluteus medius, and the deep 6 external rotators. Tsai and coworkers[21] demonstrated that hip strength in general and left hip abductor strength was greater in elite golfers.[21] Watkins and colleagues[22] demonstrated the importance of trunk and hip muscles in stabilizing and controlling the loading response for max power and accuracy in golfers.

Muscle dynamic stabilization and endurance seems to be the key to a healthy back. Because the majority of athletic movement patterns involve a twisting or rotational movement, the only mechanism to control those forces is a cocontraction or dynamic stabilization. A study that performed 3-dimensional trunk loadings, especially tasks involving axial twist moments, resulted in complex patterns of muscle activity.[23] The above study found that axial twisting involves substantial cocontraction of rectus abdomens and erector spinae muscles, despite their limited potential to generate twisting moments.[23–26] Presumably, the apparent excess lumbar muscle cocontractions noted above are used in part for stiffening the spine.[27,28] Stiffening of the spine via cocontraction of spinal muscles protects the spinal segments while rotational power is developed in the pelvis, hips, lower legs. Chaudhari and coworkers[29] demonstrated that professional baseball pitchers that had greater Lumbopelvic control had greater velocity, better control, and more endurance.

The following tests can be used to determine trunk torsional control. The push-up test (**Fig. 1**) and the single leg bridge test (**Fig. 2**) are good tests to determine torsional trunk control. Trunk muscular endurance tests include lateral musculature test (side bridge) (**Fig. 3**), flexor endurance test (**Fig. 4**) and back extension test (**Fig. 5**).

To achieve cocontraction of muscle and promote endurance, McGill and coworkers[19] advocate abdominal bracing, isometric loading times, and exercises that involve high repetitions with low resistance. Abdominal bracing involves cocontraction of all the abdominals and the extensors, while the spine is held in neutral. Isometric holds for different muscle groups that surround the trunk have been advocated by several references noted above.[17,19,27] The hip and pelvis muscle strength is essential to protect the trunk. Exercises that isolate the posterior lateral hip muscles are essential to hip strength. Strength testing and exercise for the posterior fibers of gluteus medius and gluteus minimus are performed side lying with abduction and extension movement of the lower limb (**Fig. 6**). Strengthening of the external rotators (deep 6)

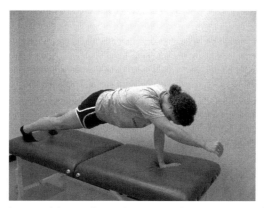

Fig. 1. One arm push-up position to determine torsional trunk control of the upper trunk.

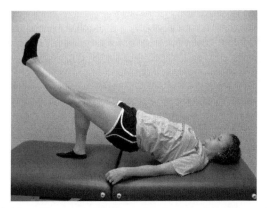

Fig. 2. Single Leg Bridge—Torsional stability or trunk control for hips and lower trunk.

can be performed in several positions, over the side of the table with the hip and knee at right angles (**Fig. 7**) or with the use of a pulley rotation device (**Fig. 8**). Hip extension strengthening is performed lying prone with the knee bent to 90° and a neutral spine (**Fig. 9**).

CREWING

Low back pain is one of the most common injuries seen in crewing.[30] The rowing stroke places a significant load on the lumbar spine and, combined with the high training volume commonly seen in elite rowers, increases the likelihood of injury. Hosea and coworkers[31] found that rowers spend approximately 70% of the stroke cycle in a flexed position of the spine. As previously mentioned, Kong and colleagues[10] demonstrated that the disc pressure, forces on the lumbar ligaments, and load across the facet joints increased with progressive spine flexion and a load in the hands. During the rowing stroke, the average compressive loads were found to be 3919 N for men and 3330 N for women with the peak compressive loads being 6066 N for men and 5031 N for women.[31] Reid and McNair[32] estimated that during a training session, rowers will commonly go through 1800 cycles of lumbar flexion.

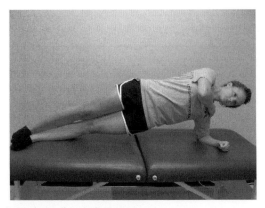

Fig. 3. Side bridge lateral muscles endurance test.

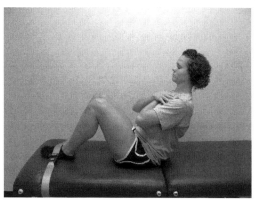

Fig. 4. Flexors muscles endurance test.

Maurer and coworkers[33] found that 41% of asymptomatic elite adolescent rowers demonstrated at least 1 abnormality on magnetic resonance imaging scan. These findings included disc changes (31.8%) and stress reaction of the pars interarticularis (27.3%). Because of the high muscular demands placed on the low back during rowing, proper lumbar strength and endurance is of the utmost importance in preventing low back injury in this population. Roy and colleagues[34] found that muscle fatigue may increase the incidence of low back pain in rowers. With back extensor muscle fatigue, there will be a resultant increase in lumbar flexion and increased loads on the lumbar spine.[35] Proper treatment programs to rehabilitate or to prevent low back injury in the rower should, therefore, begin with a thorough assessment of the endurance of the lumbar musculature. Any inherent loss of lower extremity flexibility that will affect the lumbopelvic rhythm will also lead to decreased dynamic stability of the spine and a decreased ability to dissipate forces along the spinal column.

GOLF

Low back pain is the most common injury reported in golf in both the amateur and the professional populations.[36–39] Loss of spinal stabilization will lead to increased load

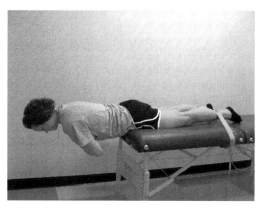

Fig. 5. Extensor muscles endurance test.

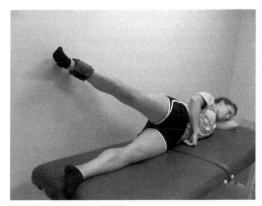

Fig. 6. Strength test and strengthening exercise for the posterior fibers of gluteus medius—side lying with abduction and extension.

transmission away from the muscular components toward the ligaments, disc, and bony structures of the spine. In golfers, the repetitive rotational movements can lead to instability and pain. There are differences among the amateur and professional golfers with regard to swing mechanics, trunk rotation strength, range of motion of the lead hip, and overall hip strength.[21,39–42] Vad and colleagues[39] attribute the modern golf swing as a primary cause of low back pain because of the twisting of the spine during the backswing and derotation and hyperextension during the downswing and follow through. Amateur golfers develop higher torque in the lumbar spine than elite golfers.[37,43] Lindsay and Horton[40] tested trunk rotation strength and endurance in healthy normal and elite golfers with and without low back pain. They found no significant difference in peak torque (strength) between the groups but did find significantly less endurance during the follow through phase in the golfers with low back pain. Biering and Sorenson[17] also found that poor back endurance rather than isometric back strength was more indicative of future back pain. The coordinated stability of the spine through complex, repeated rotational movements must be a

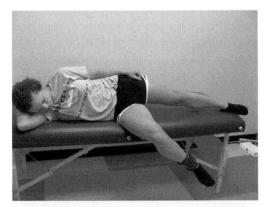

Fig. 7. Strengthening exercise for the hip external rotators. Subject is side lying with the hip and knee at right angles. Resistance can be used on the ankle with and ankle weight.

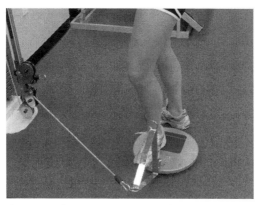

Fig. 8. External rotation strengthening with the use of a pulley rotation device. The trunk in neutral and the hip slightly flexed.

balance between strength and endurance of the hip and core. As the literature shows, golfers can demonstrate good isometric strength and poor endurance at the same time.[40] A common presentation of the golfer with low back pain generally includes weakness of the hip abductors and external rotators, decreased lumbar endurance, and tightness of the hip flexors. Watkins and colleagues[22] showed the importance of the trunk and hip muscles in stabilizing and controlling the loading response for maximum power and accuracy in golfers. Failure to properly stabilize the hip and spine will lead to spinal instability and subsequently may lead to spinal pathology and pain. In the sport of golf, this dynamic spinal stabilization must be maintained over the course of many swings throughout a golf game. Therefore, lumbar and core endurance is critical to protection of the spine in golf.

FOOTBALL

In the United States, football is one of the most popular sports played by young athletes and leads all other sports in the number of injuries sustained.[44] Low back

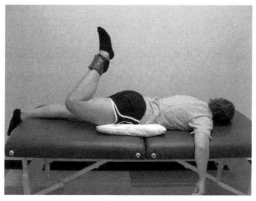

Fig. 9. Hip extension strengthening is performed lying prone with the knee bent to 90° and a neutral spine.

pain in youth football is more prevalent than what is seen in the National Football League. Looking at the 2011 opening season injury report of all 32 teams, 14 of the 187 injuries are listed as back injuries and, of those 14 players, 6 were either on the defensive or offensive lines.[45] A study that looked at the predictive value of prior injury on careers in professional American football found that a history of spondylolisthesis did not significantly reduce the chance of playing in the league for any position, whereas a history of spondylolysis had a significant effect for running backs.[46]

Spondylolysis is encountered most frequently in adolescents. It most commonly involves the lower lumbar spine, with particularly high prevalence among athletes involved in certain sports or activities such as football.[47] Because of this higher incidence of spondylolysis and other traumas to the spine, the incidence of degenerative disc disease and facet degeneration is greater in the football population than in the general population.[48] Another study found that having a spondylolysis was the most significant risk factor for low back pain in high school and college football players.[49]

The authors believe that the higher incidence of spodylolysis and other lumbar spine issues in football players is caused by the excessive compressive, torsional, and shearing forces produced in the spine secondary to improper conditioning, leading to muscle imbalances. As previously mentioned, the trunk muscles are designed to stabilize, which means they restrict spinal movements by cocontractions, whereas the pelvis and hip muscles generate the power. Inadequate training of all of the above muscle groups will result in a "dysfunctional" and destabilized spine.

Spinal stability can be maintained in a neutral position with little emphasis on strength and greater prominence on sustained contractions or endurance. Football is strongly associated with explosive power and strength. To achieve powerful and strong athletes, the ensuing conditioning and strength training is based on explosive and heavy weight lifting. The majority of football players do not receive the proper endurance training for their local and global stabilizers of the spine. The strength training needs to be focused on hip extensors, external rotators, and abductors to negate muscle imbalances that usually include hip weakness of the above muscle groups and hip flexor tightness or increased strength. In fact, the increased incidence of low back pain in some athletes has been related to increased strength of the lumbar flexors creating a muscle imbalance of flexor-to-extensor ratios.[50] Hip flexor tightness can cause an anterior tilt of the pelvis, which has also been associated with low back pain. Strength of the abdominal muscles can counteract the pelvic tilt. However, abdominal strength is usually lacking and, therefore, unable to counteract the pelvic tilt. This anterior tilt can then cause increased compressive and shear forces through the T12–L5 segments from which the Psoas muscle originates.[50]

The exercises that should be part of a football player's conditioning and rehabilitation program include the side bridge, the single leg bridge, prone bridge, lunges, and all 4's arm/leg lift. The side bridge (see **Fig. 3**) has been shown to elicit good electromyography (EMG) activity in the longissimus thoracis, lumbar multifidus, external obliques, rectus abdominus, and the gluteus medius.[49] The single leg bridge (see **Fig. 2**) has been shown to elicit good EMG activity of the longissimus thoracis, lumbar multifidus, gluteus medius, and gluteus maximus.[49] The prone bridge has been shown to elicit good activity of the external obliques and rectus abdominus.[49] The All 4's arm/leg lift has been shown to elicit good EMG activity in the longissimus thoracis, lumbar multifidus, gluteus medius, gluteus maximus, and hamstrings.[49] Lastly, lunges while holding a weight in 1 hand and keeping the trunk and shoulders stiff has been shown to cause increased activity within the contralateral iliocostalis and quadratus lumborum,[15] 2 critical stabilizers of the trunk.

Together, these exercises will target the majority of the global and local dynamic stabilizers of the spine and the support musculature of the hip. This will allow for the proper stiffening of the spine in all 6 functional patterns.

SOCCER

Spinal injuries in soccer are not reserved to just the elite or semiprofessional; they have been reported in pediatric, adolescent, and adult soccer players. Rassi and colleagues[51] found spondylolysis in pediatric and adolescent soccer players, and 43% of the patients noted pain with the forward kick. Another study found that the incidence of spondylolysis was at 30% in the soccer-playing population, which was 5 times the national average.[52] One study out of Europe found that elite soccer players had a higher incidence of osteophytes and that forwards specifically had decreased disc height in the lumbar spine.[53] Reducing injuries and improving performance in soccer is very much dependent on neuromuscular control.

It cannot be emphasized enough that dynamic stabilization exercises need to be the essence of training for competitive soccer players. Arend and Lemmink[54] defined dynamic stability as the capability of the neuromusculoskeletal system to maintain or resume an upright position of the trunk in the presence of disturbances. Trunk and hip stability are maintained primarily by well-coordinated neuromuscular control, which can be defined as a dynamic process of maintaining balance.[54] In a soccer game, the surroundings are rapidly changing, which brings about internal and external perturbation forces. Decreased core stability is associated with a higher incidence of lower extremity injuries and low back pain in a physical contact sport, such as soccer. Neural muscular control is crucial in maintaining stability of the trunk and hip to reduce injuries and improve performance. Several studies have found that deficient trunk and hip neuromuscular control predisposes athletes to low back and lower extremity injuries.[55–60] Arend and Lemmink[54] demonstrated that reaction times are shorter in soccer players compared with less-active nonplayers. The above study found that reflex delays of soccer players were shorter for perturbations in the sagittal plane but not in the frontal plane, which may reflect the lumbar spine's natural propensity for sagittal plane movements during soccer activities.[54] Muscles acting in the sagittal plane encounter a greater challenge in providing core stability, whereas frontal plane stability is more controlled by passive tissues.[54]

OVERHEAD ATHLETE: BASEBALL AND TENNIS

In overhead athletes, the creation of power to hit or throw a ball is a coordinated movement through the kinetic chain. Energy must be created and transferred from the lower extremity up through the trunk to the arm and ultimately delivered to the ball with proper sequencing and force production. Any loss of mobility, stability, strength, endurance, or neuromuscular control along the kinetic chain continuum will lead to a decrease in force production and increased potential for injury. The repetitive nature of these sports, combined with the extremes of spinal range of motion and speed at which the spine must move, sets these athletes up for potential overuse injuries to the spine and its surrounding musculature. Injury rates for Major League Baseball[61] from 2002 to 2008 demonstrated an overall incidence rate of 11.7% for injuries to the spine and core musculature. In tennis, incidence rates of 31% to 50% for low back pain[62–65] have been reported. Injuries in the spine in the overhead athlete commonly include disk pathology, facet injury, costovertebral joint pathology, spondylosis, and muscle strains.

According to Watkins and colleagues,[66] the rib cage is responsible for 30% of the stability of the thoracic spine in axial rotation. Often, baseball pitchers will complain of costovertebral pain within the thoracic spine, which could have several different etiologies. A specific case of a college baseball pitcher complaining of chest pain and difficulty breathing was a consequence of faulty pitching mechanics and hip and trunk muscle deficits, which resulted in rib facet and costovertebral joint dysfunction. In the late cocking phase of pitching, between foot contact and extreme shoulder external rotation, there is maximum pelvic rotation, increased trunk rotation, and angular velocities.[67] External rotation of the leg allows the foot to point toward home plate and facilitates transmission of the pelvic and trunk rotations into the lower limb. In this case, the pitcher did not externally rotate his lower limb at foot contact; instead, the foot made contact with the ground in a closed position. Therefore, the transmission of the trunk and pelvic rotations into the lower limb were limited. The lack of distribution of rotation forces through the pelvis into the lower limb prolonged rotation of the thoracic spine, resulting in increased strain to the thoracic rib facets and costovertebral joints. The reproduction of the athletes' pain within the upper and middle thoracic spine segments was elicited upon passive testing of the costovertebral articulations, indicating a hypomobility. Mobilization of the restricted segments, strengthening of the posterior lateral hip muscles, and changing the pitching mechanics resolved this problem.

Putnam[68] demonstrated that core stability was also necessary to allow for optimal transfer of force from the lower extremity through the trunk to the upper extremity. Kibler and coworkers[69] described the role of the core to provide proximal stability for distal mobility. This conception of proximal stability is especially important in the overhead athlete. Oliver and Keeley[70] examined the gluteal muscle group activity in high school baseball pitchers and found that there is a need for greater control of gluteal activation throughout the pitching motion. Chaudhari and colleagues[29] found that professional baseball pitchers with greater lumbopelvic control had better in-game pitching performance and were able to pitch significantly more innings than those with poorer control. The concept of core stability in the overhead athlete includes the strength of the hip abductors, extensors, and external rotators as well as strength and endurance of the stabilizing musculature of the spine. The treating clinician must also look at neuromuscular control and functional balance as it applies to each sport.

SUMMARY

Athletes consistently recruit or transfer high levels of repetitive force through the spine. Proper force transmission from the legs to the hips and pelvis and through the trunk is vital. Hip and pelvis joint restrictions and muscle strength deficits coupled with poor endurance of the trunk muscle will lead to spinal instability, which is habitually described in symptomatic athletes. A rehabilitation program that targets the unstable base first, and then progresses to strengthening of the pelvis and hips and targets control of movement in a sport-specific approach, should result in pain reduction, skill enhancement, and a safe return to play.

REFERENCES

1. White AA, Panjabi MM. Clinical Biomechanics of the Spine. 3rd edition. Philadelphia: Lippincott Williams & Wilkins; 1990.

2. Richardson C, Hodges P, Hides J. Therapeutic Exercise for Lumbopelvic Stabilization: a motor control approach for the treatment and prevention of low back pain. 2nd edition. Oxford: Churchill Livingstone; 2004.

3. McGill SM, Yingling VR, Peach JP. Three-dimensional kinematics and trunk muscle myoelectric activity in the elderly spine—a database compared to young people. Clin Biomech (Bristol, Avon) 1999;6:389–95.

4. Pearcy M, Portek I, Shepherd J. Three-dimensional x-ray analysis of normal movement in the lumbar spine. Spine 1984;9:294–7.

5. Bogduk N. In: Clinical anatomy of the lumbar spine and sacrum. 32rd edition. London (UK): Churchill Livingstone; 1997. p.1–261.

6. Cossette JW, Farfan HF, Robertson GH, et al. The instantaneous center of rotation of the third lumbar intervertebral joint. J Biomech 1971;2:149–53.

7. Gertzbein SD, Holtby R, Tile M, et al. Determination of a locus of instantaneous centers of rotation of the lumbar disc by moire fringes. A new technique. Spine 1984;9:409–13.

8. Pearcy MJ, Bogduk N. Instantaneous axes of rotation of the lumbar intervertebral joints. Spine 1988;13:1033–41.

9. Ochia RS, Inoue N, Renner SM, et al. Three-dimensional in vivo measurement of lumbar spine segmental motion. Spine 2006;18:2073–8.

10. Kong WZ, Goel VK, Gilbertson LG, et al. Effects of muscle dysfunction on lumbar spine mechanics: a finite element study based on a two motion segments model. Spine 1996;21(19):2197–206.

11. Potvin JR, O'Brien PR. Trunk muscle co-contraction increases during fatiguing, isometric, lateral bend exertions: possible implications for spine stability. Spine 1998;23(7):1998.

12. Solomonow M, Baratta R, Zhou B, et al. Electromyogram co-activation patterns of the elbow antagonist muscles during slow kinetic movement. Exp Neurol 1988;100: 470–7.

13. Thelen DG, Schultz AB, Ashton-Miller JA. Co-contraction of lumbar muscles during the development of time-varying triaxial moments. J Orthop Res 1995;13:390–8.

14. Watkins R, Watkins R, Williams L, et al. Stability provided by the sternum and rib cage in the thoracic spine. Spine 2005;30:1283–6.

15. McGill S. Ultimate Back Fitness and Performance. 4th edition. Waterloo (ON): Wabuno Publishers; 2009.

16. Bergmark A. Stability of the lumbar spine. A studying mechanical engineering. Acta Ortho Scand 230;20–4:1989.

17. Biering-Sorensen F. Physical measurements as risk indicators for low back trouble over a one year period. Spine 1984;9:106–9.

18. Luoto S, Hellovaara M, Hurri H, et al. Static back endurance and the risk of low back pain. Clin Biomech 1995;1:323–4.

19. McGill SM, Grenier S, Bluhm M, et al. Previous history of LBP with work loss is related to lingering affects in biomechanical, physiological, personal, and psychosocial characteristics. Ergonomics 2003;46(7):731–46.

20. Marras WS, Lavender SA, Leurgans SE, et al. The role of dynamic three dimensional trunk motion in occupationally related low back disorders: the effects of workplace factors, trunk position and trunk motion characteristics on the risk of injury. Spine 1993;18:617–28.

21. Tsai YS, Sell TC, Myers JB, et al. The relationship between hip muscle strength and golf performance. Med Sci Sports Exerc 2004;36:S9.

22. Watkins RG, Uppal GS, Perry J, et al. Dynamic electromyographic analysis of trunk musculature in professional golfers. Am J Sports Med 1996;24(4):535–8.

23. Thelen D, Ashton-Miller J, Schultz A. Lumbar muscle activities in rapid three-dimensional pulling tasks. Spine 1996;21(5):605–13.

24. McGill SM. Electromyographic activity of the abdominal low back musculature during the generation of isometric and dynamic axial trunk torque. J Orthop Res 1991;9:91–103.

25. Pope MH, Andersson GBJ, Broman H, et al. Electromyographic studies of the lumbar trunk musculature during the development of axial torques. J Orthop Res 1986;4:288–97.

26. Thelen DG, Schultz AB, Ashton-Miller JA. Co-contraction of lumbar muscles during the development of time-varying triaxial moments. J Orthop Res 1995;13:390–8.

27. Crisco JJ, Panjabi MM. The intersegmental and multisegmental muscles of the lumbar spine: a biomechanical model comparing lateral stabilizing potential. Spine 1991;16:793–9.

28. McGill S. Low back disorders: evidence-based prevention and rehabilitation. 2nd edition. Champaign: Human Kinetics; 2007.

29. Chaudhari A, McKenzie C, Borchers J, et al. Lumbopelvic control and pitching performance of professional baseball pitchers. J Strength Conditioning Res 2011;10:2127–32.

30. Perrin A. Rowing injuries. Conn Med 2010;8:481–4.

31. Hosea T, Boland A, McCarthy K, et al. Rowing injuries. Post graduate advances in sports medicine University of Pennsylvania: Forum Medicum Inc, 1989;3:1–16.

32. Reid D, McNair P. Factors contributing to low back pain in rowers. Br J Sports Med 2000;34:321–5.

33. Maurer M, Soder R, Baldisserotto M. Spine abnormalities depicted by magnetic resonance imaging in adolescent rowers. Am J Sports Med 2011;39:392–7.

34. Roy S, DeLuca C, Snyder-Mackler L, et al. Fatigue, recovery and low back pain in varsity rowers. Med Sci Sports Exerc 1990;22:463–9.

35. Caldwell J, McNair P, Williams M. The effects of repetitive motion on lumbar flexion and erector spinae muscle activity in rowers. Clin Biomech (Bristol, Avon) 2003;8:704–11.

36. Batt M. Golfing injuries: an overview. Sports Med 1993;16:64–71.

37. Batt M. A Survey of golf injuries in amateur golfers. Br J Sports Med 1992;26:63–5.

38. McCarroll J, Gioe T. Professional golfers and the price they pay. Physician Sports Med 1982;10:64–70.

39. Vad V, Bhat A, Basrai D, et al. Low back pain in professional golfers. Am J Sports Med 2004;2:494–7.

40. Lindsay D, Horton J. Trunk rotation strength and endurance in healthy normals and elite male golfers with and without low back pain. N Am J Sports Phys Ther 2006;1:80–9.

41. Cole M, Grimshaw P. Trunk muscle onset and cessation in golfers with and without low back pain. J Biomechanics 2008;41:2829–33.

42. Cole M, Grimshaw P. Electromyography of the trunk and abdominal muscles in golfers with and without low back pain. J Sci Med Sport 2008;11:174–81.

43. McCarroll J, Rettig A, Shelbourne K. Injuries in the amateur golfer. Physician Sports Med 1990;18:122–6.

44. Comstock RD, Knox C, Gilchrist J. Center for Disease Control Morbidity and Mortality Weekly Report September 29, 2006;55(38):1037–40.

45. Brophy RH, Lyman S, Chehab EL, et al. Predictive value of prior injury on career in professional American football is affected by player position. Am J Sports Med 2009;37(4):768–75.

46. Leone A, Cianfoni A, Cerase A, et al. Lumbar spondylolysis: a review. Skeletal Radiol 2011;40(6):683–700.
47. Gerbino PG, d'Hemecourt PA. Does football cause an increase in degenerative disease of the lumbar spine? Sports Med Rep 2002;1(1):47–51.
48. Iwamoto J, Abe H, Tsukimura Y, et al. Relationship between radiographic abnormalities of lumbar spine and incidence of low back pain in high school and college football players: a prospective study. Am J Sports Med 2004;32(3):781–6.
49. Ekstrom RA, Donatelli R, Carp K. Electromyographic analysis of core trunk, hip, and thigh muscles during 9 rehabilitation exercises. J Orthop Sports Phys Ther 2007; 37(12):754–62.
50. Carlson C. Axial back pain in the athlete: pathophysiology and approach to rehabilitation. Curr Rev Musculoskelet Med 2009;2:88–93.
51. Rassi G, Takemitsu M, Woratanarat P, et al. Lumbar spondylolysis in pediatric and adolescent soccer players. Am J Sports Med 2005;33(11):1688–93.
52. Sakai T, Sairyo K, Suzue N, et al. Incidence and etiology of lumbar spondylolysis: review of the literature. J Orthop Sci 2010;15(3):281–8.
53. Oztürk A, Ozkan Y, Ozdemir RM, et al. Radiographic changes in the lumbar spine in former professional football players: a comparative and matched controlled study. Eur Spine J 2008;17(1):136–41.
54. Arend JB, Borghuis J, Koen AP, et al. Core muscle response times and postural reactions in soccer players and nonplayers. Med Sci Sports Ex 2010;10:108–14.
55. Pedersen MT, Randers MB, Skotte JH, et al. Recreational soccer can improve the reflex response to sudden trunk loading among untrained women. J Strength Cond Res 2009;23(9):2621–6.
56. Cholewicki J, Silfies SP, Shah RA, et al. Delayed trunk muscle reflex responses increase the risk of low back injuries. Spine 2005;30(23):2614–20.
57. Gill KP, Callaghan MJ. The measurement of proprioception in individuals with and without low back pain. Spine 1998;23(3):371–7.
58. Zazulak BT, Hewett TE, Reeves NP, et al. Deficits in neuromuscular control of the trunk predict knee injury risk: a prospective biomechanical–epidemiologic study. Am J Sports Med 2007; 35(7):1123–30.
59. O'Sullivan P, Dankaerts W, Burnett A, et al. Lumbopelvic kinematics and trunk muscle activity during sitting on stable and unstable surfaces. J Orthop Sports Phys Ther 2006;36(1):19–25.
60. Cholewicki J, Silfies SP, Shah RA, et al. Delayed trunk muscle reflex responses increase the risk of low back injuries. Spine 2005;30(23):2614–20.
61. Posner M, Cameron K, Wolf J, et al. Epidemiology of Major League Baseball injuries. Am J Sports Med 2011;39:1676–80.
62. Kibler B, Safran M. Tennis injuries. Med Sport Sci 2005;48:120–37.
63. Safran M, Hutchinson M, Moss R, et al. A comparison of injuries in elite boys and girls tennis players. Transactions of the 9th Annual Meeting of the Society of Tennis Medicine and Science. Indian Wells, CA, 1999.
64. Hellstrom M, Jacobsson B, Sward L, et al. Radiologic abnormalities of the thoracolumbar spine in athletes. Acta Radiol 1990;31:127–32.
65. Sward L, Hellstrom M, Jacobsson B, et al. Anthropometric characteristics, passive hip flexion, and spinal mobility in relation to back pain in athletes. Spine 1980;15:376–82.
66. Watkins R 4th, Watkins R 3rd, Williams L, et al. Stability provided by the sternum and rib cage in the thoracic spine. Spine (Phila Pa1976) 2005;30(11):1283–6.

67. Aguinaldo AL, Buttermore J, Chambers H. Effects of upper trunk rotation on shoulder joint torque among baseball pitchers of various levels. Appl Biomech 2007;23(1):42–51.
68. Putnam C. Sequential motions of body segments in striking and throwing skills: Descriptions and explanations. J Biomech 1993;26:S125–35.
69. Kibler B, Press J, Sciascia A. The role of core stability in athletic function. Sports Med 2006;36:189–98.
70. Oliver G, Keeley D. Gluteal muscle group activation and its relationship with pelvis and torso kinematics in high-school baseball pitchers. J Strength Cond Res 2010;24: 3015–22.

Sport-Specific Biomechanics of Spinal Injuries in Aesthetic Athletes (Dancers, Gymnasts, and Figure Skaters)

Pierre A. d'Hemecourt, MD[a,*], Anthony Luke, MD[b,c]

KEYWORDS

- Dance • Figure skating • Gymnastics • Spinal biomechanics

KEY POINTS

- The interaction of the spine and pelvis is crucial in aesthetic sports. For instance, improper attempts to increase hip turnout in the dancer may lead to hyperlordosis of the lumbar spine with subsequent stress injury.
- The gymnast may manifest a combination of weak lower abdominal and gluteal muscles with tight psoas and erector spinae muscles. This may result in an anterior pelvic tilt and posterior element stress.
- Core and lower extremity strength and flexibility are crucial for the aesthetic athlete to avoid spinal stress injuries.
- Nutritional concerns are a significant worry with any of these activities that stress highly visible body exposure. Preparticipation and ongoing screening for nutritional intake should be part of most dance programs.

Although there are similarities and common themes in the biomechanics of lumbar injuries in sports, there are some distinct characteristics of aesthetic athletes (dance, figure skating, and gymnastics) that lead to different injury patterns. In collision and contact sports there is more direct spinal loading and trauma, whereas in throwing athletes there are significant rotational forces that are applied across the torso and spine. Aesthetic or artistic athletes involve extreme movements that are practiced

The authors have nothing to disclose.
[a] Primary Care Sports Medicine, Division of Sports Medicine, Children's Hospital Boston, 300 Longwood Avenue, Boston, MA 02115, USA; [b] Department of Clinical Orthopaedic Surgery, UCSF Medical Center, University of California San Francisco, San Francisco, CA, USA; [c] Primary Care Sports Medicine and UCSF Human Performance Center, UCSF Orthopedic Institute, 1500 Owens Street, San Francisco, CA 94158, USA
* Corresponding author.
E-mail address: pierre.dhemecourt@childrens.harvard.edu

Clin Sports Med 31 (2012) 397–408
http://dx.doi.org/10.1016/j.csm.2012.03.010
0278-5919/12/$ – see front matter © 2012 Elsevier Inc. All rights reserved.

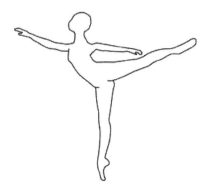

Fig. 1. The arabesque.

repetitively from an early age, which can be in all six directions of motion, depending on the discipline. In addition, many maneuvers often involve simultaneous extreme hip and lumbar spine motion.

Athletes in aesthetic sports are more commonly female, starting in early prepubescence. In the growing athlete, there is an abundance of growth cartilage about the spine, which is predisposed to injury. The nature of the artistic sports includes a great deal of spine hyperextension, increased mobility, flexibility, and axial loading from jumping and landing. Many of these maneuvers are performed repetitively during training. Arabesque and attitude a derrière are two maneuvers in which the leg is posterior while maintaining an upright posture on a single leg (**Fig. 1**), which are athletically challenging and aesthetically beautiful. Frequently performed in dance, this is also commonly seen in gymnastics and figure skating.

In dance, lumbar injuries are more common in younger rather than older dancers.[1] Back injuries are reported less frequently than extremity injury in dancers but range from 12% to 23%.[2,3] Similarly in gymnastics, extremity injuries are more common but back injuries show prevalence rates in 25% to 86%.[4–6] Back pain in singles figure skating has been reported in 12.7%.[7] To understand causes, rehabilitation from injury, and directions for injury prevention, the physical demands of the sport must be understood.

SPINAL MOTION IN ARTISTIC ATHLETES
Dance

Ideally, classic ballet attempts to maintain a very stable and stiff core or "center" while allowing the extremities to move gracefully. However, certain postures may render a more precarious lumbopelvic motion. The basic foot positions in dancers are demonstrated in **Fig. 2**. A full 180° turnout is considered to be the most aesthetically pleasing posture. This would be functional external rotation of 90° per leg and is best demonstrated in turnout a la seconde (**Fig. 3**). Here, the hip should align over the knee which should be directly over the second toe. Other significant turnout maneuvers include plie' and grand plié', in which the dancer prepares to jump by squatting from this position.

It has been demonstrated that the hip joint can attain only about 60° of turnout.[8,9] The remainder is achieved at the foot and knee. Hip anteversion is the most significant determinant of external rotation of the hip. This is defined as the angle of the neck of the femur relative to the long shaft of the femur (**Fig. 4**). The more anteverted hip will

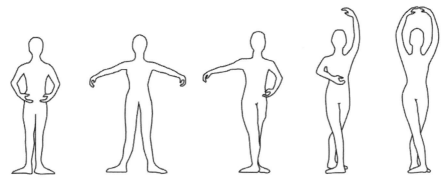

Fig. 2. The classic ballet positions, from left to right: first position, second position, third position, fourth position, and fifth position.

appear more in-toed with less ability for turnout. This is less aesthetically appealing to the dancer. Other structures about the hip that may inhibit hip external rotation include the ileofemoral ligament (Y ligament of Bigelow). In hyperflexible dancers, this may allow more turnout than anticipated by the level of anteversion. The bony alignment may be influenced by prolonged training before the age of 11 but not after.[10,11]

When the dancer is limited in external rotation there are several ways to compensate to increase turnout. However, this may increase the risk of injury both in the lower extremities and in the spine. The dancer may achieve this by rolling the foot in (pronation) as well as "screwing the knee" by externally rotating the tibia while the knee is bent.[12] Finally, by rotating the pelvis forward, the iliofemoral ligament is relaxed and the femoral head is in the more capacious posterosuperior acetabulum.[13] This anterior pelvic tilt places the lumbar spine in a more lordotic posture and places more stress and shear across the lumbar spine.[14]

Other causes of lordosis also occur in dancers. Classic ballet involves a number of motions with the back in full extension often with arabesque and attitude a derrière when the leg is posterior while maintaining an upright posture on a single leg. With

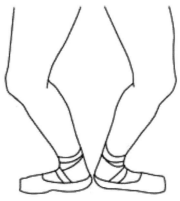

Fig. 3. Turnout a la seconde.

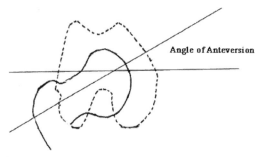

Angle of Anteversion

Fig. 4. Hip anteversion.

fatigue, an anterior pelvic tilt may occur. This is commonly due to weak abdominal and gluteal muscles with tight thoracolumbar fascia.[15,16] A tight psoas muscle has also been associated with increased lordosis. Landing from a jump with an anterior pelvic tilt may further increase lumbar compression. Male dancers are also adversely affected if this anterior pelvic tilt is maintained while performing lifts such as a "pas de deux" when dancers partner in maneuvers such as a lift.

Several other factors may increase lumbar lordosis and recurrent strain. A raked stage is one that is less common with the newer constructions. These stages are lower toward the audience and secondarily increase lumbar lordosis when the dancer faces the audience.[17,18] Similarly, heeled shoes may also increase lordosis. Finally, a genu recurvatum may also secondarily increase lumbar lordosis.

Gymnastics

Gymnastics requires multiple events in the athlete. Female gymnasts must perform on the floor, the vault, the uneven bars, and the beam. For males, six events must be mastered: the horizontal bar, parallel bars, vault, rings, floor, and pommel horse. During the floor and vault activities, there is tremendous transfer of forces from the upper to the lower extremities, with force transferred to the spine. Similar to dance, there are postures that also require lumbar lordosis.[19] With dismounts, impact forces occur that may be directed to the lumbar spine, especially if there is an anterior pelvic tilt. Increased forces are also noted across the spine with both extremes of hyperextension as well as suspension from the rings or parallel bars.[20] The traction forces can be great during swinging events such as the high bar or the uneven bars, predisposing gymnasts to lumbar injury.[19]

The handspring, vault, and walkover maneuvers caused the highest vertical and lateral impact forces to the spine.[21] The back handspring and back walkover produced the greatest amounts of lumbar hyperextension while bridging, front handsprings, and some vaulting maneuvers accentuate lumbar hyperextension. When performing front and back walkovers and during the back handspring, the maximum amount of lumbar hyperextension occurred very close to the time that impact force was sustained by either the hands or the feet.[21]

A case series of seven young competitive female gymnasts who had back injuries showed that back pain in gymnasts can be associated with abnormalities such as anterior and middle column abnormalities, including vertebral compression fractures, Schmorl's nodes, disc degeneration, and disc herniation.[22] Gymnasts can still have a weak core or an imbalance between their core muscles, despite their relatively good general limb strength and lower extremity flexibility, which can result in mechanical lower back pain.

This anterior pelvic tilt may be perpetuated in the gymnast by what has been described as the "crossed pelvic syndrome."[23] The syndrome depicts the combination of tight and overactive iliopsoas and thoracolumbar fascia along with weakness of the lower abdominal muscles and gluteus maximus. The resultant vector of forces is a forward flexion of the pelvis and secondary posterior element stress, especially during extension drills. This is also seen in the other aesthetic athletes.

Rhythmic gymnastics is an art form that combines gymnastics, ballet, and dance while handling one or two apparatuses such as ropes, ribbons, or balls. These athletes display a more excessive range of spinal and hip motion. There is a greater emphasis on artistic turnout to 180° similar to dance, and this is often accompanied by a jump. The extremes of motion to the spine are unparalleled in any sport. Most of these athletes display signs of generalized ligamentous laxity.

Figure Skating

Increased forces to the lumbar spine may be caused by several factors in figure skaters. In freestyle skating, the boot is somewhat rigid, allowing minimal ankle dorsiflexion, especially during the stroking phase. The skater may incur some secondary genu recurvatum as well as hyperlordosis to maintain aesthetic posture.[24] Specific spin moves often force the skater into various positions that hyperextend the spine. For example, a camel spin is executed when the skater extends the leg and lands into arabesque while rotating. The "Biellman" involves spinning while pulling leg above head from behind with the leg in full hyperextension (**Fig. 5**).

INJURY PATTERNS

Aesthetic sports involve challenging skills, which makes the spine vulnerable to injuries. The biomechanical mechanism of injuries for the lumbar spine include a

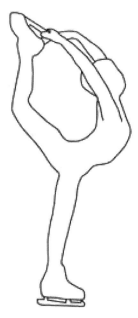

Fig. 5. The Biellman spin.

torsional injury, which is the most common.[25] This can occur from overload in axial torsion or is more often due to several minor episodes. Pathologically under rotational load, the disc annulus can be stretched and torn off its attachment to the vertebral endplate; one facet joint can be compressed and articular surface is damaged; and ligaments of other facet joint undergo traction injury. Second, a compression injury[25] can lead to axial overload, for example, during a fall. Repeated axial loads are highest at the lowest joint of the spine. Therefore, the L5 level is usually at greatest risk. Falls on the ice, in the gym, or on the stage can result in fractures of the endplate, which are difficult to see on radiographs, while the facet joint and annulus are not injured. More commonly, loss of disc thickness may become a chronic problem with subsequent development of arthritis in facet joints. With repetitive compression, a burst disc with herniation of disc contents into canal is rare. Tensile stresses are an additional mechanism and are produced through excessive motion on the spine and are common in artistic sports. Direct trauma is the least likely injury mechanism, though it may lead to fractures of the transverse or spinous processes.

Spondylolysis and spondylolisthesis are common associations with dance and other sports involving hyperextension as well as torsional forces. Spondylolysis is a fracture of the pars interarticularis whereas spondylolisthesis is a forward slippage of one vertebra over the next. This is discussed further in other article by Haus and Micheli elsewhere in this issue. This is most commonly seen at L5. In the general population, the prevalence is 4.4% in the first grade and reaches about 6% in the adult but has been reported up to 11%.[26] There is an approximately fourfold increase in the dancing population.[14] There is a wide spectrum of prevalence reports ranging from 15% and above in gymnasts.[27] Spondylolysis has also been recognized in figure skating.[28] These athletes will usually present with activity related pain, particularly with extension such as a back handspring or lay back spin. Pain is usually reproducible with lumbar hyperextension.

Other abnormalities that may mimic spondylolysis are sacroiliac strain and facet joint inflammation. In a dancer with an anterior pelvic tilt during stance, the dancer may utilize the gluteus to attempt to perform a posterior tilt known as tucking. With the ileum locked forward due to the planted feet, this may cause some posterior rotation of the sacrum and possibly sacroiliac dysfunction. Sacroiliac dysfunction is more commonly associated with asymmetric landing. This is well recognized in a figure skater who is wearing a stiffer boot.[29] With this impact, the boot allows little ankle motion and forces are directly increased at the sacroiliac joint. Similarly, a gymnast may incur asymmetric forces at the pelvis when landing from the vaults, beam, pommel horse, bar, or rings. These athletes will present with pain at the sacral sulcus and sacroiliac ligaments. Another less common but potential cause of pain that may mimic sacroiliac dysfunction is the piriformis. This is one of the small external rotators of the hip along with obdurator internus, gemellus superior, and inferior and quadratus femoris. In dancers, these small external rotators may play a significant role in the turnout, with the gluteus maximus involved in more global motion.[11,30] These athletes will present with buttock pain aggravated by activity, particularly with turnout. Prolonged sitting or standing may also cause pain, which may radiate to the posterior thigh. In these athletes, the piriformis is quite palpable and usually tender. Symptoms may be aggravated with forced internal rotation of the hip (Freiberg's test) and resisted hip abduction in the seated position (Pace's test).

In the adolescent spine, Scheuermann's kyphosis may occur with sports that also accentuate flexion activities, such as gymnastics.[31] This is defined as an excessive kyphosis of greater than 45° with three consecutive vertebrae wedged by more than 5° each. This is associated with vertebral endplate and disc changes.[32] An atypical form of Scheuermann's kyphosis is described with similar endplate and disc changes in the thoracolumbar juncture and is associated with pain in artistic athletes.[33] The pain is usually aggravated by gymnastic activity and demonstrates tenderness at the site of accentuated spinal angulation.

Discogenic pain is uncommon in younger athletes but certainly occurs in older athletes. With dance, one significant risk factor is the axial load that occurs with partnering and lifts.[34] Disc changes have been demonstrated in gymnasts and correlate well with the level of activity and hours performed.[5] These changes were identified in 9% of pre-elite, 43% of elite, and 63% of Olympic-level gymnasts. These may manifest with nonradiating back pain that is worse with flexion and sitting activities as well as at rest. Radiation may occur with nerve root inflammation.

Tanchev has described an increased prevalence of scoliosis in the rhythmic gymnast and Warren has discussed this in the ballet dancer.[35,36] It is unclear whether this is secondary to asymmetric forces across the spine or if the intense prepubertal training may affect the hormonal balance, affecting spinal curvature.

REHABILITATION CONCERNS
Core Stability

Core stability exercises remain one of the cornerstones of rehabilitation of spinal disorders in artistic athletes. Despite relatively good general body strength and flexibility, gymnasts may still demonstrate weak or imbalanced core muscles, which can be a risk factor for injury.[37] Mechanical low back pain can often be associated with inhibition of the abdominal and gluteus muscles, with overactivation of the erector spinae and iliopsoas muscles.

General models of spinal stabilization have been proposed. The Panjabi model of spinal stability includes the neural control subsystem, active subsystem (spinal muscles), and the passive subsystem (spinal column).[38] A significant decrease in the capacity of the stabilizing system of the spine to maintain the intervertebral neutral zones within physiologic limits can result in pain and disability.[38] Spinal musculature can be divided into local and global muscle systems.[39] Specific focus is recommended toward the local muscle stabilization system composed of the deep muscles, which make the major contribution to spinal stability, being closer with shorter muscle lengths to help control intersegmental motion. These smaller muscles also seem to play a proprioceptive role.[40] Multifidus is active in all antigravity activity (involved in posture) and its role is to finely adjust the spine.[41] Transversalis abdomis (TA) attaches to lumbar vertebrae via the thoracolumbar fascia, and when it contracts the intraabdominal pressure increases[42] and applies tension in the thoracolumbar fascia. Activation studies of the abdominal muscles show that TA activates before the prime movers of the hip and other trunk muscles.

Gluteal Muscles

A common source of hip pain and lower leg dysfunction in aesthetic athletes is the result of hip abductor weakness. The gluteus medius abducts and pulls the ilium away from sacrum to help keep the hip from dropping during gait. If it is weak, the lower leg adducts and internally rotates and increases stress on the tensor fascia lata. Gluteus medius weakness has been associated with patellofemoral pain, iliotibial pain, and medial tibial stress syndrome. The gluteus maximus moves with the hamstring to extend the hip and acts in conjunction with the contralateral and ipsilateral erector spinae muscles. The gluteals affect the position of the ilium extrinsic pelvic stabilizers (contraction rotates the ilium posteriorly).[43] The hamstrings, if shortened, posteriorly rotate the ilium, or can promote an anteriorly rotated ilium if they are relatively weak.

Weak hamstrings relative to quadriceps can affect proper lumbopelvic rhythm and distribution of forces on the lumbar spine.[44] Iliopsoas, which is made up of the iliacus, psoas major, and psoas minor, maintains the angle of anteversion of the pelvis and lateral stability of the spine with ipsilateral side bending and contralateral rotation of vertebrae. The abdominals may be stretched if there is significant anterior rotation of the ilium, which affects force absorption and stability at the lumbar spine and pubic symphysis.[43]

Flexibility

Artistic athletes often demonstrate hypermobility. Excessive flexibility in the vertebral column can predispose these athletes to instability and low back pain. Kujala and colleagues suggest that excessive training cannot increase lumbar spine extension.[45] They compared maximal lumbar flexion and extension in young ballet dancers, athletes (gymnasts and figure skaters), and sedentary controls in a 3-year longitudinal study. The intervention included flexibility training with the aims of maximizing lumbar sagittal mobility between T12 and S2 measured by traces of the back surface curvature in maximal flexion and maximal extension. Further, with degenerative changes in the lumbar spine, the range of motion will decrease. Therefore, excessive training to improve motion on extension of lumbar spine is not suggested. However, stretching to maintain adequate range of motion as well as maintain good flexibility of the hip flexors and hamstrings are recommended for good lumbopelvic positioning and control. In an expanded study group, Kujala and colleagues also demonstrated that low individual physiologic maximum of lower segment lumbar extension mobility was predictive of more low back pain and may cause overloading of the low back among athletes performing frequent maximal lumbar extension.[46]

Conditioning

During rehabilitation, continuing similar tasks in the respective practices is often worthwhile in artistic sports. Dancers more commonly can participate in modified dance classes to protect recovering injuries and at the same time prevent deconditioning and loss of neuromuscular training.[47] Similarly, gymnasts and skaters can continue with more traditional training often outside the gym or rink while rehabilitating from injury.

NUTRITIONAL CONCERNS

Athletes in artistic sports often train for long hours early in the morning or after classes. Some young gymnasts may be practicing up to 18 to 20 hours per week. Dancers can report similar hours or greater. With irregular and long schedules, nutrition is a challenge and not routinely a major focus for these athletes. In addition, there is a high risk for disordered eating leading to the female athlete triad, which is the presence of disordered eating, irregular periods or amenorrhea (loss of periods for more than 6 months), and osteoporosis. Aesthetic sports account for a high proportion of athletes with disordered eating.[48]

Calorie Intake

During artistic sports, athletes must have enough fuel to maintain their amount of activity. Whereas the average adult may consume 1800 to 2500 kilocalories per day, athletes and dancers need more. Energy intakes of elite figure skaters were reported as 2329 kcal/day for men and 1545 kcal/day for women, which were below recommended values for sex and age.[49] Ziegler and colleagues recommended that dietary professionals address the increased energy needs of elite athletes by recommending energy-dense foods. Unfortunately, the energy intake of teenage female competitive figure skaters is worse. The same authors found energy intake over the three seasons did not vary significantly (mean preseason, 1678 kcal/day; competitive season, 1630 kcal/day; off-season, 1673 kcal/day; $P>.05$). During the competitive season, 78%, 50%, and 44% of the skaters had intakes of less than 67% of the recommended dietary allowance (RDA) for folate, iron, and calcium, respectively.[50] Comparing gymnasts versus controls in Italy, 55 gymnasts reported better dietary habits than 55 age-matched controls. Both groups, however, reported low levels of calcium, phosphorus, iron, and zinc and energy intake deficits.[51]

Calcium and Vitamin D

Greater than 90% of peak bone mass is most likely present by 18 years of age. There are current concerns that aesthetic athletes are deficient in both vitamin D and calcium. In a survey study of 18 Australian elite gymnasts aged 10 to 17 years, 15 were found to have vitamin D levels below 75 nmol/L (30 ng/mL) and 6 were below 50 nmol/L (20 ng/mL), which is consistent with significant deficiency.[52] Thirteen of the athletes had dietary calcium intakes below those recommended for their age. Their daily dietary calcium intakes averaged 823 mg (range, 240–1740 mg). Increased dietary calcium/dairy products, with and without vitamin D, significantly increases total body and lumbar spine bone mineral density in children with low baseline intakes.[53] Vitamin D insufficiency may be defined as serum 25-(OH)D concentration of less than 30 ng/mL. Another study of young athletes in Israel showed the mean serum 25-(OH)D concentration was 25.3 ± 8.3 ng/mL, with a prevalence of vitamin D insufficiency that was higher among dancers (94%) compared to other athletes (73%).[54]

There is some evidence that calcium supplementation in athletes can have positive effects overall.[55,56] Oral supplementation with at least 400 mg of calcium per day for at least 2 years demonstrated increases total body bone density by 2.05% and in the lumbar spine and hip by approximately 1.6% each in postmenopausal women.[57] A randomized trial showed that adding 800 mg/day calcium to the diets of young distance runners of average age 23.7 years with intake of 1000 mg/day prevents cortical but not trabecular bone loss compared to placebo.[58] More studies need to be performed on artistic athletes and dancers because they are already at high risk.

Iron

Iron is another mineral that is commonly deficient in young athletes and nonathletes, and the can occur in males as well as females.[59] One study estimated that 3.3% of ballet dancers had iron deficiency anemia (hemoglobin <14.0),[59,60] which is in the same approximate range as other athletes, both male and female.[61] Thirty-six percent of male gymnasts suffered from low ferritin level (<20 ng/mL), which was double that of non gymnasts (19%). Thirty percent of females in both athlete and nonathlete populations had low ferritin levels.[59] The authors suggest that adolescent athletes of both genders in particular are prone to nonanemic iron deficiency, which might compromise their health and athletic performance.[59]

SUMMARY

Young aesthetic athletes require special understanding of the athletic biomechanical demands peculiar to each sport. The performance of these activities may impart specific biomechanical stresses and subsequent injury patterns. The clinician must understand these aspects as well as the spinal changes that occur with growth when many of these injuries often occur. Further, athletes, parents, coaches, and health care providers must be sensitive to the overall aspects of the athlete, including nutrition, overtraining, adequate recovery, proper technique, and limiting repetition of difficult maneuvers to minimize injuries.

REFERENCES

1. Bejjani F, Kaye G, Cheu J. Performing artists'occupational disorders and related therapies. In: DeLisa JA, editor. Rehabilitation medicine: principles and practice. 3rd edition. Philadelphia: Lippincott-Raven; 1998. p. 1627–59.
2. Nilsson C, Leanderson J, Wykman A, et al. The injury panorama in a Swedish professional ballet company. Knee Surg Sports Traumatol Arthrosc 2001;9(4):242–6.
3. Solomon R, Solomon J, Micheli LJ, et al. The "cost" of injuries in a professional ballet company: a five-year study. Med Probl Perform Art 1999;14(4):164–9.
4. Caine D, Nassar L. Gymnastics injuries. Med Sport Sci 2005;48:18–58.
5. Goldstein JD, Berger PE, Windler GE, et al. Spine injuries in gymnasts and swimmers: an epidemiologic investigation. Am J Sports Med 1991;19:463–8.
6. Hutchinson MR. Low back pain in elite rhythmic gymnasts. Med Sci Sports Exerc 1999;31:1686.
7. Dubravcic-Simunjak S, Pecina M, Kuipers H, et al. The incidence of injuries in elite junior figure skaters. Am J Sports Med 2003;31:511.
8. Hamilton WG, Hamilton LH, Marshall P, et al. A profile of the musculoskeletal characteristics of elite professional ballet dancers. Am J Sports Med 1992;20(3): 267–73.
9. Khan K, Roberts P, Nattrass C, et al. Hip and ankle range of motion in elite classical ballet dancers and controls. Clin J Sport Med 1997;7(3):174–9.
10. Sammarco GJ. The dancer's hip. Clin Sports Med 1983;2(3):485–98.
11. Clippinger K. Biomechanical considerations in turnout. In: Solomon R, Solomon J, Minton SC, editors. Preventing dance injuries. 2nd edition. Champaign (IL): Human Kinetics; 2005. p. 75–102.
12. Motta-Valencia K. Dance-related injury. Phys Med Rehabil Clin N Am 2006;17:697–723.
13. Coplan J. Ballet dancer's turnout and its relationship to self-reported injury. J Orthop Sports Phys Ther 2002;32(11):579–84.
14. Tsirikos AI, Garrido EG. Spondylolysis and spondylolisthesis in children and adolescents. J Bone Joint Surg [Am] 2010;92(6):751–9.
15. Micheli LJ. Back injuries in dancers. Clin Sports Med 1983;2:473–84.
16. Gelabert R. Dancers' spinal syndromes. J Orthop Sports Phys Ther 1986;7:180–91.
17. Evans RW, Evans RI, Carvajal S. Survey of injuries among West End performers. Occup Environ Med 1998;55:585.
18. Evans RW, Evans RI, Carvajal S, et al. A survey of injuries among Broadway performers. Am J Public Health 1996;86(1):77–80.
19. Kruse D, Lemmen B. Spine injuries in the sport of gymnastics. Curr Sport Med Rep 2009;8(1):20–8.
20. Bruggeman GP. Biomechanics in gymnastics. Med Sport Sci 1987;25:142–76.
21. Hall SJ. Mechanical contribution to lumbar stress injuries in female gymnasts. Med Sci Sports Exerc 1986;18(6):599–602.
22. Katz DA, Scerpella TA. Anterior and middle column thoracolumbar spine injuries in young female gymnasts: report of seven cases and review of the literature. Am J Sports Med 2003;31(4):611–6.

23. Jull G, Janda V. Muscles and motor control in low back pain. In: Twomey T, Taylor JR, editors. Physical therapy for the low back: clinics in physical therapy. New York: Churchill Livingstone; 1987. p. 253–78.

24. Fortin J, Harrington L, Langenbeck D. The biomechanics of skating. Phys Med Rehab 1997;11(3):627–48.

25. Watkins RG (Kerlan-Jobe Clinic). The spine in sports. St. Louis: CV Mosby; 1996. p. 16–7.

26. Beutler WJ, et al. The natural history of spondylolysis and spondylolisthesis: 45-year follow-up evaluation. Spine 2003;28(10):1027–35 [discussion: 1035].

27. Standaert C, Herring S. Spondylolysis: a critical review. Br J Sports Med 2000;34: 415–22.

28. d'Hemecourt PA, Gerbino PG, Micheli LJ. Back injuries in the young athlete. Clin Sports Med 2000;19(4):663–79.

29. Porter E, Young C, Niedfeldt M, et al. Sport-specific injuries and medical problems of figure skaters. Wisc Med J 2007;106(6):330–4.

30. Kirschner J, Foye P, Cole J. Piriformis syndrome, diagnosis and treatment. Muscle Nerve 2009;40:10.

31. Hollingworth P. Back pain in children. Br J Rheumatol 1996;35:1022–8.

32. Sorensen K. Scheuermann's juvenile kyphosis: clinical appearances, radiography, aetiology and prognosis. Copenhagen: Munksgaard; 1964.

33. Sward L. The thoracolumbar spine in young elite athletes: current concepts on the effects of physical training. Sports Med 1992;13:357–64.

34. Zhang Y, Guo T, Wu S. Clinical diagnosis for discogenic low back pain. Int J Biol Sci 2009;5(7):647–58.

35. Tanchev PI, Dzherov AD, Parushev AD, et al. Scoliosis in rhythmic gymnasts.Spine 2000;25:1367–72.

36. Warren MP, Brooks-Gunn J, Hamilton LH, et al. Scoliosis and fractures in young ballet dancers: relation to delayed menarche and secondary amenorrhea. N Engl J Med 1986;314;1348–53.

37. Kruse D, Lemmen B. Spine injuries in the sport of gymnastics. Curr Sports Med Rep 2009;8(1):20–8.

38. Panjabi MM. The stabilizing system of the spine. Part 1. Function dysfunction, adaptation and enhancement. J Spinal Disord 1992;5:383–9.

39. Bergmark A. Stability of the lumbar spine: a study in mechanical engineering. Acta Orthop Scand 1989;230(S):20–4.

40. Cristo JJ, Panjabi MM, Yamammoto I, et al. The intersegmental and multisegmental muscles of the spine: a biomechanical model comparing lateral stabilizing potential. Spine 1991;7:793–9.

41. McGill SM. Kinetic potential of the lumbar trunk musculature about three orthogonal orthopaedic axes in extreme postures. Spine 1991;16:809–15.

42. Cresswell AG, Grundstrom A, Thorestensson A. Observations on intra-abdominal pressure and patterns of abdominal intra-muscular activity in man. Acta Physiol Scand 1992;144:409–18.

43. Prather H. Pelvis and sacral dysfunction in sports and exercise. Phys Med Rehab Clin North Am 2000;11(4):805–36.

44. Koutedakis Y, Frischknecht R, Murthy M. Knee flexion to extension peak torque ratios and low back injuries in highly active individuals. Int J Sports Med 1997;18:290–5.

45. Kujala UM, Oksanen A, Taimela S, et al. Training does not increase maximal lumbar extension in healthy adolescents. Clin Biomech [Bristol, Avon] 1997;12(3):181–4.

46. Kujala UM, Taimela S, Oksanen A, et al. Lumbar mobility and low back pain during adolescence: a longitudinal three-year follow-up study in athletes and controls. Am J Sports Med 1997;25(3):363–8.
47. Gottschlich LM, Young CC. Spine injuries in dancers. Curr Sports Med Rep 2011; 10(1):40–4.
48. Thomas JJ, Keel PK, Heatherton TF. Disordered eating attitudes and behaviors in ballet students: examination of environmental and individual risk factors. Int J Eat Disord 2005;38(3):263–8.
49. Ziegler P, Nelson JA, Barratt-Fornell A, et al. Energy and macronutrient intakes of elite figure skaters. J Am Diet Assoc 2001;101(3):319–25.
50. Ziegler P, Sharp R, Hughes V, et al. Nutritional status of teenage female competitive figure skaters. J Am Diet Assoc 2002;102(3):374–9.
51. D'Alessandro C, Morelli E, Evangelisti I, et al. Profiling the diet and body composition of subelite adolescent rhythmic gymnasts. Pediatr Exerc Sci 2007;19(2):215–27.
52. Lovell G. Vitamin D status of females in an elite gymnastics program. Clin J Sport Med 2008;18(2):159–61.
53. Huncharek M, Muscat J, Kupelnick B. Impact of dairy products and dietary calcium on bone-mineral content in children: results of a meta-analysis. Bone 2008;43(2):312–21.
54. Constantini NW, Arieli R, Chodick G, et al. High prevalence of vitamin D insufficiency in athletes and dancers. Clin J Sport Med 2010;20:368–71.
55. Lanou AJ, Berkow SE, Barnard ND. Calcium, dairy products, and bone health in children and young adults: a reevaluation of the evidence. Pediatrics 2005;115(3): 736–43.
56. Winzenberg T, Powell S, Shaw KA, et al. Effects of vitamin D supplementation on bone density in healthy children: systematic review and meta-analysis. BMJ 2011;342: c7254.
57. Shea B, Wells G, Cranney A, et al and Osteoporosis Methodology Group and The Osteoporosis Research Advisory Group. Meta-analyses of therapies for postmeno-pausal osteoporosis. VII. Meta-analysis of calcium supplementation for the prevention of postmenopausal osteoporosis. Endocr Rev 2002;23(4):552–9.
58. Winters-Stone KM, Snow CM. One year of oral calcium supplementation maintains cortical bone density in young adult female distance runners. Int J Sport Nutr Exerc Metab 2004;14(1):7–17.
59. Constantini NW, Eliakim A, Zigel L, et al. Iron status of highly active adolescents: evidence of depleted iron stores in gymnasts. Int J Sport Nutr Exerc Metab 2000; 10(1):62–70.
60. Weight LM, Klein M, Noakes TD, et al. "Sports anemia"—a real or apparent phenom-enon in endurance-trained athletes? Int J Sports Med 1992;13(4):344–7.
61. Clement DB, Lloyd-Smith DR, Macintyre JG, et al. Iron status in Winter Olympic sports. J Sports Sci 1987;5(3):261–71.

Overview of Spinal Interventions

Daniel V. Colonno, MD[a],*, Mark A. Harrast, MD[b,c],
Stanley A. Herring, MD[d,e,f]

KEYWORDS

- Athletes • Spinal injections • Epidural injections • Facet interventions
- Sacroiliac injections

KEY POINTS

- A role exists for spinal interventional procedures in carefully selected athletes to maximize functional recovery and return to play.
- Spinal interventions in athletes should not be considered in isolation; but rather as part of a comprehensive rehabilitation program.
- When interventional procedures are warranted; they should be performed according to existing guidelines where possible and with systems in place to maximize patient safety and to consistently monitor for response.
- When returning an athlete to play after ESI, we recommend careful serial evaluation; and athletes should not return to play with any significant objective neurologic deficits.

Back pain is a common complaint among athletes. The incidence of back pain in athletes is as high as 30% and a sports related cause is identified in 6% to 13% of spinal trauma.[1] Athletes with back and neck pain not only differ from the general population in terms of epidemiology and etiology, but they are also distinctly motivated to recover. In addition to likely underreporting of back and neck symptoms compared with the general population,[2,3] athletes typically seek the fastest possible solution and return to play option. Not surprisingly, interventional spinal procedures, such as epidural steroid injections (ESIs), zygapophyseal joint (z-joint) injections, and sacroiliac joint (SIJ) injections, have become increasingly popular and represent an appealing treatment option for athletes and physicians alike.

The authors have nothing to disclose.
[a] Department of Rehabilitation Medicine, University of Washington, Box #356490, 1959 NE Pacific Street, Seattle, WA 98195, USA; [b] Seattle Marathon, 325 9th Avenue, Seattle, WA 98104, USA; [c] UW Medicine Sports and Spine, Box #359721, 325 Ninth Avenue, Seattle, WA 98104, USA; [d] Spine, Sports and Musculoskeletal Medicine, UW Medicine Health System, Box #359721, 325 Ninth Avenue, Seattle, WA 98104, USA; [e] Seattle Sports Concussion Program, 325 9th Avenue, Seattle, WA 98104, USA; [f] Orthopaedics and Sports Medicine, University of Washington, 325 9th Avenue, Seattle, WA 98104, USA
* Corresponding author.
E-mail address: colonno@uw.edu

Clin Sports Med 31 (2012) 409–422
doi:10.1016/j.csm.2012.03.004
0278-5919/12/$ – see front matter © 2012 Elsevier Inc. All rights reserved.

sportsmed.theclinics.com

Even though spinal injections have long been in the armamentarium of spine practitioners, their clinical use has drastically increased over the last 15 years. Based on Medicare data, there was a 271% increase in the use of lumbar ESIs between 1994 and 2001 with a corresponding increase in inflation-adjusted cost of $151 million.[4] One can predict a similar increase in the rate of injections in non-Medicare patients as well. Clearly, there has not been a similar increase in the incidence of spinal pain, a fact that serves to underscore that spinal interventions are increasingly being utilized as a mainstay of care for these patients. A variety of reasons can be postulated for what may be considered overuse of these interventions, ranging from treating spinal disorders as only a physical problem to the financial rewards associated with interventional care. The additional motivations and incentives inherent to the athletic population create further risk for misallocation. A systematic understanding of interventional spinal procedures is necessary to appropriately use these treatment options.

In the athletic population, interventional procedures may offer the potential for earlier return to play, but there is a notable lack of well-designed, placebo-controlled studies concerning these interventions in the general population and particularly among athletes. Furthermore, the risk of additional injury and the long-term outcomes among athletes who return to play after pain-relieving procedures are not well understood or studied. Despite the limitations of the current literature, a reasonable approach to the use of spinal injections among athletes can be developed with the goals of improving clinical outcomes and providing safe return to play.

LUMBAR EPIDURAL STEROID INJECTION
Rationale for the Use of ESI in Radicular Pain from Disk Herniation

The exact incidence of radicular pain in athletes is unknown. In the general population, the lifetime incidence of lumbar radicular pain from herniated nucleus pulposus (HNP) is 13% to 40% with an annual incidence of 1% to 5% peaking in the fourth to fifth decades.[5] Athletes, particularly those whose sport involves repetitive and powerful lumbar flexion or rotation, could be at greater theoretical risk for HNP than the general population. The L4–5 and L5–S1 levels are the most common levels for HNP. Overall, the prognosis for radicular pain from HNP is favorable. The natural history of this condition, however, can be challenging for the athlete seeking rapid return to play. Approximately 80% of HNPs improve with conservative care,[6] with 75% noting improvement within 4 to 6 weeks, 60% fully recovered at 3 months, and 75% fully recovered at 6 months.[7] Significantly, however, up to 30% of patients continue to have pain for one year or longer.[7] Resolution of HNP on imaging likely trails clinical improvement with 50% to 80% of HNP showing greater than 50% reduction in size within 1 to 2 years and the largest extrusions having the greatest likelihood of complete resolution.[8] The natural history of radicular pain from HNP is such that a significant portion of an athlete's season is likely to be affected, and thus treatments to shorten the duration of symptoms and alleviate pain are of great potential value.

Radicular pain is thought to occur as a result of both mechanical nerve compression and a chemoinflammatory response. In the athlete, mechanical compression, such as that from HNP, can cause local structural changes to nerve roots leading to demyelination, axonal transport block, vascular changes, intraneural edema, and stimulation of an inflammatory reaction.[9] However, mechanical compression by itself may not produce pain in every patient, even when compressive pathology is evident on advanced imaging. Alternatively, one can have classic radicular pain without neural impingement on magnetic resonance imaging. This is attributable to the chemoinflammatory response in the setting of HNP. An annular tear exposes the highly antigenic nucleus pulposus, triggering an inflammatory cascade that contributes to localized neural edema, altered nerve function, and sensitization.[9] Multiple sensitizing chemicals and inflammatory mediators have been identified at the site of disc injury.[10,11] Although the exact role of each substance is not known, placement of autologous nucleus pulposus around the dorsal root ganglion does cause sustained nerve discharges consistent with nociception.[11] This chemoinflammatory reaction may sensitize nerve endings such that even minor irritation may produce radicular pain in sensitized nerve roots.

Given the chemoinflammatory contribution to pain, corticosteroids provide a rational treatment approach. Although the complete mechanisms are not understood, corticosteroids are thought to decrease inflammation through inhibition of prostaglandins in the arachidonic acid cascade, which may improve microcirculation through decreasing capillary permeability, nerve root edema, and ischemia.[12,13] Steroids also directly inhibit the excitation of pain-generating c-fiber neurons.[11] Theoretically, ESIs place a higher concentration of corticosteroid at the site of pathology compared with more systemic oral therapy while limiting systemic side effects. Moreover, some animal models report possible synergistic effects of local anesthetics with steroids for improving inflammation after HNP and improving intraneural blood flow in a compressed nerve root.[13,14]

There is reasonable support for the use of fluoroscopically guided ESI for the treatment of radicular pain associated with HNP. There is evidence showing earlier relief from pain, decreased need for surgical intervention, and facilitation of an active therapy program.[9,15–21] Neither severity of symptoms nor characteristics of disc herniations on advanced imaging have been shown to correlate strongly with response to ESI. In one study, the type and size of disc herniation did not predict outcome after ESI; however, centrally located herniations and lower grade nerve root compression did predict a positive response.[22] The use of ESI in the athlete with radicular pain from HNP has not been studied but likely has a role in expediting return to play, particularly when ESI is applied judiciously and to a select patient population. Extrapolating from functional gains observed in the general population, it is reasonable to posit that athletes who achieve relief or radicular pain after ESI may return to sport earlier. Clearly, an athlete with sensory or motor deficits from radiculopathy should not return to the field, but for those with radicular pain only, ESI may represent a valuable treatment adjunct. Each decision regarding the use of ESI should be tailored to the individual athlete and clinical scenario with a focus on safety and long-term health.

Rationale for Use of ESI in Discogenic Pain

Discogenic pain (intrinsic disc pain) may result from the same local chemoinflammatory process described above. Exposure of the antigenic nucleus pulposus and sensitization of the annular or ligament nerve endings theoretically lead to this response. Discogenic pain may result from degenerative disc, annular tear, or HNP, although the latter is more likely to cause extrinsic disc pain from nerve root irritation.[13] In general, back pain from degenerative conditions, including disc degeneration, is far less likely in the athlete than in the general population primarily because of natural history and typical age of onset. Micheli and Wood[23] found a 48% incidence of discogenic back pain in the general population versus an 11% incidence in young athletes. Such incidence data, however, must be interpreted with caution, as athletes are potentially less willing to report symptoms than the general population. In a study of Olympic athletes at the Sydney games, Ong[2] reported a greater prevalence and degree of lumbar disc degeneration than in the general population. Compared with the use of ESI in radicular pain, less literature exists to support the use of ESI for discogenic pain. Given the likely role of a chemoinflammatory response in discogenic pain, however, a trial of ESI would be reasonable in select refractory cases with recognition that conclusive evidence is lacking for both the general and athletic populations.

Contraindications to ESI

ESIs, particularly lumbar ESIs, are generally safe. Absolute contraindications to lumbar ESI include uncompensated coagulopathy, infection, history of severe allergic reaction to any of the injected materials, local malignancy, acute spinal cord compression, and inability to obtain informed consent. Lumbar ESI should also be avoided in the setting of uncontrolled diabetes or congestive heart failure. Fluoroscopy is contraindicated in pregnancy. Particular care should be taken regarding the temporary discontinuation of anticoagulant and antiplatelet medications such as warfarin, ticlopidine, and clopidogrel. Because athletes are generally less likely to be taking these medications, particular guidelines are not discussed here but should be reviewed before ESI in the appropriate setting. Although not absolute contraindications, factors that negatively affect outcomes should be considered on a case-by-case basis before ESI. For example, worse outcomes have been reported in smokers, chronic pain syndrome, axial-only pain, diffuse pain, opioid dependence, and in patients with ongoing disability claims.[24] Similarly, athletes may have very unique motivations for pursuing spinal interventions, and these should be weighed carefully in the risk-benefit analysis before ESI. Although ESI is generally low risk, significant adverse outcomes can occur as discussed further below. The overall safety of the athlete is paramount despite pressure to return to play or other incentives.

Frequency/Timing/Steroid Selection

There is no consensus among experts or within the literature regarding the frequency, timing, or steroid selection for ESI in the athletic population. Despite its general popularity, no basis for a series of 3 injections exists and no definitive determination about the most appropriate frequency of injections has been made.[25] Most studies indicate that an average of 1 to 3 injections is needed to achieve significant improvement.[13] For transforaminal ESI, most subjects averaged 2 injections to reach 70% improvement.[19] The International Spine Intervention Society (ISIS) guidelines recommend no more than 4 injections in a 6-month period.[26] Others argue to limit injection to 3 per year to decrease the risk of systemic side effects.

Injections should be performed with at least 2 weeks between procedures, as it may take 2 weeks for the steroid to take full effect. If the athlete has significant partial improvement, then a repeat injection may be indicated. If there is no improvement, but radiculopathy is still suspected, a repeat injection with a different steroid or different approach is warranted. In general, there are 3 distinct fluoroscopic approaches for accessing the epidural space of the lumbar spine: transforaminal, interlaminar, and caudal. Transforaminal injections (**Fig. 1**) offer the most specific means of targeting a particular nerve root level. They are, therefore, the generally accepted injection of choice for radicular pain, although definitive evidence of superior efficacy is lacking.[27,28] Medication is introduced into the "safe triangle" at the superior aspect of the intervertebral foramen, thereby avoiding the radicular arteries and delivering medication directly to the exiting nerve root. With an interlaminar technique, the epidural space is accessed by piercing the ligamentum flavum in the interlaminar space. An interlaminar approach may be indicated in the setting of an anatomic or technical challenge, for instance, after lumbar fusion. Caudal injections

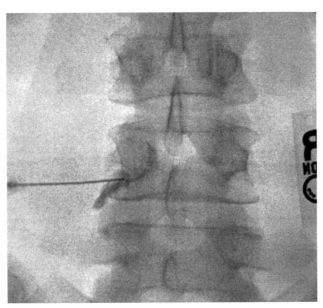

Fig. 1. Fluoroscopic image of a transforaminal epidural steroid injection shows epidural dye flow.

are administered via the sacral hiatus with needle advancement rostrally to the level of S3. A larger volume of injectant is used with more diffuse spread of medication. This affords the least amount of target specificity but may be a useful approach for lower lumbar and lumbosacral pain generators. If excellent improvement with initial or with repeat injection is observed, rehabilitation should be maximized, and the athlete may be cautiously returned to play.

Risks

Complications from lumbar epidural steroid injection are rare. Complications can result from the procedure itself or from the injectant. Procedural complications include hematoma, intravascular injection, infection, dural puncture, air emobolism, and vasovagal syncope. Serious infection is rare with a reported incidence of 0.01% to 0.1% and most often results from inadequate sterile technique.[29] Reported types of infection include meningitis, epidural abscess, vertebral osteomyelitis, and discitis.[29] Epidural hematomas are also rare with a reported incidence of 1 in 150,000 epidural injections performed on patients with normal clotting function. Intravascular uptake occurs in 8% of all lumbar injections.[29] There have been no reported severe effects of intravascular injection of contrast or local anesthetic. There have been multiple reports, however, of paraplegia resulting from the intravascular injection of particulate steroids into the artery of Adamkiewicz. There have been no reported complications of intravascular injection of nonparticulate steroids. Risk of intravascular uptake is further reduced when using the combination of live fluoroscopy with contrast and digital subtraction angiography.[30] Nerve damage from nerve puncture and intraneural hematoma is also a theoretical risk but is unlikely to occur in an awake patient. Dural puncture is rare but is more likely to occur with interlaminar ESI. Dural puncture alone caries no serious risk, but may cause a spinal headache. Intrathecal injection of local anesthetic causes variable levels of spinal block, and intrathecal injection of any substance, particularly corticosteroid, may lead to arachnoiditis.[29] Vasovagal syncope occurs in 1% to 2% of lumbar ESI (LESI) and in 8% of cervical ESI.

Serious complications related to the injectant are rare. Hypersensitivity or anaphylactic reactions occur most commonly with contrast but may also occur with local anesthetic. Corticosteroids have systemic side effects, such as the elevation of blood glucose in diabetics an average of 106 mg/dL on the evening of injection and increased levels for 3 days.[31] Caution should be taken in patients with congestive heart failure, as fluid retention can occur. There is also the potential for hypothalamic-pituitary-adrenal axis suppression lasting up to 4 weeks.

Benefits of Lumbar ESI

In the general population, consensus opinion regarding the efficacy of LESI has been difficult to achieve for various reasons related to heterogeneous study design, patient selection, injection technique, and outcome measures. Consensus does exist across review articles in that LESI likely provides short-term relief of radicular pain. Variable evidence exists for longer-term pain relief, disability, axial pain, and surgery avoidance. Few studies exist comparing the progression to surgery in patients treated with ESI versus those not receiving ESI. Theoretically, LESI offers a temporizing measure to help patients through acute flares, thereby avoiding surgical intervention (ie, for pain management). There is also some prognostic value with LESI. A greater than 80% immediate improvement in leg symptoms and greater than 50% relief for at least 1 week after ESI predicts greater than 50% relief with surgical decompression.[32]

Most of the randomized, controlled trials regarding LESI have relied on self-reported decrease in pain and disability as the primary outcome. In a placebo-controlled study, Vad and coworkers[19] compared transforaminal epidural steroid injection (TFESI) with saline trigger point injection and found that in patients with leg pain greater than back pain from HNP for at least 6 weeks, significantly more patients treated with TFESI declared at least 50% pain relief and at least 5-point improvement on the Roland-Morris Disability Index than those treated with trigger point injection (84% vs 48%). The study was not blinded, and raw data and baseline characteristics were not provided.

Karppinen compared TFESI with transforaminal saline injections and found that in patients with clinical evidence of radicular leg pain, those treated with either steroids or saline showed significant improvement over time with greater improvement in the steroid group at 2 weeks. Limitations included technical quality of injection (lower-than-expected local anesthetic effect) and only 1 injection allowed. This study does bring to light the possible therapeutic effect of saline as a washout of chemoinflammatory mediators in the epidural space.

Ng and colleagues[33] compared TFESI with transforaminal injection of bupivacaine only in patients with chronic radicular pain from HNP or lumbar stenosis. They found decreased pain and disability at 6 and 12 weeks in both groups, with shorter duration of symptoms being the only predictor of better outcome. Several studies compare TFESI with other approaches, but interpretation of each is limited by methodologic concerns. Akerman and Ahmad[27] used strict selection criteria for 90 patients with S1 radiculopathy and randomly assigned patients to TFESI, interlaminar epidural steroid injection (ILESI), or caudal ESI. Oswestry disability scores were similarly improved for all groups, whereas pain improvement was reported to be better for TFESI, attributed to more anterior spread of medication. Pain scores were not reported, however, making clinically relevant differences difficult to discern.

In a small sample of 31 patients, Thomas and colleagues[28] found that fluoroscopically guided TFESI improved pain greater than blind ILESI, which is of no surprise given the high miss rate with blind injections. Kolsi and coworkers[34] found that both fluoroscopically guided TFESI and ILESI provide similar improvement at 2 weeks, but follow-up beyond 2 weeks was not reported. Finally, Candido and colleagues[35] compared ILESI and TFESI in patients with low back pain and unilateral radicular symptoms and found no significant differences in visual analog scale scores, but significant crossover limits interpretation of this outcome. There are still no high-quality, prospective, controlled studies specifically evaluating the efficacy of fluoroscopically guided ILESI or caudal ESI. The available controlled studies with and without fluoroscopy still do tend to support some relative short-term pain relief from ILESI or caudal ESI, with variable long-term benefit beyond 4 weeks.

No studies exist regarding the efficacy of LESI in athletes. Extrapolating from the existing literature in the general population, however, it is reasonable to conclude that LESIs are likely to provide short-term pain relief and improved function in athletes with radicular pain from HNP as well as in athletes with discogenic pain. This may allow the appropriately selected athlete to return to sport earlier. Although no definite evidence exists to support a particular return to play algorithm after ESI in the athlete, the authors propose the following general approach: before proceeding with ESI and considering return to play, the specific rules and regulations pertinent to the athlete's sport and its governing body should be clarified. For example, NCAA and Olympic athletes require therapeutic use exemptions for ESIs.

If, after ESI, neurologic examination abnormalities exist, the athlete should not return to play. With pain only and a normal neurologic examination after injection, return to play is most likely safe; however, risks of return to play should be considered carefully within the individual context and with involvement of parents, athletic trainers, and coaches where appropriate. Decisions should account for the demands of the individual sport and position. If and when an athlete is appropriate for return to play, rehabilitation should proceed in a graduated fashion, progressing toward sport-specific activities. Additionally, the athlete's maintenance training programs should emphasize core conditioning and proper athletic technique.

ZYGAPOPHYSIAL JOINT INJECTIONS, MEDIAL BRANCH BLOCKS, AND RADIOFREQUENCY NEUROTOMY
Rationale for Use in Zygapophyseal Joint Mediated Pain

Although historically controversial, zygapophyseal or facet joints are now generally accepted as pain generators. The 2 posterior joints along with the intervertebral disc make up the functional unit of the spine. Histologic studies have found that zygapophyseal joint (z-joint) capsules have multiple forms of innervation and contain chemical mediators, such as substance P, calcitonin, and neuropeptide Y.[36] This suggests the presence of nociceptive afferent and sympathetic efferent fibers.[36] Each zygapophyseal joint is diarthrodial with a distinct joint capsule that can accommodate 1 to 1.5 mL of fluid. The z-joints are generally innervated by medial branches of the dorsal ramus, although exceptions exist at several levels. Interventional approaches for z-joint pain include diagnostic medial branch blocks (MBBs) followed by radiofrequency neurotomy as well as intra-articular injections.

The exact incidence of lumbar zygapophyseal joint pain in the athlete is not known. In the general population, z-joint–mediated pain has been estimated to account for 15% to 40% of low back pain.[36] Theoretically, z-joint joint pain may represent a relatively higher percentage of back pain in athletes, particularly in sports involving repetitive lumbar extension or axial rotation. This has been suggested in adolescent tennis players with 70% of asymptomatic elite teenage tennis players showing at least 1 level of facet arthropathy.[37] It is important to recall, however, that approximately 50% of adolescent athletes with low back pain have symptoms attributable to spondylolysis and that this pain is often exacerbated with lumbar extension.[23] Spondylolysis or other bony stress injury should be excluded in this age group before pursuing diagnostic or therapeutic interventions for z-joint–mediated pain.

Diagnostic blocks are generally the accepted standard for the diagnosis of z-joint–mediated pain. It remains unclear, however, whether medial branch blocks or intra-articular z-joint injections provide a more accurate diagnosis.[38] Nevertheless, many agree that because MBBs are easier to perform and involve anesthetization of the nerves to be lesioned, they are the preferred diagnostic block when considering radiofrequency denervation. The rate of false-positive blocks has been reported to be 25% to 40% and independent of the type of block used.[38] False-negative blocks, or failure to anesthetize the targeted facet joint, have been reported in 11% of cases.[38] It is prudent to perform double blocks or blocks on 2 separate occasions given the high rates of false-positives and false-negatives.[38] This is rarely done in clinical practice because of a lack of definitive literature. In the setting of the athlete with back pain and suspected z-joint pathology, diagnostic blocks likely have legitimate value and should be performed as part of a comprehensive workup before dennervation. The use of bone scan with SPECT (single photon emission computed tomography) is sometimes used to detect z-joint pathology likely to respond to interventional procedures. In a study by Dolan and coworkers[39] the percentage of scan-positive patients who reported improvement after injection was significantly greater than in the scan-negative control group, with 95% and 79% of scan-positive patients indicating improvement at 3 and 6 months, respectively.[39]

The use of inta-articular steroid injection in the setting of z-joint–mediated pain is controversial regarding long-term treatment effectiveness. Few randomized, controlled trials comparing steroid with placebo exist, and there is no clear consensus in favor of intra-articular steroid injection. Based on clinical experience, it is likely that intra-articular z-joint injections (**Fig. 2**) have a legitimate role in a carefully selected subset of patients with z-joint–mediated pain and active inflammation. In the athletic population, intra-articular z-joint injections should be considered when other etiologies have been excluded, conservative management has failed, and when the specific z-joint level is suspected with a high degree of accuracy. There is no literature regarding the outcomes of intra-articular z-joint injections in athletes; however, clinical experiences suggest they can be useful in carefully selected patients as discussed above.

Radiofrequency dennervation (RFD) also represents a controversial treatment option for z-joint pain, in large part because of the controversy regarding the utility of diagnostic and prognostic blocks but also because of indeterminate evidence regarding efficacy. Multiple studies evaluating RFD have claimed a positive benefit, but these studies have lacked sufficient control groups. In the existing controlled trials, inconsistent study design and technical discrepancies have limited generalizability. In the only prospective study to evaluate radiofrequency outcomes in patients selected based on response to serial local anesthetic blocks, Dreyfuss and colleagues[40] reported that 87% of 15 patients obtained at least 60% pain relief 12 months status post RFD, with 60% of these patients achieving at least 90% relief.[40]

In the general population, most authors agree that radiofrequency dennervation is an effective treatment option for z-joint pain. In the athletic population, insufficient

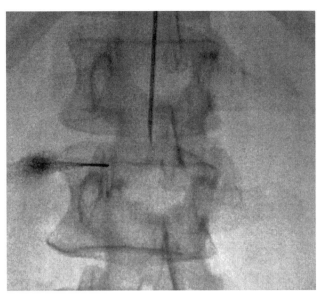

Fig. 2. Fluoroscopic image of an intra-articular facet joint injection shows intra-articular dye pattern.

literature exists to reach meaningful consensus. Vad and coworkers[41] studied radiofrequency ablation in 12 baseball pitchers not responding to conservative management and who had at least 50% pain relief with intra-articular injections or medial branch blocks. A total of 83% were able to return to their prior level of performance at a mean of 1.3 years after radiofrequency dennervation. Given that medial branch regeneration typically occurs 8 to 12 months after RFD, it is unclear from this study what effect can be attributed to RFD as opposed to favorable natural history and spontaneous recovery. As with intra1articular z-joint injections, radiofrequency dennervation is likely useful in a small subset of athletes who do not respond to conservative therapy with well-localized lesions and a positive response to diagnostic blocks.

Risks

Complications from intra-articular z-joint injections and medial branch blocks are rare and are generally similar to those described above for epidural steroid injections. Radiofrequency ablation may produce focal transient numbness or dysesthesia that generally resolves quickly.[38] The most common complication after RFD for z-joint pain is neuritis, which occurs in approximately 5% of cases.[42] Burns are rare with radiofrequency ablation, but may occur due to electrical faults, insulation breaks, or generator malfunction.[38] In addition to the potential complications above, radiofrequency ablation of the medial branches leads to subsequent initial dennervation of the lumbar multifidi at that level, but significant long-term segmental atrophy has not been found.[43] The biomechanical effect of this dennervation has remained controversial in the general population, and the effect on athletic performance has not been studied.

Sacroiliac Joint Injections

The sacroiliac joint (SIJ) may be responsible for up 20% of low back pain in the general population.[44,45] Although sacroiliac joint dysfunction (SIJD) remains controversial in terms of definition, evaluation, and treatment, the SIJ has generally been accepted as a potential pain generator (Brolinson). SIJD is thought to be a common cause of low back pain in athletes because of the high mechanical demand placed on the spine and pelvis during athletic competition. SIJD in athletes, however, has not been well studied, and incidence and prevalence among athletes has not been established. This is in large part due to difficulties in establishing specific definitions of SIJD and a lack of a confirmatory diagnostic gold standard. In a study of elite rowers, for example, SIJD was found to have a prevalence of 54.1%.[46] In this study, however, SIJD was defined via the standing flexion test followed by palpation of anatomic landmark, highlighting the lack of clear criteria for establishing this diagnosis. In theory, SIJD can develop in any sport, placing biomechanical stress through the lumbar spine and pelvis; although, as mentioned above, no epidemiologic data exist to compare one sport with another.

The role of SIJ injection (**Fig. 3**) for diagnostic purposes has been well established. Many practitioners consider intra-articular fluoroscopically guided injection to be the "gold standard" for diagnosis of SIJD, but this remains somewhat controversial. Some of the controversy surrounding this issue pertains to what SIJD truly means. SIJD encompasses a number of biomechanical factors that affect the SIJ, the surrounding ligaments, and the muscles that act on the pelvis. Thus, with SIJD, the SIJ may not be the sole "pain generator." Even when the SIJ itself is highly suspected as the source of pain, inflammation may not be present, weakening the rational for corticosteroid injection. The goal of an SIJ injection is to deposit steroid into the joint space; however, extravasation of injectant is common and reduces the diagnostic specificity. The prevalence of ventral tears of the SIJ capsule in patients with low back pain is 16% to 42%.[47–49] The injected solution may block surrounding neurologic structures, such as the sacral plexus, the L5 spinal nerve root, or the first

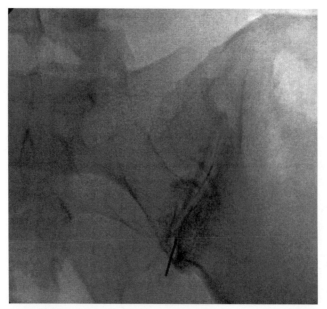

Fig. 3. Fluoroscopic image of an intra-articular sacroiliac joint injection shows intra-articular and periarticular dye flow.

sacral foramen (Fortin), further limiting specificity. In non–placebo-controlled studies, SIJ injections have confirmed SIJ pain in 13% to 30% of patients with chronic low back pain.[48,49] In a study by Katz and colleagues,[50] using greater than 75% relief for at least 10 days as criteria, the SIJ was found to be the definitive source of pain in 32% of postlumbosacral fusion patients.

Another controversial issue regarding SIJ injections is that there is no agreed-upon level of response to injection that is considered diagnostic. There is general consensus; however, that pain relief from an anesthetic SIJ injection helps confirm the diagnosis of SIJD. SIJ injection must be performed under fluoroscopy to ensure penetration of the joint capsule. Without fluoroscopy, it is unlikely that the injectant will reach the intra-articular target. Injections without imaging have been found to be intra-articular in only 22% of subjects.[51] Even with fluoroscopy, the joint can be difficult to reach because of its thick capsule and irregular articulation. Contrast is typically injected before the injection of local anesthetic and steroid to confirm intra-articular location and prevent intravascular flow. Local anesthetic is then injected with a typical volume of 1.0 to 2.5 mL.

Intra-articular corticosteroid injections are frequently used to treat suspected SIJD. To date, however, only 4 randomized, controlled trials and 14 observational reports on the efficacy of intra-articular SIJ injection have been performed.[52] Because there is no gold standard for diagnosis of SIJD, patient selection has been problematic in these studies. Patient selection is frequently based on history or physical examination or a single diagnostic block. Despite limitations in the literature, lasting improvement in pain and disability with an SIJ injection has been shown in patients who had relief after a single diagnostic block.[52,53] Therapeutic injections of the SIJ often lead to significant pain relief in well-selected patient populations.[52] Intra-articular injections are most effective, but there is also evidence that periarticular injections may provide some benefit. The available studies have primarily evaluated patients in the setting of spondyloarthropathy, with less clear evidence in patients without spondyloarthropathy. Controversy also remains regarding the true target of an injection for SIJ pain. As discussed above, the joint space itself may be the source of pain, but periarticular soft tissue structures, such as the sacroiliac, sacrotuberous, and sacrospinal ligaments, may also be pain generators.[52] As with any steroid injection, risks include hematoma, infection, allergic reaction, hyperglycemia, and fluid retention. When the sacroiliac joint is the suspected pain generator in an athlete based on history and physical examination and conservative management has not led to improvement, a diagnostic block with therapeutic steroid injection can be performed. Based on the current literature, there is a limited role of SIJ injections in treating sacroiliac joint dysfunction in athletes.

Several other procedures have been developed to alleviate refractory pain in the setting of SIJD. These include lateral and medial branch blocks as well as neurotomy. The extent to which the SIJ can be denervated by these procedures is unclear, and these interventions likely denervate the posterior SIJ and not the anterior portion of the joint. Evidence to support the utility of these procedures is lacking, and further research is necessary.

SUMMARY

Athletes represent a specific subgroup of highly motivated patients with a unique set of social and psychological incentives. Demands placed on the lumbosacral system are high, and athletes may be particularly prone to the pathology discussed above. For this reason, it is crucial to consider the athlete as a functional whole operating in concert with intrinsic and extrinsic factors and to consider the lumbosacral system within the context of the complete kinetic chain. Spinal interventions should never be considered in isolation but rather as part of a comprehensive rehabilitation program targeting psychosocial as well as biomechanical opportunities.

When interventional procedures are warranted, they should be performed according to existing guidelines regarding indication, patient selection, and technique where possible and with systems in place to maximize patient safety and to consistently monitor for response. Each of the interventions discussed above should be performed with fluoroscopic guidance, given the lack of accuracy without fluoroscopy, and generally be reserved for athletes not responding to conservative care.

When returning an athlete to play after ESI, we recommend careful serial evaluation as well as involvement of appropriate family members, athletic trainers, and coaches in the decision-making process. Athletes should not return to play with any significant objective neurologic deficits. In appropriate athletes, return to play should occur with graduated and comprehensive rehabilitation as discussed above.

Because evidence concerning the interventions discussed in this article is often lacking, clinical judgment is paramount regarding their allocation. The interventions explored above likely do provide viable treatment adjuncts in the carefully selected athlete but are not without risk. Athlete safety and global well being should guide any decision to pursue interventional treatment options.

REFERENCES

1. Trainor T, Trainor M. Etiology of low back pain in athletes. Curr Sports Med Rep 2004;3:41–6.
2. Ong A, Anderson J, Roche J. A pilot study of the prevalence of lumbar disc degeneration in elite athletes with lower back pain at the Sydney 2000 Olympic Games. Br J Sports Med 2003;37:263–6.
3. Lundin O, Hellstrom M, Nilsson I, et al. Back pain and radiological changes in the thoracolumbar spine of athletes: a long term follow-up. Scand J Med Sci Sports 2001;11:103–9.
4. Friedly J, Chan L, Deyo R. Increase in lumbosacral injections in the Medicare population. Spine 2007;32:1754–60.
5. Frymoyer J. Back pain and sciatica. N Engl J Med 1988;318:291–300.
6. Bush K, Cowan N, Katz D, et al. The natural history of sciatica associated with disc pathology. A prospective study with clinical and independent radiologic follow-up. Spine 1992;17:1205–12.
7. Koes B, Tulder M, Peul W. Diagnosis and treatment of sciatica. BMJ 2007;334:1313–7.
8. Saal JA, Saal JS, Herzog RJ. The natural history of lumbar intervertebral disc extrusions treated non-operatively. Spine 1990;15:683–6.
9. Barr KPHarrast MALow back pain.Physical medicine and rehabilitation. In: Braddom RL, editor. 3rd edition. Philadelphia: Elsevier Inc; 2007. p. 888–90.
10. Harrington JF, Messier AA, Bereiter D, et al. Herniated lumbar disc material as a source of free glutamate available to affect pain signals through the dorsal root ganglion. Spine 2000;25:29–36.
11. McLaine RF, Kapural L, Mekhail NA. Epidural steroid therapy for back and leg pain: mechanisms of action and efficacy. Spine 2005;5:191–201.
12. Harrast MA. Epidural steroid injections for lumbar spinal stenosis. Curr Rev Musculoskelet 2008;1:32–8.
13. Friedrich M, Harrast MA. Lumbar epidural steroid injections: indications, contraindications, risks, and benefits. Curr Sports Med Rep 2010;9:43–9.

14. Huston CW. Cervical epidural steroid injections in the management of cervical radiculitis: interlaminar versus transforaminal. A review. Curr Rev Musculoskelet 2009;2:30–42.

15. Lutz GE, Vad VB, Wisneski RJ. Fluoroscopic transforaminal lumbar epidural steroid injections: an outcome study. Arch Phys Med Rehabil 1998;79:1362–6.

16. Riew KD, Yin Y, Gilula L, et al. The effect of nerve-root injections on the need for operative treatment of lumbar radicular pain: a prospective, randomized, controlled double-blind study. J Bone Joint Surg Am 2000;82-A:1589–93.

17. Riew KD, Park JB, Cho YS, et al. Nerve root blocks in the treatment of lumbar radicular pain: a minimum 5-year follow up. J Bone Joint Surg Am 2006;88:1722–5.

18. Karppinen J, Malmivaara A, Kurunlahti M, et al. Periradicular infiltration for sciatica: a randomized controlled trail. Spine 2001;26:1059–67.

19. Vad VB, Bhat AL, Lutz GE, et al. Transforaminal epidural steroid injections in lumbar radiculopathy: a prospective randomized study. Spine 2002;27:11–6.

20. Weiner BK, Fraser RD. Foraminal injection for lateral lumbar disc herniation. J Bone Joint Surg 1997;79B:804–7.

21. McQuay HJ, Moore A. Epidural steroids for sciatica. Anaesth Int Care 1996;24:284–5.

22. Choi SJ, Song JS, Kim C, et al. The use of magnetic resonance imaging to predict the clinical outcome of non-surgical treatment for lumbar intervertebral disc herniation. Korean J Radiol 2007;8:156–63.

23. Micheli LJ, Wood R. Back pain in young athletes. Significant differences from adults in causes and patterns. Arch Pediatr Adolesc Med 1995;149:15–8.

24. Abram SE. Treatment of lumbosacral radiculopathy with epidural steroids. Anesthesiology 1999;91:1937–41.

25. Novak S, Nemeth WC. The basis for recommending repeating epidural steroid injections for radicular low back pain: a literature review. Arch Phys Med Rehabil 2008;89:543–52.

26. Bogduk N. Lumbar transforaminal injection of corticosteroids. In: International spine interventions society. Practice guidelines for spinal diagnostic and treatment procedures. San Francisco (CA): International Spine Interventions Society; 2004. p. 187.

27. Akerman WE, Ahmad M. The efficacy of lumbar epidural steroid injections in patients with lumbar disc herniations. Anesth Analg 2007;104:1217–22.

28. Thomas E, Cyteval C, Abiad L, et al. Efficacy of transforaminal versus interspindous corticosteroid injection in discal radiculalgia—a prospective, randomized, double-blind study. Clin Rheumatol 2003;22:299–304.

29. Goodman BS, Posecion LWF, Mallempati S, et al. Complications and pitfalls of lumbar interlaminar and transforaminal epidural injections. Curr Rev Musculoskelet Med 2008;1:212–22.

30. Smuck M, Fuller BJ, Choido A, et al. Accuracy of intermittent fluoroscopy to detect intravascular injection during transforaminal epidural steroid injections. Spine 2008;33:E205–10.

31. Gonzalez P, Laker SR, Sullivan W. The effects of epidural betamethasone on blood glucose in patient with diabetes mellitus. PMR 2009;1:340–5.

32. Derby R, Kine G, Saal JA. Response to steroid and duration of radicular pain as predictors of surgical outcome. Spine 1992;17(Suppl):S176–83.

33. Ng L, Chaudhary N, Sell P. The efficacy of corticosteroids in periradicular infiltration for chronic radicular pain: a randomized, double-blind, controlled trial. Spine 2005;30:857–62.

34. Kolsi I, Delecrin J, Berthelot JM, et al. Efficacy of nerve root versus interspinous injections of glucocorticoids in the treatment of disk-related sciatica. A pilot, prospective, randomized, double blind study. Joint Bone Spine 2000;67:113–8.

35. Candido KD, Raghavendra MS, Chinthagada M, et al. A prospective evaluation of iodinated contrast flow patterns with fluoroscopically guided lumbar epidural steroid injections: a lateral parasagittal interlaminar approach versus the transforaminal approach. Anesth Analg 2008;106:638–44.

36. Beresford ZM, Kendall RW, Willick SE. Lumbar facet syndromes. Curr Sports Med Rep 2010;9:50–6.

37. Alyas F, Turner M, Connell D. MRI findings in the lumbar spines of asymptomatic, adolescent, elite tennis players. Br J Sports Med 2007;41:836–41.

38. Cohen SP, Raja SN. Pathogenesis, diagnosis, and treatment of lumbar zygapophyseal (facet) joint pain. Anesthesiology 2007;106:591–614.

39. Dolan AL, Ryan PJ, Arden NK, et al. The value of SPECT scans in identifying back pain likely to benefit from facet joint injection. Br J Rheumatol 1996;35:1269–73.

40. Dreyfuss P, Baker R, LeClaire R, et al. Radiofrequency facet joint denervation in the treatment of low back pain: a placebo-controlled clinical trial to assess efficacy. Spine 2002;27:556–7.

41. Vad VB, Cano WG, Basrai D, et al. Role of radiofrequency denervation in lumbar zygapophyseal joint synovitis in baseball pitchers: a clinical experience. Pain Physician 2003;6:307–12.

42. Kornick C, Kramarich SS, Lamer TJ, et al. Complications of lumbar facet radiofrequency denervation. Spine 2004;29:1352–4.

43. Dreyfuss P, Stout A, Aprill C, et al. The significance of multifidus atrophy after successful radiofrequency neurotomy for low back pain. PMR 2009;1:719–21.

44. Dreyfuss P, Dreyer S, Griffin J, et al. Positive sacroiliac screening tests in asymptomatic adults. Spine 1994;19:1138–43.

45. Brolinson PG, Kozar AJ, Cibor G. Sacroiliac joint dysfunction in athletes. Curr Sports Med Rep 2003;2:47–56.

46. Timm KE. Sacroiliac joint dysfunction in elite rowers. J Orthop Sports Phys Ther 1999; 29:288–93.

47. Fortin JD, Washington WJ, Falco FJ. Three pathways between the sacroiliac joint and neural structures. AJNR Am J Neuroradiol 1999;20:1429–34.

48. Shwarzer AC, Aprill CN, Bogduk N. The sacroiliac joint in chronic low back pain. Spine 1995;20:31–7.

49. Foley BS, Buschbacher RM. Sacroiliac joint pain. Anatomy, biomechanics, diagnosis, and treatment. Am J Phys Med Rehabil 2006;85:997–1006.

50. Katz V, Shofferman J, Reynolds J. The sacroiliac joint: a potential cause of pain after lumbar fusion to the sacrum. J Spinal Disord Tech 2003;16:96–9.

51. Rosenberg JM, Quint TJ, de Rosayro AM. Computerized topographic localization of clinically- guided sacroiliac joint injections. Clin J Pain 2000;16:18–21.

52. Kennedy DJ, Shokat M, Visco CJ. Sacroiliac joint and lumbar zygapophyseal joint corticosteroid injections. Phys Med and Rehab Clin North Am 2010;21:835–42.

53. Slipman CW, Lipetz JS, Plastaras CT, et al. Fluoroscopically guided therapeutic sacroiliac joint injections for sacroiliac joint syndrome. Am J Phys Med Rehabil 2001;80:425–32.

Back Pain in the Pediatric and Adolescent Athlete

Brian M. Haus, MD[a], Lyle J. Micheli, MD[b],*

KEYWORDS

- Back pain • Young athletes • Acute injuries • Overuse injuries

KEY POINTS

- Back pain is becoming more common in young athletes, due in part to injuries sustained during organized sports.
- The spectrum of clinical entities is different from that in adults, and in young athletes, back pain usually arises from either an acute traumatic event or from chronic overuse.
- Acute injuries include thoracolumbar fractures, spinal cord injury without radiographic abnormality, acute disc herniation, apophyseal ring fractures, and muscular sprains.
- Problems associated with overuse include spondylolysis, spondylolisthesis, degenerative disc disease, hyperlordotic mechanical back pain, and atypical Scheurmann disease.
- It is important to remember that an infection, a neoplasm, or a rheumatologic condition may be mistaken for a sports injury.

Although back pain in adults is very common, its incidence among pediatric patients is variable, depending on age and level of activity. Classically, it was believed that children rarely have back pain,[1] and that in comparison to adults, a child with a backache is more likely to have a serious underlying disorder such as a neoplasm, discitis, or osteomyelitis. Although this may be the case in an inactive child or one younger than 10 years of age,[2] recent evidence demonstrates that the prevalence of back pain in older children and adolescents may be much higher than previously thought. By late adolescence, the incidence of low back pain in may be as high 24% to 36%.[3,4]

The increased incidence of back pain in adolescents is likely related to the increasing level of participation in organized sports. In 2008, an estimated 44 million preadolescents and adolescents participated in organized sports in the United States.[5] Because of the competitive emphasis of organized sports, young athletes are now specializing in fewer sports and training and playing with greater intensity. As a

The authors have nothing to disclose.
[a] Division of Sports Medicine, Department of Orthopaedic Surgery, Children's Hospital Boston, 319 Longwood Avenue, Boston, MA 02115, USA; [b] Division of Sports Medicine, Children's Hospital Boston, Harvard Medical School, 319 Longwood Avenue, Boston, MA 02115, USA
* Corresponding author.
E-mail address: michelilyle@aol.com

Clin Sports Med 31 (2012) 423–440
http://dx.doi.org/10.1016/j.csm.2012.03.011
0278-5919/12/$ – see front matter © 2012 Published by Elsevier Inc.

result of increased repetitive training in these sports, the risk of sustaining injuries, and, in particular, overuse injuries, is now much greater. Sports injuries occur from either an acute traumatic event or from chronic overuse due to repetitive training and microtrauma. Children's overuse injuries were rarely encountered before the advent of organized sports training; however, they are now a major source of morbidity in children and adolescents. In fact, epidemiologic data now show that sports injuries exceed infectious diseases as a cause of children's morbidity in Canada.[6]

Acute and overuse injuries of the back are an important subset of injuries in adolescents. Repetitive trauma and hyperextension during sports can cause young athletes to be susceptible to clinical or subclinical injuries that can lead to acute or chronic back pain. Unfortunately, despite the increasing incidence of back pain in adolescents, these injuries can be missed by the clinician unaware of the common diagnosis in adolescent athletes. Injuries occurring in the adolescents differ in etiology and prevalence from those occurring in adults. A recent study found that in adults, 48% of patients with low back pain have discogenic etiologies, whereas 47% of low back pain in adolescents is due to spondylolysis and 25% to hyperlordosis.[7] Further, in contrast to back pain in the nonactive general adolescent population, which most often has a nonspecific cause,[8] back pain in young athletes is usually due to an identifiable diagnosis. Because of the increasing frequency of back pain, it is important that clinicians understand that pediatric and adolescent athletes are a distinct at-risk population with a unique set of differential diagnoses. Using a sport-specific history and a careful systematic physical exam, combined with the appropriate imaging techniques, clinicians can usually make an accurate diagnosis. Correctly identifying common and uncommon diagnoses in young athletes will prevent further disability and allow earlier return to sports.

ANATOMY AND BIOMECHANICS

Spinal injuries are particularly prevalent during adolescence, when the spinal column undergoes structural and flexibility transformations associated with accelerated growth. These changes occur within the growth tissues in the vertebral bodies and neural arch. During growth, these become the weakest part of the spinal column and stand the greatest risk of injury during force transfer.[9]

The spine consists of a triple joint complex comprising the intervertebral disc and bilateral facet joints, which together form a triangular base for support, motion, and force transfer. It is divided into anterior and posterior columns. In competitive adolescent athletes, the spine is at risk for injury because it transfers forces between the upper and lower extremities during rapid and forceful movements. Injury occurs when the spine and its supporting structures cannot withstand compression, distraction, or shear forces during movement in an acute or overuse situation. Forced forward flexion causes disc compression and injury. Loaded hyperextension can contribute to pars fractures, and rotational forces stress the facet joints.

The anterior column includes the vertebral body, the intervertebral disc, and the anterior and posterior longitudinal ligaments. Within the vertebral body of children, there is a superior and an inferior epiphyseal growth plate, each with a contiguous ring apophysis. The cartilaginous portions of these epiphyses develop into the vertebral end-plate, which can be a source of weakness in the spinal column and is susceptible to injury during growth. The anterior and posterior longitudinal ligaments are important stabilizers in the pediatric spine, as they protect against hyperextension and hyperflexion.

The posterior column consists of the neural arch, facet joints, spinal process, and pars interarticularis. The posterior arch has three primary growth centers, one in the spinous process and one in each pedicle bilaterally. Ossification proceeds in a posterior direction and may be incomplete on the superior aspect of the pars interarticularis, predisposing to stress fracture from the abutting inferior articular facet above.[10] The posterior epiphyses usually closes by age 8, whereas the anterior epiphyses do not close until age 18.[11] If an asymmetric force is placed on the two spinal columns, this temporal difference in epiphyseal growth arrest may contribute to the development of deformity in adolescent athletes.

Although the intervertebral disc is a more frequent site of injury in adults, it is nonetheless involved in an important minority of injuries in immature athletes. Its changing morphology during growth creates different injury patterns than those seen in adults. The disc is a fibrocartilaginous structure composed of an outer layer, the annulus fibrosis, and an inner layer, the nucleus pulposus. The nucleus pulposus is 88% water with a high polysaccharide content, a composition that allows it to act as the primary absorber of compressive forces in the spine. When compressive forces are transmitted outward to the annulus fibrosis, there can be different consequences in the immature versus adult spine. This is due the fact that, in the immature spine, the cartilaginous end-plate is attached to the ring apophysis and the annulus fibrosis. Here, compressive forces are transferred into distractive forces to the weaker cartilaginous end-plate, resulting in either an avulsion of the apophysis with the attached annulus or a disc herniation into the vertebral body at the apophysis (limbus vertebrae). This is in contrast to the adult spine, in which such forces lead to rupture of the annulus fibrosis and subsequent herniation of the nucleus pulposus.

The lower spine and pelvic ring are connected by the sacroiliac joint. The sacroiliac joint is a diarthrodial joint that remains flat until puberty and then develops corrugations that lead to ankylosis later in life. The sacroiliac joint transfers forces from the lower extremity to the trunk. With hip flexion, there is an ipsilateral posterior pelvic rotation and subsequent increased sacroiliac joint compression. Fortunately, the sacroiliac joint is not commonly injured in pediatric athletes. However, sacral stress fractures should be included in the differential diagnosis of lower back pain, especially in female athletes.[12]

RISK FACTORS
Overuse Injuries

Until recently, most young athletes had been participating recreationally in many sports; now they are participating more intensively in fewer, more organized sports. As a result of increased training in these sports, repetitive microtrauma is the main causative factor leading to spinal injuries in athletes. Cyclic loading of shear, tensile, and compressive forces can exceed tissue elasticity and result in failure and subsequent injury. This threshold may be surpassed by total volume of hours per week or in excessive single-session drills of the same motion.

Growth

The morphology of the growth plate renders it susceptible to injury during sports. Growth cartilage is less resistant to deforming forces than either ligament or bone. Bone is also susceptible to fracture, as bone mineralization is delayed after linear skeletal growth during the adolescent growth spurt.[13,14] The dissociation between skeletal growth and mineralization during puberty makes the skeleton more susceptible to fracture because the elastic modulus and the strength of bone are a function of the density of the bone.[15,16] In addition, periods of rapid growth cause substantial increases in muscle–tendon tightness about the joints, with subsequent loss of flexibility and increasing potential for injury. In the spine, a combination of all of these factors leads to increased risk of injury in the growing athlete. Compressive forces can rupture the cartilaginous end-plate, causing Schmorl nodes to form, or the ring apophysis to produce limbus vertebrae. Conversely, tensile stresses can result in apophysitis or apophyseal avulsions. Sports in which athletes are exposed to repetitive asymmetric forces, as in gymnastics, may contribute to spinal curve deformity.

Anthropomorphic Factors

Malalignment of the lower extremities and pelvis can result in improper transfer of ground forces to the lower trunk. Weak lower abdominal muscles and tight hip flexors may contribute to increased lumbar lordosis, which can increase the compressive load to the posterior elements of the spine. Athletes who participate in sports that require excessive lower lumbar flexion have an increased risk of having low back pain.[17] In addition, abnormalities in pelvic and sacral morphology increase the local shearing forces in the lumbar spine and can contribute to the development of injury in the form of spondylolysis and spondylolisthesis.[18]

Sex-Specific Factors

Data regarding differences in risk of injury based on gender are limited and are based on pathologic entity and by sport. Spondylolysis was historically believed to be two to three times more common in boys than in girls,[19] but more recent data suggest equal prevalence.[20] However, there is an increased incidence of spondylolysis in some female-dominated sports such as ballet, figure skating, and gymnastics. Spondylolisthesis appears to occur more frequently in girls.[21–23] The overall rate of scoliosis is higher in girls than in boys.[24] Sacral stress fractures are more predominant in female long-distance runners, likely due to a catabolic response to overtraining, associated with the "female athletic triad." Bone homeostasis is regulated, in part, by nutritional and hormonal balance. In female athletes with negative caloric balance from overtraining, estrogen production decreases, which may predispose to lower bone density and an associated increased risk of stress fracture.

Sports-Specific Factors

Particular sports render pediatric athletes prone to back injuries. Repetitive hyperextension causes direct macrotrauma or repetitive microtrauma to the posterior spine, and is a major risk factor particularly in gymnastics,[25] football lineman,[26] figure skating,[27] and dance. Young athletes participating in gymnastics for more than 15 hours per week, for example, have an increased risk of spine injury.[28] The prevalence of back injuries in football linemen may be as high as 50%.[29] Baseball players, bowlers, and swimmers are susceptible to disc pathology secondary to repetitive rotational motions. Sports that involve flexion and axial loading, such as weight lifting, snowboarding, rowing, and collision sports, place the athlete at risk for sustaining fractures and herniated discs.[30,31]

CLINICAL EXAMINATION
History

To determine the etiology of a young athlete's back pain, it is important to obtain a thorough clinical history. The history should include a review of the specific sports the athlete plays, as well as the playing position, level of conditioning, and training volume. The mechanism of injury, and the nature and severity of the pain, including the character, location, duration, and aggravating movements, should be evaluated.

Pain that is made worse by extension suggests posterior element involvement whereas pain aggravated by flexion movements or the Valsalva maneuver suggests discogenic involvement. Mechanical back pain is usually felt in the lower back, whereas nerve compression pain is usually felt in the legs. Changes in neurologic status, including bowel and bladder habits, should be assessed for herniated nucleus pulposus or limbus vertebrae. Response to medications, including acetaminophen and nonsteroidal anti-inflammatory drugs (NSAIDs), should be noted. Constitutional symptoms associated with a serious pathologic condition include night pain, recent weight loss, and fever. It is important to obtain a nutritional history, especially in female athletes. A history of an eating disorder, menstrual irregularity, and osteoporosis—the "female athlete triad"—places the patient at increased risk for stress fractures.[20]

Physical Examination

A well-performed and thorough physical examination is an essential element in obtaining an accurate diagnosis in the pediatric athlete. The examination begins by observing the patient's body habitus and gait pattern. Cachexia or pallor may indicate an underlying malignancy or nutritional disorder. A comprehensive gait examination can identify motor weakness, a lumbar shift, and pain intensity. For that reason, it is also important to test for the ability to heel-to-toe walk, which helps assess gross motor strength of the L4 and S1 nerve roots. After this is completed, the patient should be examined in the standing position, in an examination gown to allow proper visualization of spinal alignment. Coronal and sagittal alignment should be evaluated to look for scoliosis, kyphosis, hyperlordosis, or flat back syndrome, as well as any pelvic obliquity or leg length deficiency.

Testing range of motion in the lumbar spine can elicit a provocative painful response, an important clue that can be beneficial in attaining a correct diagnosis. Maneuvers include forward flexion, extension, side bending, and rotation. Back pain with extension may indicate posterior element pathology; the specificity of this test is increased while performing it with a single-leg stance (stork testing) because it can localize the pain to a unilateral location. Pain with forward flexion may indicate an injury with a discogenic origin.

Palpation of the lumbar spine may also elicit important clues to the etiology of back pain. Spinous process tenderness may indicate ligamentous injury, fracture, or apophysitis. A palpable step-off deformity may indicate a fracture or a spondylolisthesis. A complete palpatory examination should include the sacroiliac joints, piriformis fossa, and greater trochanters.

A complete neurologic exam including formal manual motor and sensory testing and deep tendon reflexes is essential. With the patient sitting, patellar tendon (L4) and Achilles tendon (S1) reflexes can be tested. Motor function testing of the extensor hallucis longus (L5), quadriceps (L3–4), and hip flexors (L2–3) should also be performed, as well as a sensory examination in the T12–S1 dermatomes. Tension signs for nerve root compression should be tested in the supine position, including the straight leg raise test, femoral nerve stretch test, and Lasegue sign. Abnormal Babinski and abdominal reflexes are also tested to investigate for upper motor neuron pathology. Pain with flexion–abduction–external rotation may indicate sacroiliac inflammation. The relative tightness of the hip flexors is assessed with the Thomas test and the hip extensors with the straight leg raise popliteal angle test, whereas tightness of the hip external rotators can be determined with rotation assessment. Tight hamstrings can contribute to the cause of lower back pain, but they can also be the result of spondylolisthesis.

ACUTE INJURIES
Thoracolumbar Fractures

Fortunately, thoracolumbar trauma is relatively rare in the pediatric population, representing fewer than 8% of all spine fractures in those younger than 8 years of age.[32] However, the adolescent population is more prone to thoracolumbar fractures,[31] with sports injuries accounting for approximately 21% of them.[31] Athletes participating in sports that involve axial loading such as diving and snowboarding have an especially high risk for these injuries, as do contact sports that involve blunt trauma, such as hockey and wrestling.

Acute evaluation and treatment of an athlete with a suspected spinal injury should begin by following Advanced Trauma Life Support protocols, including the implementation of strict spine precautions as well as maintaining proper immobilization on a spine board for transport to prevent additional injury. A secondary survey should be also be performed, including inspection of the spine for tenderness and step-offs, and a complete neurologic examination. Although the clinical examination is an imperative part of evaluating an athlete with a spine injury, it is only 81% sensitive and 68% specific for accurately detecting a spinal fracture.[33]

For this reason, all pediatric and adolescent patients with a history of thoracolumbar trauma should also be assessed with screening radiographs. Standard AP and lateral radiographs are helpful in identifying the presence of a fracture or dislocation and for determining the stability of the spine. In the presence of fracture, spinal stability is determined using Denis' three-column classification system.[34] The spine is divided into three columns: the anterior, middle, and posterior columns. The anterior column contains the anterior longitudinal ligament (ALL) and the anterior half of the vertebral body and annulus fibrosis. The middle column contains the posterior half of the vertebral body and annulus fibrosis and the posterior longitudinal ligament (PLL). The posterior column consists of the posterior ligamentous complex and bony elements. When two of the columns are disrupted, the fracture is unstable.

If an unstable fracture is suspected, a computed tomography (CT) scan of the chest/abdomen/pelvis should be performed. CT scan is helpful in assessing canal compromise and better characterizes the integrity of the osseous structures. Because this stepwise approach may be inefficient in the setting of an acute traumatic situation, it has been suggested that CT scan replace screening radiographs in the initial evaluation of a patient with a suspected thoracolumbar fracture. Advocates of this management report that the CT scan is more sensitive[35] and that an accurate diagnosis can be obtained much faster.[36] Although this approach may be reasonable in adults, these methods have not yet been properly studied in pediatric populations. For this reason, the standard of care for children should still be to obtain screening radiographs initially. If a neurologic deficit is present, magnetic resonance imaging (MRI) can provide important information about spinal cord injury and damage to the surrounding ligaments. MRI is best utilized when soft-tissue injuries, such as herniated discs, neuroforaminal encroachments, hematomas, spinal cord edema, or posttraumatic spinal cord cysts, are suspected.

Whereas thoracolumbar fractures are more common in the adolescent population, cervical fractures and spinal cord injury without radiographic abnormality (SCIWORA) are more common in the children with an immature spine. In addition, while children younger than 9 years of age are less likely to have spinal injury, they have a higher incidence of neurologic injury.[37,38] The immature spinal column is more elastic than in the adult, and can therefore accommodate more motion and displacement before a fracture or ligamentous rupture occurs. However, the spinal cord is not as elastic, and displacement therefore results in SCIWORA in 30% to 40% of spinal cord injuries in pediatric patients. SCIWORA is an unstable injury, and given the lack of radiographic findings, it is especially critical to understand that 23% of patients with SCIWORA have a delayed onset of neurologic deficit ranging from 6 to 72 hours after injury.[39] Patients who are at high risk for SCIWORA should be admitted for careful observation. Unfortunately, there are currently no clear guidelines or evidence that identifies which types of patients are at risk for neurologic deterioration.[37]

Fortunately, most thoracolumbar fractures in children are stable fractures that are not associated with neurologic injury. The most common include posterior element fractures (spinous process, transverse process fractures) and compression fractures, representing 23% and 49% of fractures, respectively, in the pediatric population.[31] These fractures usually heal uneventfully and are not associated with cessation of growth. Restoration of vertebral body height in compression fractures with less than 30° of angulation can be expected in patients with open physes. Most of these stable fractures are treated successfully with bed rest and activity restriction, followed by a thoracolumbosacral orthosis for 4 to 12 weeks.[40] However, compliance with prolonged bed rest and rigid brace wear my be difficult in pediatric patients, and treatment with short periods of bed rest and gradual resumption of activities is successful for many fractures.[31] Sports activity is restricted during this period, and the athlete is allowed to return to sports after a period of gradual rehabilitation, evidence of radiographic union, and resolution of pain.

Burst fractures represent a minority of thoracolumbar fractures in children. The injury occurs when an axial load crushes one or both of the vertebral end-plates and subsequently pushes the nucleus pulposus and/or ring apophysis into the vertebral body, causing it to fracture and collapse.[33] The injury disrupts the anterior and middle columns, and the normal sagittal alignment of the spine may subsequently become kyphotic. Retropulsion of fracture fragments from the vertebral body can also protrude into the spinal canal and cause neurologic injury. These fractures are important in the child not only because they are associated with instability and neurologic deficits, but also because improper management can cause physeal arrest and progressive sagittal or coronal spinal deformity.[41] Absolute indications for surgical stabilization include fracture-dislocations or protruding vertebral body or end-plate fracture fragments, herniated discs, or hematomas causing neurologic compromise. In contrast to thoracolumbar injuries in adults, in children, the percentage of canal compromise does not necessary correlate with the risk of spinal cord injury. Instead, the level of injury is more predictive, with thoracic fractures more likely to cause neurologic compromise.[42] The immature spine has a larger canal diameter with respect to the spinal cord, which may, in part, explain the lower incidence of neurologic injury despite significant retropulsion of bone fragments in children.[43,44]

The management of burst fractures in neurologically intact patients is a source of debate regarding both adults and children. Classic surgical indications include those fractures with greater than 40% canal compromise, 40% loss of height, or 20% kyphotic deformity.[45,46] More recent studies, however, have shown no difference in the incidence of postinjury kyphosis in adults treated operatively versus nonoperatively. In addition, patients treated nonoperatively have improved clinical outcomes and less disability.[47] Similar long-term studies in children have shown only small amounts of improvement in the degree of kyphosis with surgical management, and no improved clinical outcomes in comparison to those treated nonoperatively.[41,48]

Acute Disc Herniation

Although the true prevalence of lumbar disc herniation is unknown, discogenic pathology, including disc herniation, causes 11% of lumbar pain in pediatric athletes.[7] The overwhelming majority of pediatric patients with disc herniations are older than the age of 12.[49] The L4–5 and L5–S1 discs are the most common locations for herniated nucleus pulposus, representing 92% of cases in adolescents.[50] Most herniations are centrolateral and remain subligamentous.

Athletes who participate in collision sports and weightlifting are at increased risk for lumbar disc herniation due to increased axial forces exerted on the spine during activities that require extreme flexion and extension. However, although trauma is often cited as the primary causative factor of disc herniation in adolescents,[51,52] there is growing evidence suggesting that this is true only in the setting of a preexisting spinal deformity.[50,53] Between 30% and 70% of adolescents with acute disc herniation also have vertebral anomalies, such as scoliosis, transitional defects (lumbarization and sacralization), schisis, and canal narrowing.[50] Patients with these anomalies can exert eccentric biomechanical loading during sports, and may be prone to early disc degeneration and subsequent herniation. In addition, early disc disease may have a familial[54] and genetic relationship.[55] There also appears to be an increased incidence of acute disc herniations in patients with growth cartilage abnormalities of the lumbar spine, such as Schmorl nodes and Scheuermann disease.[56]

In adolescents, pain is located in the low back, buttock, posterior thigh, and/or leg. One study suggested that the primary complaint in adolescents with herniated discs is low back along with leg pain (82%), with 13% complaining of lumbar pain alone and 5% complaining of leg pain alone.[48] Overt neurologic deficits are rare in pediatric and adolescent patients. The physical examination should include gait analysis, as well as lumbar range of motion, which is often abnormal. Pain and apprehension may occur with lumbar flexion and Valsalva maneuver. The straight leg test is positive in approximately two thirds of patients with MRI evidence of lumbar nerve root compression.[57] It has frequently been noted that children or adolescents with herniated discs often have more dramatic physical findings but relatively less pain complaints, in contrast to adults. Adolescent patients with a disc herniation may also assume a scoliotic posture as a compensatory attempt to relieve nerve root irritation.[58] A rectal examination should be performed in the setting of saddle anesthesia or bladder symptoms to rule out cauda equina syndrome. MRI remains the best modality to assess for a herniated disc.

Nonsurgical management is the first line of treatment for herniated discs in the adolescent athlete. The usual method of management includes a short period of relative rest, NSAIDs, and physical therapy, followed by progressive return to activities. A rigid hyperlordotic brace worn for 3 months or an epidural corticosteroid injection may be helpful in alleviating symptoms and preventing recurrence. Unfortunately, some studies suggest that adolescents, as opposed to adults, are less responsive to conservative treatment.[59,60] This is attributed mainly to the high elasticity of the disc material in adolescents in comparison to adults.[61] One study suggests that as few as 40% of adolescents with herniated lumbar discs respond to conservative management, and that recurrence is common.[62] For the minority of patients with persistent pain and severe limitations, or progressive neurologic deficits including cauda equina syndrome, surgery may be necessary. Adolescents do very well with surgery in the short term, with most reports suggesting a greater than 90%

successful relief of symptoms.[60,63] However, the revision rate 10 and 20 years after surgery is approximately 20% and 26%, respectively.[64]

After surgical or nonsurgical treatment, athletes should have progressive rehabilitation before returning to sports. Therapy should be directed at core-strengthening, sport-specific training, and lumbar stretching. Athletes can be generally expected to return to activity 3 to 6 months after nonsurgical treatment and 6 to 12 months after surgical treatment.

Apophyseal Ring Fractures

An apophyseal ring fracture, or limbus fracture, is a fracture seen almost exclusively in adolescents who are still skeletally immature. The apophyseal ring ossifies at age 4 to 6 years and fuses at age 18. Along with the posterior longitudinal ligament, it is firmly attached to the annulus fibrosis. The osteo–cartilagenous junction between the vertebral body and the apophyseal ring is comparatively weaker, and after compressive or traction force, the attachment of the annulus fibrosis at this junction can be avulsed and displaced posteriorly into the spinal canal. Chronic stress or overuse microtrauma may also cause a limbus fracture. Similar to herniated nucleus pulposus, congenital anomalies of the lumbosacral spine may be associated with apophyseal ring fractures in adolescents, including lumbarization, sacralization, and spinal dysraphsim.[61] Irregularities in the end-plate cartilage may also be implicated in apophyseal ring fractures, synonymous with slipped capital femoral epiphysis.[65] In fact, there may be an association with obesity, as the increased weight places excessive stresses on the lumbar spine.[66] Adolescent athletes who are involved in a sport such as weightlifting or gymnastics are particularly at risk. Apophyseal ring fractures occur most commonly at the L4–5 level, accounting for more than 90% of cases.[60,67]

On examination, the patient may have tenderness and spasm of the paraspinal musculature. The physical examination findings may be similar to those of herniated nucleus pulposus, including pain with coughing, sneezing, or spinal flexion. Straight leg testing and nerve tension signs are usually positive. Although a bony avulsion can sometimes be seen on a lateral radiograph, CT is the diagnostic study of choice. MRI is not as sensitive for detection of apophyseal ring fractures due to poor visualization of bone.[68]

The treatment of apophyseal ring fractures is similar to that of herniated nucleus pulposis, initially activity modification and NSAIDs. Surgery is reserved for patients with cauda equina syndrome or neurologic deficit.

Strains, Sprains, and Contusions

Strains, sprains, and contusions are common injuries in athletes and the diagnosis one of exclusion. Sprains represent the stretching of ligaments beyond their elastic limit and strains are tearing of the muscle during concentric and eccentric loading. Contusions occur after blunt impact to the soft tissues and will often lead to hematoma formation, swelling, and pain. Athletes may have spasm and palpable, localized tenderness over the area of injury. Diagnostic imaging is negative, except in the case of MRI, in which hematoma or edema in the soft tissues may be seen. The management of each is icing, activity modification and NSAIDs initially, followed by progressive rehabilitation with physical therapy to increase flexibility and strength.

OVERUSE INJURIES
Spondylolysis and Spondylolisthesis

Spondylolysis refers to a defect of the pars interarticularis, the narrow part of the vertebrae between the inferior or superior articular processes of the facet joints. The injury occurs as a result of an acute traumatic overload, or more commonly, due to chronic cyclic loading of the inferior articular facet onto the pars interarticularis of the inferior vertebrae during repetitive hyperextension.[69] Differing biomechanical theories have also been suggested as the cause of spondylolysis, including that the pars interarticularis may fail through excessive traction forces[70] and that abnormalities of the sacral growth plate may also play a role.[71] Because pediatric and adolescent athletes subject their lower backs to forceful and repetitive forces, they are at much higher risk of obtaining spondylolysis than inactive children. Spondylolysis is the primary cause of back pain in athletes, and accounts for as much as 47% of back pain.[7] Athletes who participate in such sports as football, rugby, ballet, diving, and gymnastics have the highest rates of spondylolysis.[7] A specific traumatic event is identified in as many as 40% of cases.[72] The injuries may be unilateral or bilateral, and they occur most commonly at L5.

Spondylolisthesis describes the forward translation of one vertebra relative to the next caudal vertebral segment; it occurs most commonly at the L5–S1 motion segment. Spondylolisthesis has multiple etiologies and the Wiltse Classification is the most commonly used method of characterizing its causes: dysplastic (I), isthmic (II), degenerative (III), traumatic (IV), and pathologic (V). Isthmic spondylolisthesis is the most common subtype and is associated with bilateral pars injuries in spondylolysis. Slipping of one vertebra on another can occur after an acute macrotraumatic overload, or as a result of progression from a stress fracture. Dysplastic spondylolisthesis is an important minority of spondylolisthesis because it has the highest risk of neurologic damage. Congenital dysplasia of the lumbosacral facets and sacrum can allow pathologic anterior translation of the L5 vertebral body in the setting of intact posterior elements, which can ultimately compress the L5 and sacral nerve roots. There is a significantly higher frequency of progression in the dysplastic type (32%) than in the isthmic type (4%).[73]

Spondylolysis is relatively common in the general population, although most are asymptomatic. In a prospective study of 500 children followed for 45 years beginning in first grade, the prevalence of pars interarticularis lesions was 4.4% among 6-year-olds and 6% among adults.[74] Fifteen percent of those with a spondylolysis had progression to spondylolisthesis.

Risk factors for developing spondylolysis include a family history and a preexisting developmental spine defect.[75,76] Spondylolysis was historically believed to be two to three times more common in boys than in girls,[18] but more recent data suggest equal prevalence.[19] There is an increased incidence of spondylolysis in some female-dominated sports such as ballet, figure skating, and gymnastics. Spondylolisthesis appears to occur more frequently in girls.[20–22] The rates of both are two to three times higher in children of European descent than in those of African descent.[77]

The athlete typically presents with low back pain or, occasionally, pain that radiates to the buttock or posterior thigh. Although acute injury may precipitate the onset of pain, insidious onset is more common. The pain is worse with activity, especially hyperextension. If there is an associated high-grade slip, the pain is often severe. On physical examination, bilateral hamstring tightness is common, and hyperextension with a one-leg stance exacerbates the pain. A palpable step-off may be present. Paresthesia, neurologic deficit, and tension signs may be present in the presence of spondylolisthesis. Patients with chronic spondylolysis may develop neurologic symptoms in the L5 nerve distribution. In spondylolysis, gait is often normal, but in a high-grade spondylolisthesis with neurologic deficits, the gait will be impaired.

Radiographic workup starts with AP and lateral radiographs. Oblique radiographs can also be obtained for confirmation of the diagnosis. However, although the oblique view may show the "scotty dog" sign (a break in the neck of the dog represents a defect in the pars interarticularis), the study is only 32% sensitive.[78] In the case in which radiographs are negative for spondylolysis, but clinical suspicion is high, the most sensitive test is single-photon emission computed tomography (SPECT).[79] SPECT may also be an indicator of osseous healing potential, as increased signal intensity correlates with metabolically active bone.[80] MRI may also be useful in detecting a pars interarticularis lesion, especially at detecting bone marrow edema in a pre-lysis lesion.[81] Early detection of stress reaction may prevent the development of pars defects.[82] Once a spondylolysis is diagnosed, healing is best followed with a CT scan. CT scan can be employed to classify lesions as early, progressive, and chronic.[83]

The initial management of spondylolysis is conservative, with activity modification and restriction from sports for a 3- to 6-month period. Physical therapy is also indicated to decrease lumbar lordosis, to strengthen core musculature, and to stretch hamstring contractures. A lumbar brace is also recommended by some to decrease lumbar lordosis and to alleviate stresses on the pars interarticularis. A modified Boston brace molded in 0° to 15° of flexion is worn 24 hours a day for 3 months and then during sports activity for the following 3 months. Return to sports is allowed once pain free range of motion is obtained. This treatment regimen has shown to have good or excellent clinical results in 78% of patients,[84] with 72% to 89% successfully returning to sports.[85,86] The use of a spinal orthosis remains controversial; however, as similar results have been reported without bracing.[87] A recent meta-analysis of the nonoperative treatment suggests that 84% of patients treated nonoperatively will have a successful clinical outcome after 1 year and that bracing does not seem to influence this outcome.[88] No Level I or II studies have yet been performed comparing bracing and nonbracing treatment regimens.[88] Healing is believed to occur in most unilateral lesions, half of bilateral lesions, and rarely in chronic lesions.[81] In most patients, formation of a fibrous union appears to offer acceptable stability in the short term. Proponents of brace treatment argue that the bony union rate is higher, especially when also combined with transcutaneous electrical bone stimulation.[20]

Surgical treatment is reserved for patients with a progressive spondylolisthesis (grade III or higher), neurologic deficit, or painful nonunion and persistent back pain despited nonsurgical treatment. Patients with dysplastic spondylolisthesis are most likely to require surgical treatment relative to other forms of spondylolisthesis.[89,90] The gold standard for surgical management of lesions at L5 is in situ fusion with autogenous bone graft. L4, and proximal lesions are treated with direct repair. Methods for achieving union include posterior wiring of the transverse process and spinous process, pedicle screw-and-hook techniques, or Buck translaminar interfragmentary screws. Results from Buck fusion are the most studied in the literature, with a 88% of patients achieving painless union[91] and 82% returning to sports.[92]

Degenerative Disc Disease

Whereas discogenic pathology is the primary cause in nearly half of adults with back pain,[7] in inactive adolescents, it is the cause of only a small minority of cases. Adolescent athletes, however, have a relatively higher incidence of back pain attributable to discogenic causes, representing as many as 11% of cases.[7] Repetitive hyperflexion and extension loading on the lumbar disc during sports can lead to end-plate irregularities and the formation of Schmorl nodes, as well as annular tearing, disc protrusion, and end-plate fractures. An association between participation in competitive sports and early lumbar disc degeneration has also been demonstrated in multiple studies. There appears to be an increased prevalence of disc degeneration in sports with more frequent trunk rotation[93] including gymnastics,[94] soccer,[95] and weightlifting.[90] An MRI comparison of college athletes with nonathletes showed a higher degree of disc degeneration, most significantly in baseball players and swimmers.[20]

The adolescent growth spurt appears to be the most vulnerable time for injuries to the lumbar intervertebral disc, as degenerative changes on MRI are relatively uncommon before this time.[31] A long-term outcomes study of young athletes showed that most of the degenerative abnormalities seen in the lumbar discs at 15 years follow-up were already present in comparative MRI scans taken in late adolescence and early adulthood.[96] These findings suggest that most of these injuries occured during the adolescent growth spurt.

Discogenic pain is often nonspecific in its presentation. Athletes may complain of aching low back pain that is worse with forward flexion. On examination, patients often have decreased flexibility in the lumbar spine and hamstrings, and thoracic hypokyphosis and lumbar hypolordosis may be present as well. Some patients may stand with a scoliotic posture in an attempt relieve discogenic pain. MRI will often show early degenerative changes including disc signal reduction, loss of height, bulging, apophyseal abnormalities, and modic changes.

The mainstay of treatment for young athletes with degenerative disc disease is nonsurgical. Activity modification, restriction from sports, and NSAIDs are usually successful in managing back pain. A corset brace is also sometimes helpful in relieving back pain in the short term. Physical therapy is directed at increasing trunk strength and lumbar and hamstring flexibility, and a sport-specific training program can help the athlete with a gradual return to sports. Microdiscectomy may be necessary in patients who fail nonsurgical treatment.

Lordotic Low Back Pain

Lordotic low back pain is the second most common type of low back pain in pediatric and adolescent athletes, representing approximately one fourth of cases.[7] Lordotic back pain is associated with decreased flexibility during the adolescent growth spurt. During this phase, the accelerated growth of the spine causes tightening of the thoracolumbar fascia, interspinous ligaments, and tendinous attachments on the spine. Athletes who exert repetitive hyperextension to their lower back while playing sports can develop traction apophysitis, impingement of the spinous processes, and pseudoarthrosis of the transitional vertebrae.

Patients usually complain of low back with activity. On examination, pain is reproduced with provocative hyperextension of the lower back and usually the hamstrings are very tight. Radiographs may show an apophyseal avulsion or incomplete segmentation of a vertebra at the transitional zone, consistent with a pseudarthrosis. Lordotic low back pain is diagnosis of exclusion after other etiologies are ruled out. Bertolotti syndrome may also be seen as a cause of extension pain in young athletes.[97]

Treatment involves physical therapy emphasizing antilordotic, hamstring, and peripelvic stretching. The athlete gradually returns to sports once symptoms resolve. Those patients who do not respond to physical therapy may benefit from antilordotic bracing. Corticosteroid injections into inflamed facets or transitional pseudoarthrosis may be helpful as well.

Scheurmann Kyphosis

Scheurmann kyphosis, or juvenile kyphosis, is the most common cause of structural kyphosis in the adolescent. Hyperkyphosis of greater than 40° occurs within the thoracic spine, usually between T7 and T9, due to anterior wedging of multiple vertebrae. The diagnosis is made on a lateral radiograph in which there are at least three consecutive vertebrae with wedging of 5° or more. In addition, there are typical vertebral end-plate changes and Schmorl nodes, as well as apophyseal ring fractures. Juvenile kyphosis is diagnosed between the ages of 13 and 17 and is more common in boys. It is rare in patients younger than 10 years.

Patients with juvenile kyphosis may complain only of a cosmetic deformity; it is painless in approximately 80% of patients. Higher demand athletes, however, may complain of back pain with activity. Examination of the patient reveals a round back appearance in the thoracic spine that is most prominent with forward flexion and is not reducible with hyperextension or by lying supine. This is in contrast to postural kyphosis, which is usually reducible with hyperextension. Thoracic kyphosis may be accompanied by a compensatory hyperlumbar lordosis, which is associated with a much higher rate of back pain, as well as an increased risk of spondylolysis. Patients often have hamstring and thoracolumbar fascia tightness.

The treatment of juvenile kyphosis is somewhat controversial. Some advocate that Scheurmann kyphosis is a self-limited condition with a benign course, which does not need any treatment. However, thoracolumbar braces are often used to stabilize progression of the deformity in the skeletally immature patient with a kyphosis of 50° or more. When worn for 12 to 24 months until maturity, the Milwaukee and DuPont braces may limit progression of the deformity, and in some cases may also lead to improvement.[98]

Surgical management is limited to a low percentage of patients. In patients with persistent pain and curves greater than 75°, spinal fusion may be recommended. Rigid curves of greater than 55° are treated with anterior release and interbody fusion followed by posterior fusion with compression instrumentation. Those patients whose kyphosis corrects to less than 55° with hyperextension can often be treated by posterior-only approaches.

Atypical Scheurmann Kyphosis

Atypical Scheuermann disease is an uncommon, but important, cause of back pain in adolescents. Similar to persons with Scheuermann kyphosis, patients have vertebral wedging; however, the deformities occur at the thoracolumbar junction and proximal lumbar spine rather at than the thoracic spine. This condition is often associated with sagittal malignment, so-called flat back syndrome, which presents as lumbar hypolordosis and thoracic hypokyphosis. End-plate changes, Schmorl nodes, and apophyseal ring fractures may occur, but frequently involve only one vertebra. The condition is caused by repetitive flexion injury of the thoracolumbar vertebrae. Management is focused at activity modification from the aggravating activity and extension-based physical therapy. Lordotic bracing is sometimes used.

SUMMARY

Clinicians taking care of athletes are likely to see many young patients complaining of back pain. The young athlete places significant repetitive stresses across the growing thoracolumbar spine, which can cause acute and overuse injuries that are unique to this age and patient population. Fortunately, by using a careful and systematic approach, with a sport-specific history, careful physical exam, and proper imaging, most problems can be properly identified. Although it is important to always remember that rare and more serious problems such as a neoplasm or infection may be a source of pain in the athletic patient, most problems are benign and can be treated conservatively. Accurate diagnosis and management of back pain not only can prevent long-term deformity and disability, but it can also allow young athletes to return to doing what they love to do most: play sports.

REFERENCES

1. Turner PG, Hancock PG, Green JH, et al. Back pain in childhood. Spine 1989;14: 812–4.
2. Mirovsky Y, Jakim I, Halperin N, et al. Non-specific back pain in children and adolescents: a prospective study until maturity. J Pediatr Orthop 2002;11:275–8.
3. Olsen TL, Anderson RL, Dearwater SR, et al. The epidemiology of low back pain in the adolescent population. Am J Public Health 1992; 82:606–9.
4. Watson K, Papageorgiou A, Jones G, et al. Low back pain in school children: occurrence and characteristics. Pain 2002;97:87–92.
5. National Council of Youth Sports. Report on trends and participation in organized youth sports. Available at: http://www.ncys.org/publications/2008-sports-participation-study.php. Accessed April 22, 2012.
6. Pipe A. Consternation amidst perspiration: sport medicine and children. Presented at the annual meeting of the Canadian Orthopaedic Association, Winnipeg, Manitoba, Canada, June, 1993.
7. Micheli LJ, Wood R. Back pain in young athletes: significant differences from adults in causes and patterns. Arch Pediatr Adolesc Med 1995;199:15–8.
8. Bhatia NN, Chow G, Timon SJ, et al. Diagnostic modalities for the evaluation of pediatric back pain: a prospective study. J Pediatr Orthop 2008;28:230–3.
9. Salter RB, Harris WR. Injuries involving the epiphyseal plate. J Bone Joint Surg [Am] 1963;45:587–622.
10. Sagi H, James G, Jarvis M, et al. Histomorphic analysis of the pars interarticularis and its association with isthmic spondylolysis. Spine 1998;23:1635–40.
11. Labrom RD. Growth and maturation of the spine from birth to adolescence. J Bone Joint Surg [Am] 2007;89(Suppl 1):3–7.
12. Micheli LJ, Curtis C. Stress fractures in the spine and sacrum. Clin Sports Med 2006;25:75–88.
13. Krabbe S, Christiansen C. Effects of puberty on rates of bone growth and mineralization: with observations in male delayed puberty. Arch Dis Child 1979;54:950–3.
14. Bailey DA, Wedge JH, McCulloch RG, et al. Epidemiology of fractures of the distal end of the radius in children as associated with growth. J Bone Joint Surg [Am] 1989;71A: 1225–31.
15. Carter DR, Hayes WC. Bone compressive strength: the influence of density and strain rate. Science 1976;194:1174–6.
16. Carter DR, Spengler DM. Mechanical properties and composition of cortical bone. Clin Orthop 1978;135:192–217.
17. Kujala UM, Taimela S, Oksanen A, et al. Lumbar mobility and low back pain during adolescence: a longitudinal three-year follow-up study in athletes and controls. Am J Sports Med 1997;25(3):363–8.
18. Marty C, Boisaubert B, Descamps H, et al. The sagittal anatomy of the sacrum among young adults, infants, and spondylolisthesis patients. Eur Spine J 2002;11:119–25.

19. Roche MB, Rowe GG. The incidence of separate neural arch and coincident bone variations: a summary. J Bone Joint Surg [Am] 1952;34(2):491–4.
20. D'Hemecourt PA, Gerbino PG II, Micheli LJ. Back injuries in the young athlete. Clin Sports Med 2000;19(4):663–79.
21. Loud KJ, Micheli LJ. Common athletic injuries in adolescent girls. Curr Opin Pediatr 2001;13(4):317–22.
22. McTimoney CA, Micheli LJ. Managing back pain in young athletes. J Musc Med 2004; 21(2):63–9.
23. Wiltse LL, Jackson DW. Treatment of spondylolisthesis and spondylolysis in children. Clin Orthop Relat Res 1976;117:92–100.
24. Omey ML, Michelu LJ, Gerbino PG II. Idiopathic scoliosis and spondylolysis in the female athlete: tips for treatment. Clin Orthop Relat Res 2000;372:74–84.
25. Cirillo JV, Jackson DW. Pars interarticularis stress reaction, spondylolysis, and spondylolisthesis in gymnasts. Clin Sports Med 1985;4:95–110.
26. Micheli LJ, Kasser JR. Painful spondylolysis in a youngfootball player. In: Hochschuler SH, editor. The spine in sports. Philadelphia: Hanley and Belfus; 1990. p 327–30.
27. Michell LJ, McCarthy C. Figure skating. In: Watkins RG, editor. The spine in sports. St. Louis (MO): Mosby-Yearbook; 1996. p. 557–64.
28. Micheli LJ. Back injuries in gymnastics. Clin Sports Med 1985;4:85–93.
29. Mundt DJ, Kelsey JL, Golden AL, et al. An epidemiologic study of sports and weight lifting as possible risk factors for herniated lumbar and cervical discs. Am J Sports Med 21(6):854–60.
30. Watkins RG. Lumbar disc injury in the athlete. Clin Sports Med 2002;21(1):147–65.
31. Baranto A, Hellstrom M, Cederlund CG, et al. Back pain and MRI changes in the thoracolumbar spine of top athletes in four different sports: a 15-year follow-up study. Knee Surg Sports Traumatol Arthrosc 2009;17(9):1125–34.
32. Dogan S, Safavi-Abbasi S, Theodore N, et al. Thoracolumbar and sacral spinal injuries in children and adolescents: a review of 89 cases. J Neurosurg 2007;106 (6 Suppl): 426–33.
33. Junkins EP, Stotts A, Santiago R, et al. The clinical presentation of pediatric thoracolumbar fractures: a prospective study. J Trauma 2008; 65(5):1066–71.
34. Denis F. The three column spine and its significance in the classification of acute thoracolumbar spinal injuries. Spine 1983;8:817–31.
35. Hauser CJ, Visvikis G, Hinrichs C, et al. Prospective validation of computed tomographic screening of the thoracolumbar spine in trauma. J Trauma 2003;55:228–34.
36. Berry GE, Adams S, Harris MB, et al. Are plain radiographs of the spine necessary during evaluation after blunt trauma? Accuracy of screening torso computed tomography in thoracic/lumbar spine fracture diagnosis. J Trauma 2005;59:1410–3.
37. Hadley MN, Zabramski JM, Browner CM, et al. Pediatric spinal trauma: review of 122 cases of spinal cord and vertebral column injuries. J Neurosurg 1988;68:18–24.
38. Ruge JR, Sinson GP, McLone DG, et al. Pediatric spinal injury: the very young. J Neurosurg 1988;68:25–30.
39. Hamilton MG, Myles ST. Pediatric spinal injury: review of 174 hospital admissions. J Neurosurg 1992;77:700–4.
40. Clark P, Letts M. Trauma to the thoracic and lumbar spine in the adolescent. Can J Surg 2001;44:337–45.
41. McPhee IB. Spinal fractures and dislocations in children and adolescents. Spine. 1981;6:533–7.
42. Vander Have KL, Caird MS, Gross S, et al. Burst fractures of the thoracic and lumbar spine in children and adolescents. J Pediatr Orthop 2009;29:713–9.

43. Lalonde F, Letts M, Yang JP, et al. An analysis of burst fractures of the spine in adolescents. Am J Orthop 2001;30:115–20.
44. Dimeglio A. Growth in pediatric orthopaedics. In: Morrissy RT, Weinstein SL, editors. Lovell and Winter's pediatric orthopaedics. Philadelphia: Lippincott Williams and Wilkins; 2001. p. 33–62.
45. Domenicucci M, Preite R, Ramieri A, et al. Thoracolumbar fractures without neurosurgical involvement: surgical or conservative treatment? J Neurosurg Sci 1996;40: 1–10.
46. Schnee CL, Ansell LV. Selection criteria and outcome of operative approaches for thoracolumbar burst fractures with and without neurological deficit. J Neurosurg 1997;86(Suppl 1):48–55.
47. Wood K, Buttermann G, Mehbod A, et al. Operative compared with nonoperative treatment of a thoracolumbar burst fracture without neurologic deficit: a prospective randomized study. J Bone Joint Surg [Am] 2003;85A:773–81.
48. Parisini P, DiSilvestre M, Greggi T. Treatment of spinal fractures in children and adolescents. Spine 2002;27:1989–94.
49. Parisini P, Di Silvestre M, Greggi T, et al. Lumbar disc excision in children and adolescents. Spine 2001;26:1997–2000.
50. Epstein JA, Lavine LS. Herniated lumbar intervertebral discs in teen-age children. J Neurosurg 1964;21:1070–5.
51. Epstein JA, Epstein NE, Marc J, et al. Lumbar intervertebral disc herniation in teenage children: recognition and management of associated anomalies. Spine 1984;9:427–32.
52. Shoeter I, Entzian W. Lumbar disc protrusion in children and adolescents. Adv Neurosurg 1977;4:12–7.
53. Clarke NMP, Cleak DK. Intervertebral lumbar disc prolapse in children and adolescents. J Pediatr Orthop 1983;3:202–6.
54. Matsui H, Terahata N, Tsuji H, et al. Familial predisposition and clustering for juvenile lumbar disc herniation. Spine 1992;17:1323–8.
55. Cleveland RH, Delong GR. The relationship of juvenile lumbar disc disease and Scheuermann's disease. Pediatr Radiol 1981;10:161–4.
56. Paajanen H, Alanen A, Erkintalo BM, et al. Disc degeneration in Scheuermann's disease. Skeletal Radiol 1989;18:523–6.
57. Rabin A, Gerszten PC, Karausky P, et al. The sensitivity of the seated straight-leg raise test compared with the supine straight-leg raise test in patients presenting with magnetic resonance imaging evidence of lumbar nerve root compression. Arch Phys Med Rehabil 2007;88(7):840–3.
58. Zhu Z, Zhao Q, Wang B, et al. Scoliotic posture as the initial symptom in adolescents with lumbar disc herniation: its curve pattern and natural history after lumbar discectomy. BMC Musculoskelet Disord 2011;12:216–24.
59. Kumar R, Kumar V, Das NK, et al. Adolescent lumbar disc disease: findings and outcome. Childs Nerv Syst 2007;23:1295–9.
60. Fakouri B, Nnadi C, Boszczyk B, et al. When is the appropriate time for surgical intervention of the herniated lumbar disc in the adolescent? J Clin Neurosci 2009; 16:1153–6.
61. Gennuso R, Humphreys RP, Hoffman HJ, et al. Lumbar intervertebral disc disease in the pediatric population. Pediatr Neurosurg 1992;18:282–6.
62. Kurihara A, Kataoka O. Lumbar disc herniation in children and adolescents: a review of 70 operated cases and their minimum 5-year follow-up studies. Spine 1980;5:443–51.

63. Ebersold MJ, Quast LM, Bianco AJ Jr. Results of lumbar discectomy in the pediatric patient. Neurosurgery 1987;67:643–7.
64. Papagelopoulos PJ, Shaughnessy WJ, Ebersold MJ, et al. Long-term outcome of lumbar discectomy in children and adolescents sixteen years of age of younger. J Bone Joint Surg [Am] 1998;80(5):689–98.
65. Epstein NE. Lumbar surgery for 56 limbus fractures emphasizing noncalcified type III lesions. Spine 1992;17:1489–96.
66. Yen CH, Chan SK, Ho YF, et al. Posterior lumbar apophyseal ring fractures in adolescents: a report of four cases. J Orthop Surg 2009;17(1):85–9.
67. Dietemann JL, Runge M, Badoz A, et al. Radiology of posterior lumbar apophyseal ring fractures: report of 13 cases. Neuroradiology 1988;30:337–44.
68. Peh WC, Griffith JF, Yip DK, et al. Magnetic resonance imaging of lumbar vertebral apophyseal ring fractures. Australas Radiol 1998;42(1):34–7.
69. Labelle H, Roussouly P, Berthonnaud E, et al. The importance of spino-pelvic balance in L5–S1 developmental spondylolisthesis: a review of pertinent radiologic measurements. Spine 2005;30(6 Suppl):S27–34.
70. Labelle H, Roussouly P, Berthonnaud E, et al. Spondylolisthesis, pelvic incidence, and spinopelvic balance: a correlation study. Spine 2004;29(18):2049–54.
71. Yue WM, Brodner W, Gaines RW. Abnormal spinal anatomy in 27 cases of surgically corrected spondyloptosis: proximal sacral endplate damage as a possible cause of spondyloptosis. Spine 2005;30(6 Suppl):S22–6.
72. El Rassi G, Takemitsu M, Woratanarat P, et al. Lumbar spondylysis in pediatric and adolescent soccer players. Am J Sports Med 2005;33(11):1688–93.
73. McPhee IB, O'Brien JP, McCall IW, et al. Progression of lumbosacral spondylolisthesis. Australas Radiol 1981;25:91–5.
74. Beutler WJ, Fredrickson BE, Murtland A, et al. The natural history of spondylolysis and spondylolistheis: 45-year follow-up evaluation. Spine 2003;28(10):1027–35.
75. Albanese M, Pizzutillo PD. Family study of spondylolysis and spondylolisthesis. J Pediatr Orthop 1982;2(5):496–9.
76. Wynne-Davis R, Scott JH. Inheritance and spondylolisthesis: a radiographic family survery. J Bone Joint Surg [Br] 1979;61(3):301–5.
77. Fredrickson BE, Baker D, McHolick WJ, et al. The natural history of spondylolysis and spondylolisthesis. J Bone Joint Surg [Am] 1984;66(5):699–707.
78. Saifuddin A, White J, Tucker S, et al. Orientation of lumbar pars defects: implications for radiological detection and surgical management. J Bone Joint Surg [Br] 1998;80(2):208–11.
79. Bellah RD, Summerville DA, Treves ST, et al. Low-back pain in adolescent athletes: detection of stress injury to the pars interarticularis with SPECT. Radiology 1991;180(2):509–12.
80. Van den Oever M, Merrick MV, Scott JH. Bone scintigraphy in symptomatic spondylolysis. J Bone Joint Surg [Br] 1987;69(3):453–6.
81. Hollenberg GM, Beattie PF, Meyers SP, et al. Stress reactions of the lumbar pars interarticularis: the development of a new MRI classification system. Spine 2002;27(2):181–6.
82. Cohen E, Stuecker RD. Magnetic resonance imaging in diagnosis and follow-up of impending spondylolysis in children and adolescents. Early treatment may prevent pars defects. J Pediatr Orthop B 2005;14(2):63–7.
83. Morita T, Ikata T, Katoh S, et al. Lumbar spondylolysis in children and adolescents. J Bone Joint Surg [Br] 1995;77(4):620–5.
84. Steiner ME, Micheli LJ. Treatment of symptomatic spondylolysis and spondylolisthesis with the modified Boston brace. Spine 1985;10(10):937–43.

85. Sys J, Micheielsen J, Bracke P, et al. Nonoperative treatment of active spondylolysis in elite athletes with normal X-ray findings: literature review and results of conservative treatment. Eur Spine J 2001;10(6):498–504.

86. McCleary MD, Congeni JA. Current concepts in the diagnosis and treatment of spondylolysis in young athletes. Curr Sports Med Rep 2007;6(1):62–6.

87. Standaert CJ. Spondylolysis in the adolescent athlete. Clin J Sport Med 2002;12(2): 119–22.

88. Klein G, Mehlman CT, McCarty M. Nonoperative treatment of spondylolysis and grade I spondylolisthesis in children and young adults: a meta-analysis of observational studies. J Pediatr Orthop 2009;29(2):146–56.

89. Newman PH. A clinical syndrome associated with severe lumbo-sacral subluxation. J Bone Joint Surg [Br] 1965;47:472–81.

90. Hensinger RN, Lang JR, MacEwen GD. Surgical management of spondylolisthesis in children and adolescents. Spine 1976;1:207–16.

91. Buck JE. Direct repair of the defect in spondylolisthesis: preliminary report. J Bone Joint Surg [Br] 1970;52-B:432–8.

92. Debnath UK, Freeman BJC, Gregory P, et al. Clinical outcome and return to sport after the surgical treatment of spondylolysis in young athletes. J Bone Joint Surg [Br] 2003;85-B:244–9.

93. Hangai M, Kaneola K, Hinotsu S, et al. Lumbar intervertebral disk degeneration in athletes. Am J Sports Med 2009;37(1):149–55.

94. Sward L, Hellstrom M, Jacobsson B, et al. Disc degeneration and associated abnormalities of the spine in elite gymnasts: a magnetic resonance imaging study. Spine. 1991;16:437–43.

95. Videman T, Sarna S, Battie MC, et al. The long-term effects of physical loading and exercise lifestyles on back-related symptoms, disability, and spinal pathology among men. Spine 1995;20:699–709.

96. Tertti M, Paajanen H, Kujala UM et al. Disc degeneration in young gymnasts: a magnetic resonance imaging study. Am J Sports Med 1990;18:206–8.

97. Back JD, Wyss JF, Lutz GE. Bertolotti syndrome as a potential cause of low back pain in golfers. PM R 2011;3(8):771–5.

98. Riddle EC, Bowen JR, Shah SA, et al. The duPont kyphosis brace for the treatment of adolescent Scheuermann kyphosis. J South Orthop Assoc 2003;12(3):135–40.

Spinal Deformity in Young Athletes

Pierre A. d'Hemecourt, MD[a],*, M. Timothy Hresko, MD[b]

KEYWORDS

- Scoliosis • Kyphosis • Scheuermann kyphosis • Atypical Scheuermann kyphosis

KEY POINTS

- Scoliosis may be slightly aggravated by excessive sports but this effect is minimal. Athletes with scoliosis are treated similarly to nonathletes and are encouraged to participate in sports even if they are treated with a brace, which is often not used during sports participation.
- Kyphosis may be aggravated by some sports activities. However, postural exercises and sometimes bracing will help with this. Again, sports participation is encouraged, along with proper treatment.
- Atypical or lumbar Scheuermann disease may be more painful in presentation and require more intensive treatment and temporary sports limitation.
- When surgical interventions are needed, return to play is encouraged but the level of participation and involvement in sports with collision or extremes of motion may be curtailed on an individual basis.

INTRODUCTION

Spinal deformity represents a spectrum of disorders that commonly start in childhood or adolescence and may have ramifications of pain and deformity in adults. The term "scoliosis" describes frontal plane geometry of the spine but in reality the spinal deformity is in all three dimensions: frontal, sagittal, and axial. The resulting chest wall deformity will generate the shoulder asymmetry, scapula prominence, and rib hump seen in classic examples of scoliosis. Sagittal plane deformity in idiopathic scoliosis is associated with hypokyphosis of the thoracic spine, whereas hyperkyphosis may be an indication of atypical scoliosis seen with Chiari malformation or syrinx. Scoliosis occurs in about 2% to 3% of the general population while excessive kyphosis may be present in up to 8% of the population.[1,2] The prevalence of these abnormalities can be expected to occur at least with the same frequency in athletes. However, some sports may be associated with increased risks of these deformities, as discussed in this article.

The authors have nothing to disclose.
[a] Primary Care Sports Medicine, Division of Sports Medicine, Children's Hospital Boston, 300 Longwood Avenue, Boston MA 02115, USA; [b] Department of Orthopaedic Surgery, Harvard Medical School, Children's Hospital Boston, 300 Longwood Avenue, Boston, MA 02115, USA
* Corresponding author.
E-mail address: pierre.dhemecourt@childrens.harvard.edu

NORMAL SPINAL MATURATION

In the development of the spine, each vertebral level has three ossification centers. There is one in the anterior centrum or vertebral body. This central ossification center expands to form the superior and inferior physeal end-plates, which grow by enchondral ossification. These are responsible for vertical growth as well as some of the lateral expansion.[3] In the posterior arch, each of the lateral synchondroses has an anterior ossification center as well as one near the spinous processes. The posterior ossification centers are responsible for vertical and peripheral growth. However, posterior ossification centers close by the end of the first decade of life while the anterior growth will continue through the adolescent growth period of about 16 to 18 years of age.[4] Some speculation has been given to asymmetric closure of the lateral ossification centers as a cause for scoliosis.[5]

The "ring apophysis" forms from lateral expansion of the end-plate physis at each end of the vertebral body. As the central end-plate becomes thin, the peripheral end-plate forms the ring apophysis with tensile and compressive forces.[6,7] These appear between the ages of 8 and 12 years and fuse by adulthood.[8] Abnormal forces here may predispose to compression injuries such as Scheuermann kyphosis or the limbic vertebrae.

The sagittal spinal shape changes with growth. The newborn essentially has a "C"-shaped vertebral column. With head control, the infant soon develops a cervical lordosis, whereas with the sitting posture, the kyphosis is accentuated. Lordosis starts with standing. During the adolescent growth spurt, thoracic kyphosis and lumbar lordosis increase.[9] These may be accentuated further with intense sports such as hyperlordosis in gymnasts or hyperkyphosis in swimmers.[10,11] The normal range of thoracic kyphosis is believed to be 20° to 45°, with lordosis usually in the range of 40° to 65°. Children will often manifest a 20° curve that increases to 25° in adolescence and finally approaches 40° in adulthood with corresponding changes in lordosis to maintain a balanced sagittal profile.[12]

SCOLIOSIS

Scoliosis is classified as infantile, juvenile, or adolescent idiopathic. This is dependent on the age at presentation: infantile scoliosis before 3 years of age, juvenile scoliosis between 3 and 10 years, and adolescent scoliosis between 10 years and maturity.[13] Scoliosis is generally defined as a curve of 10° or more on a standing radiograph. Smaller curves are often referred to as spinal asymmetry. Smaller curves occur equally in males and females. As the curve reaches significance, the ratio is about 4:1 female to male. If curves larger than 25° to 30° are considered, the ratio reaches 7:1.[14,15] Genetic factors play a strong role in the development of scoliosis.[16] Adolescent idiopathic scoliosis (AIS) incidence varies and has been estimated to occur in 1.5% to 3% of the population.[17] However, in sports this may vary. In classic ballet, Warren noted a significant increased prevalence of 24% minor curve in young dancers.[18] Similarly, Tanchev noted a 10-fold increase in scoliosis frequency among rhythmic gymnasts.[19] Plausible explanations for this include the repetitive asymmetric forces across the growth cartilage of the spine, particularly in prepubertal and pubertal athletes. Warren noted the association of low body mass and intense training in premenarchal dancers. Other sports have also been associated with asymmetric torque forces contributing to a functional scoliosis. These activities include swimming, throwing, and serving.[20] In a study of elite single arm throwing sports, 80% manifested some mild thoracic curve by clinical examination.[21]

AIS may be associated with mild generalized back pain. When present, other causes such as syrinx, tethered cord, or a Chiari malformation should be considered along with more common mechanical causes of back pain such as spondylolysis and disc herniation.[22] Thus, a spinal screen magnetic resonance imaging (MRI) scan should be considered in the setting of AIS that has progressed to greater than 20 and pain. However, back pain may be seen in older adolescents with AIS.[23] Further, some athletics are associated with an increased risk of pain irrespective of scoliosis.[24,25]

Treatment

Mild to moderate scoliosis may be managed by a combination of observation, bracing, and possibly exercise depending on the degree of curvature and the skeletal maturity of the athlete. Exercise has not been shown to be an effective treatment in several larger studies comparing AIS with and without exercise.[26,27] However, the compliance with exercise was very poor in both studies. Asymmetry of paraspinal musculature and rotary strength has been demonstrated in AIS.[28–30] Further, the correction of this asymmetry has correlated with a specific exercise program.[31] Finally, several small studies have demonstrated that addressing rotary torso conditioning has a positive effect on the spinal curve.[32,33] Obviously, much more needs to be studied in this respect. Nonetheless, a well directed exercise program for core strength should be encouraged for athleticism as well as possible improvement in curvature. This would seem to be particularly true in the event of bracing where muscle motion is inhibited.

In several large studies, bracing for scoliosis has shown some positive effect.[34,35] However, in other studies, this effect has been questioned.[36,37] One problem with bracing is the lack of compliance in at least a third of treatments.[38] Nonetheless, after a review of the literature, Weinstein and Dickson concluded that bracing should be considered for curves greater than 25° in skeletally immature patients.[39] A current large multicenter prospective study, Bracing in Adolescent Idiopathic Scoliosis Trial (BrAIST), is near conclusion and may provide better data.

The first step is to determine the magnitude of the curve and the risk of progression. It has been suggested that minor scoliosis, secondary to sport involvement, may benefit from cross training, with counteracting muscular strengthening.[20] Skeletal maturity is determined by several methods. The Risser score is a sign of skeletal maturity of the ilium and correlates with curve progression.[40] For instance, even with a minor curve of 5° to 19° there is a 22% progression risk with a Risser grade 0–1 while a more advanced Risser has a 1.6% risk for curve progression.[1] Other factors that are related to increased risk of curve progression include premenarchal status and double curves.[41,42] These factors include the magnitude of the curve at presentation and the presence of double curves. A hand bone-age radiograph may also be helpful in questionable cases of skeletal maturity.

The decision on type and frequency of radiographs is based on pubertal status and physical examination. The forward bend Adams test evaluates the trunk rotation with a scoliometer. If the scoliometer reaches 7° in an immature child, a PA radiograph from C7 to the iliac crest is obtained. For curves less than 25° on radiography, observational treatment is recommended with a frequency dependent on puberty. A prepubertal athlete with a curve 10° to 14° may be reevaluated in 1 year whereas a curve from 15° to 19° should be evaluated again in 3 to 6 months with a history and scoliometer examination. In prepubertal athletes with a curve of 20° to 24°, a repeat radiograph is performed in 3 months. A curve of greater than 30° or one that manifests a progression of more than 5° should be considered for bracing.[43] This may include the Boston brace, which is worn 18 to 23 hours per day. A nighttime brace may also be utilized such as the Charleston or Providence brace. The athlete is often able to compete during the time out of the brace. However, the athlete needs to be aware that the effect of the brace is dose dependent.[44] Bracing for 18 hours seems to have the optimal effect. In curves that reach 40° to 45° in immature patients, surgical stabilization is considered. The intent is to preserve as many free segments as possible while fusing the involved spine segments in a corrected position. The return to play after stabilization is quite variable and is discussed in a separate article by Hresko and Lin elsewhere in this issue.

SAGITTAL PLANE DEFORMITY
Thoracic Kyphosis

A common form of thoracic kyphosis is Scheuermann kyphosis. It is manifested as a round back deformity with a fixed deformity and was first described by Scheuermann.[45] The etiology of this disease is unknown, but it is thought to have a hereditary component as well as a biomechanical stress factor. Sorenson defined it further in 1964 as a kyphosis greater than 45° with more than 5° of anterior wedging at three adjacent vertebrae (**Fig. 1**).[46] This should be differentiated from the more benign postural kyphosis that fully corrects on extension. The apex of the Scheuermann curve is generally between the T7 and T9 vertebrae. The changes in the vertebra also include end-plate irregularities and Schmorl nodes.

Some sports have been noted to have a high correlation with kyphosis. This has been quite notable in water skiers starting competitively at a young age.[47] It has even been noted in some dancers.[48] Among adolescents, competitive swimming has also been associated with increased kyphosis.[10,49] It is conceivable that the mechanical compressive stress applied to the anterior vertebrae potentiates the deformity.

Scheuermann kyphosis presents in the teenage years and may be more prevalent in athletes.[50] The incidence ranges from 0.4% to 8% in the general population, with the majority presenting between 10 and15 years of age.[51] There may be a 2:1 male-to-female predominance, but other studies have noted an equal ratio.[52,53] The presenting symptom may be incidental or a deformity concern noted by the parents. However, it may be associated with pain in the mid-thoracic spine, periscapular region, or lumbar spine. The pain can worsen with activity or prolonged sitting and standing. There is usually no related radiculopathy unless there is disc involvement of the neuroforamina. The primary complaint is sometimes cosmetic, with patients complaining of poor posture or a visual "hunchback." On examination the patient will have a pronounced kyphotic appearance to the thoracic spine, which is accentuated with forward flexion. Scheuermann kyphosis is a fixed deformity and differentiated from postural kyphosis with a lack of correction on hyperextension. With Scheuermann kyphosis, extension may diminish the kyphosis, but not completely eliminate it. Patients may also have an excessive lumbar lordosis and have broad, barrel chests and tight hamstrings. About 20% to 30% of patients may also have scoliosis.[54] Neurologic deficits are rare.

Radiographs will include a standing lateral thoracolumbar spine view with inclusion of C7 and the femoral heads. Hyperkyphosis of greater than 45° with three or more consecutive vertebrae wedging is diagnostic. There may be associated Schmorl nodes, end-plate changes, and intervertebral disc narrowing.

Treatment

Treatment for Scheuermann kyphosis depends on the degree of kyphosis. The majority of cases can be treated conservatively. For curves less than 50°, conservative management with stretching of the anterior chest wall and shoulders and hamstrings, extension-based strengthening, and core stabilization exercises can be effective.[55] Bracing may be recommended for those with remaining growth and a

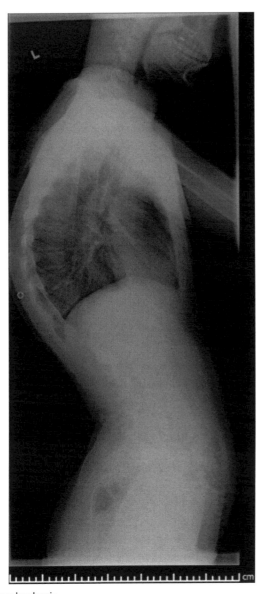

Fig. 1. Scheuermann kyphosis.

curve between 50° and 70°, especially if painful. The type of brace is dependent on the level of the apex. For curves with an apex at T7 and above a Milwaukee brace is indicated while an apex below T7 may be treated with a thoracic–lumbar–sacral orthosis (TLSO).[56] Ideally, the brace should be used 16 to 18 hours per day. By consensus, the brace is worn at night as nocturnal growth is significant and part of the day while sitting.[57] For adolescents, a Milwaukee brace (**Fig. 2**) may be challenging to accept, and if indicated the larger brace may at times be used at night while a TLSO is used for daytime wear. In compliant adolescents, initial correction in the brace may

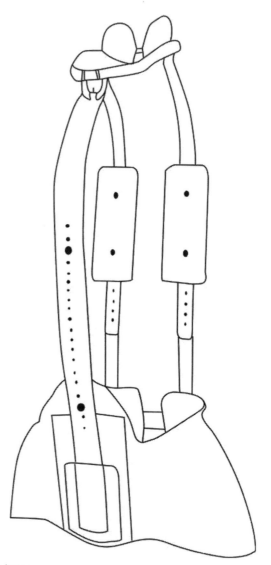

Fig. 2. Milwaukee brace.

recede but 69% of the time will maintain a mild improvement 5 years later.[58] Surgery may be indicated in rare cases in which there is a large curve, persistent pain, progressive deformity, and failed bracing.[59]

Athletics and Kyphosis

Athletes with Scheuermann kyphosis may be able to continue with their sport as tolerated. They are encouraged to maintain flexibility of their hamstrings and thoracolumbar fascia as well as strength of the spinal extensors, hamstrings, and entire core. When a brace is indicated, brace wear is encouraged for many sports. However, athletes such as swimmers and gymnasts will be able to participate in their sports activity during the allowed time out of the brace. In athletes who require surgical stabilization, return to sports may be modified. This is discussed in a subsequent article by Hresko and Lin elsewhere in this issue.

Thoracolumbar Scheuermann Disease

Thoracolumbar Scheuermann disease represents a different expression of the spectrum of thoracic Scheuermann disease. It involves the thoracolumbar spine. However, it is less well defined than thoracic Scheuermann disease and likely represents a heterogeneous group of similar end-plate, anterior Schmorl nodes and disc space narrowing. Yet, it does not necessarily meet the criteria of Sorenson. It may be more common in adolescent boys and is thought to be the result of mechanical overuse in sports.[60] However, females are commonly affected, especially in sports with extreme spinal motion such as gymnastics.[61] Lumbar Scheuermann disease generally has a more painful presentation. Blumenthal has described two types of lumbar Scheuermann disease. One type involves the typical spinal changes as described by Sorenson with a focal kyphosis at the lower thoracic–lumbar juncture. The other type manifests the end-plate changes and Schmorl nodes but without a kyphosis. This latter type is referred to as "atypical Scheuermann disease" (**Fig. 3**).[62] There is often a loss of lordosis, rendering a flat back appearance.

Thoracolumbar Scheuermann disease usually manifests as a flexion-based pain complex. Physical findings demonstrate pain on forward flexion and possibly a

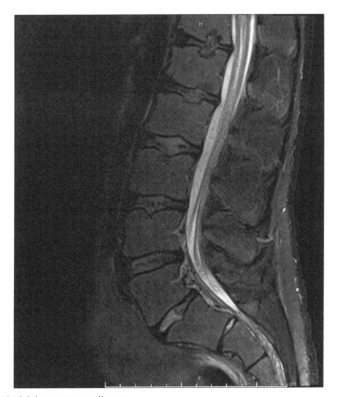

Fig. 3. Atypical Scheuermann disease.

kyphosis or flat back. Treatment for atypical Scheuermann disease is mainly conservative. Lumbar Scheuermann disease with a kyphotic deformity tends to be more painful than the nonkyphotic deformity and resistant to treatment.[63] Kyphosis is often asymptomatic in the upper thoracic location but usually symptomatic in the lower thoracic and lumbar region. Rest from sports and weightlifting alone may alleviate symptoms. Lordotic bracing with a lumbosacral orthosis or TLSO may be temporarily helpful in more severe cases. Correcting the lordosis may be very beneficial in some athletes.[64]

Athletics and Thoracolumbar Scheuermann Disease

Athletes with a kyphotic deformity of the thoracolumbar juncture may remain quite symptomatic and unable to return to sports activity. However, some athletes, such as gymnasts, will present with only the disc and end-plate changes and no kyphosis. These athletes can potentially return to full athletics.

Activity restriction, time, and physical therapy exercises may work well for some athletes. The therapy should be focused on restoring the normal lordosis as tolerated. Maintaining a tolerated cross-training program is beneficial for overall conditioning. If a brace is utilized, it should be used during the day. As the athlete is becoming pain free, a full conditioning program should be pursued.

SUMMARY

Young athletes may have a spinal deformity incidentally or potentially related to their sport. These athletes should be encouraged to continue sports participation in many instances. Brace wear is commonly used for kyphotic and scoliosis deformities. Many sports can be played in the brace. Even with sports that cannot practically be played in the brace, most bracing protocols have enough time out of brace during the day for the athlete to continue participation. However, good physical therapy for flexibility and strengthening of the spine should be continued. Even sports that potentially aggravate the deformity may be continued in these circumstances.[65]

REFERENCES

1. Lonstein JE, Carlson JM. The prediction of curve progression in untreated idiopathic scoliosis during growth. J Bone Joint Surg [Am] 1984;66:1061–71.
2. Tribus CB. Scheuermann's kyphosis in adolescents and adults: diagnosis and management. J Am Acad Orthop Surg 1998;6:36–43.
3. Moe JH. Back problems in the young athlete. J Am College Health Assoc 1968;17:126.
4. Dimeglio A. Postnatal spine growth and development: the growing spine. In: Proceedings of the Pediatric Orthopaedic Society of North America Specialty Day 2007. San Diego, CA, 2007.
5. Stokes IA, Spence H, Aronsson DD, et al. Mechanical modulation of vertebral body growth: implications for scoliosis progression. Spine 1996;21:1162–7.
6. Hindman B, Poole C. Early appearance of the secondary ossification centers. Radiology 1970;95:359–61.
7. Ogden JA. Radiology of postnatal skeletal development. XI. The first cervical vertebra. Skeletal Radiol 1984;12:12–20.
8. Loder RT, Hensinger RN. Fractures of the thoracic and lumbar spine. In: Rockwood CA Jr, Wilkins KE, Beaty JH, editors. Rockwood and Green, Fractures in Children. 4th edition. Philadelphia (PA): Lippincott-Raven; 1996. p. 1063–105. Chapter 12.
9. Akin C, Muharrem Y, Akin U, et al. The evolution of sagittal segmental alignment of the spine during childhood. Spine 2004;30(1) 93–100.

10. Wojtys EM, Ashton-Miller JA, Huston LJ, et al. The association between athletic training time and the sagittal curvature of the immature spine. Am J Sports Med 2000; 28:490–8.
11. Ohlen G, Wredmark T, Spangfort E. Spinal sagittal configuration and mobility related to low-back pain in the female gymnast. Spine 1989;14:847.
12. Fon GT, Pitt MJ, Thies ACJ. Thoracic kyphosis: range in normal subjects. AJR Am J Roentgenol 1980;134:979–83.
13. Rogala EJ, Drummond DS, Gurr J. Scoliosis: incidence and natural history. A prospective epidemiologic study. J Bone Joint Surg [Am] 1978;60A:173–6.
14. Weinstein SL. Adolescent idiopathic scoliosis: prevalence and natural history. Instr Course Lect 1989;38:115–28.
15. Brooks HL, Azen SP, Gerberg E, et al. Scoliosis: a prospective epidemiologic study. J Bone Joint Surg [Am] 1975;57:968–72.
16. Lowe TG, Edgar M, Margulies JY, et al. Etiology of idiopathic scoliosis: current trends in research. J Bone Joint Surg [Am] 2000;82A:1157–68.
17. Soucacos PN, Zacharis K, Soultanis K, et al. Risk factors for idiopathic scoliosis: review of a 6-year prospective study. Orthopedics 2000;23:833–8.
18. Warren MP, Brooks-Gunn J, Hamilton LH, et al. Scoliosis and fractures in young ballet dancers: relation delayed menarche and secondary amenorrhea. N Engl J Med 1986;314:1348–53.
19. Tanchev PI, Dzherov AD, Parushev AD, et al. Scoliosis in rhythmic gymnasts. Spine 2000;25(11):1367–72.
20. Becker TJ. Scoliosis in swimmers. Clin Sports Med 1986;5:149–58.
21. Sward L. The thoracolumbar spine in young elite athletes: current concepts on the effects of physical training. Sports Med 1992;13:357–64.
22. Schwend RM, Hennrikus W, Hall JE, et al. Childhood scoliosis: clinical indications for MRI. J Bone Joint Surg [Am] 1995;77A:46–53.
23. Ramirez M, Jonsston CE, Browne RH. The prevalence of back pain in children who have idiopathic scoliosis. J Bone Joint Surg [Am] 1997;79A:364–8.
24. Sward L, Hellstrom M, Jacobbson B, et al. Back pain and the radiologic changes in the thoracolumbar spine of athletes. Spine 1990;15:124–9.
25. Micheli LJ, Mintzer CM. Overuse injuries of the spine. In: Harries M, Williams C, Stanish WD, et al, editors. Oxford textbook of sports medicine. 2nd edition. Oxford: Oxford University Press; 1998. p. 709–20.
26. Stone B, Beekman C, Hall V, et al. The effect of an exercise program on change in curve in adolescents with minimal idiopathic scoliosis: a preliminary study. Phys Ther 1979;59:759–63.
27. Carman D, Roach JW, Speck G, et al. Role of exercises in the Milwaukee brace treatment of scoliosis. J Pediatr Orthop 1985;5:65–8.
28. Ford DM, Bagnall KM, McFadden KD, et al. Paraspinal muscle imbalance in adolescent idiopathic scoliosis. Spine 1984;9:373–6.
29. Kennelly KP, Stokes MJ. Pattern of asymmetry of paraspinal muscle size in adolescent idiopathic scoliosis examined by real-time ultrasound imaging: a preliminary study. Spine 1993;18:913–7.
30. Reuber M, Schultz A, McNeill T, et al. Trunk muscle myoelectric activities in idiopathic scoliosis. Spine 1983;8:447–56.
31. Mooney V, Gulick J, Pozos R. A preliminary report on the effect of measured strength training in adolescent idiopathic scoliosis. J Spinal Disord 2000;13:102–7.
32. Mooney V, Brigham A. The role of measured resistance exercises in adolescent scoliosis. Orthopedics 2003;26:167–71.

33. McIntire K, Asher M, Burton D, et al. Trunk rotational strength training for the management of adolescent idiopathic scoliosis (AIS). Stud Health Technol Inform 2006;123:273–80.
34. Lonstein JE, Winter RB. The Milwaukee brace for the treatment of adolescent idiopathic scoliosis: a review of one thousand and twenty patients. J Bone Joint Surg [Am] 1994;76A:1207–21.
35. Korovessis P, Kyrkos C, Piperos G, et al. Effects of thoracolumbosacral orthosis on spinal deformities, trunk asymmetry, and frontal lower rib cage in adolescent idiopathic scoliosis. Spine 2000;25(16):2064–71.
36. Dolan L, Weinstein S. Surgical rates after observation and bracing for adolescent idiopathic scoliosis: an evidence-based review. Spine 2007;32(19):91–100.
37. Noonan KJ, Weinstein SL, Jacobson WC, et al. Use of the Milwaukee brace for progressive idiopathic scoliosis. J Bone Joint Surg [Am] 1996;78A:557–67.
38. Rowe DE, Bernstein SM, Riddick MF, et al. A meta-analysis of the efficacy of non-operative treatments for idiopathic scoliosis. J Bone Joint Surg [Am] 1997;79A:664–74.
39. Dickson RA, Weinstein SL. Bracing (and screening)—yes or no? J Bone Joint Surg [Br] 1999;81B:193–8.
40. Risser JC. The iliac apophysis: an invaluable sign in the management of scoliosis. Clin Orthop 1958;11:111–9.
41. Bunnell WP. A study of the natural history of idiopathic scoliosis before skeletal maturity. Spine 1986;11:773–6.
42. Ascani C, Bartolozzi P, Logroscino CA, et al. Natural history of un-treated idiopathic scoliosis after skeletal maturity. Spine 1986;11:784–9.
43. Omey ML, Micheli LJ, Gerbino PG. Idiopathic scoliosis and spondylolysis in the female athlete. Clin Orthop 2000;372:74–84.
44. Katz DE, Durrani AA. Factors that influence outcome in bracing large curves in patients with adolescent idiopathic scoliosis. Spine 2001;26(21):2354–61.
45. Tribus CB. Scheuermann's kyphosis in adolescents and adults: diagnosis and management. J Am Acad Orthop Surg 1998;6:36–43.
46. Sorensen K. Scheuermann's juvenile kyphosis: clinical appearances, radiography, aetiology and prognosis. Copenhagen (Denmark): Munksgaard; 1964.
47. Tall RL. Spinal injury in sport: epidemiologic considerations. Clin Sports Med 1993;12:441.
48. Solomon R, Brown T, Gerbino PG, et al. The young dancer. Clin Sports Med 2000;19:717.
49. Wilson FD, Lindseth RE. The adolescent "swimmer's back." Am J Sports Med 1982;10:174.
50. Ali RM, Green DW, Patel TC. Scheuermann's kyphosis. Curr Opin Pediatr 1999;11(1):70–5.
51. Ferguson AB Jr. The etiology of preadolescent kyphosis. J Bone Joint Surg [Am] 1956;38–A(1):149–57.
52. Murray PM, Weinstein SL, Spratt KF. The natural history and long-term follow-up of Scheuermann kyphosis. J Bone Joint Surg [Am] 1993;75(2):236–48.
53. Winter R. The treatment of spinal kyphosis. Int Orthop 1991;15(3):265–71.
54. Lowe TG. Scheuermann disease. J Bone Joint Surg [Am] 1990;72(6):940–5.
55. Weiss HR. Members of SOSORT: physical exercises in the treatment of idiopathic scoliosis at risk of brace treatment: SOSORT consensus paper 2005. Scoliosis 2006;1:6.
56. Schiller J, Eberson C. Spinal deformity and athletics. Sports Med Arthrosc Rev 2008;16:26–31.

57. de Mauroy J, Weiss H, Aulisa A, et al. 7th SOSORT consensus paper: conservative treatment of idiopathic and Scheuermann's kyphosis Scoliosis 2010;5:9. Available at: http://www.scoliosisjournal.com/content/5/1/9. Accessed August, 2011.

58. Sachs B, Bradford D, Winter R, et al. Scheuermann kyphosis: follow-up of Milwaukee-brace treatment. J Bone Joint Surg [Am] 1987;69:50–7.

59. Speck GR, Chopin DC. The surgical treatment of Scheuermann's kyphosis. J Bone Joint Surg [Br] 1986;68(2):189–93.

60. Wenger DR, Frick SL. Scheuermann kyphosis. Spine 1999;24(24):2630–9.

61. Goldstein JD, Berger PE, Windler GE, et al. Spine injuries in gymnasts and swimmers: an epidemiologic investigation. Am J Sports Med 1991;19(5):463–8.

62. Blumenthal SL, Roach J, Herring JA. Lumbar Scheuermann's: a clinical classification. Spine 1987;12:929–32.

63. Djurasovic M, Glassman SD. Correlation of radiographic and clinical findings in spinal deformities. Neurosurg Clin N Am 2007;18(2):223–7.

64. Weiss HR, Werkmann M. Unspecific chronic low back pain—a simple functional classification tested in a case series of patients with spinal deformities. Scoliosis 2009;4(1):4.

65. Pizzutillo PD. Spinal considerations in the young athlete. Instr Course Lect 1993;42: 463–72.

The Young Adult Spine in Sports

Ken R. Mautner, MD[a,*], Mandy J. Huggins, MD[b]

KEYWORDS

- Low back pain • Young adult athlete • Discogenic pain • Radiculopathy

KEY POINTS

- The most common etiology of low back pain (LBP) in young athletes is internal disc disruption.
- If there are no "red flag" signs or symptoms, it is appropriate to begin conservative management without imaging.
- The natural history of acute LBP in young athletes is generally favorable.
- Rehabilitation should focus on local core stability and hip girdle strengthening.
- Interventional procedures, such as epidural steroid injection, have a role in reducing inflammation and pain associated with lumbar radicular pain for those athletes not responding to more conservative treatment.

Low back pain (LBP) has a lifetime incidence of up to 80% in the general population, and 12% to 15% of the United States population each year will visit a physician for this complaint.[1] Given those numbers, it is not surprising that LBP affects all athletes, regardless of position or level of play. In fact, the incidence of LBP in athletes has been suggested to be as high as 30%.[2]

When broken down by sport, it is thought that certain sports and/or positions predispose athletes to certain types of low back injuries. For example, a review of medical records of 199 collegiate athletes from 23 sports who had LBP indicated that female rowers, male rowers, and male football players had a higher incidence of disc herniation.[3] A study comparing college student athletes to age-matched controls suggested that baseball players and swimmers had a higher incidence of lumbar disc degeneration, whereas basketball players, runners, and soccer players did not.[4] Disk degeneration has also been shown to be more common in gymnasts[5] and weight-lifters.[6] It is also thought that offensive and defensive linemen are more at risk for discogenic problems because of their size and the repetitive forces sustained in the lumbar region.[7] In a survey of National Collegiate Athletic Association (NCAA) and

The authors have nothing to disclose.
[a] Department of Physical Medicine and Rehabilitation, Department of Orthopedics, Emory University, 59 Executive Park South, Suite 200, Atlanta, GA 30329, USA; [b] Broward Health Sports Medicine, 2300 North Commercial Pkwy, Suite 319, Weston, FL 33326, USA
* Corresponding author.
E-mail address: kmautne@emory.edu

Table 1	
LBP etiologies by age	
Age	**Etiology**
<18 y	Spondylolysis
18–50 y	Internal disc disruption
>50 y	Facet or SI joint pain

National Football League (NFL) team physicians, it was found that approximately half of athletes with isthmic spondylolisthesis (vertebral slippage due to spondylolysis) were linemen.[8] Spondylolysis, stress fracture of the pars interarticularis, is also commonly diagnosed in gymnasts, weightlifters, track and field athletes, and soccer players.[9]

Although up to 70% of acute LBP is thought to be due to sprain or strain, other etiologies exist and are typically what will present to the clinician's office.[10] The cause of LBP can be generally broken down by age. Spondylolysis has been shown to be the most common diagnosis in adolescent athletes.[11] Between the ages of 18 and 50, internal disc disruption (IDD) is the most common etiology of LBP, whereas facet joint and sacroiliac joint (SIJ) pain are more common beyond age 50 (**Table 1**). DePalma and colleagues have confirmed with diagnostic interventional procedures that the younger the patient (with the exception of adolescents), the more likely the etiology is the disc.[12] We know from previous studies and surveys that most episodes of acute LBP will resolve within 6 weeks, but recurrence rates are reported to be between 50% and 84% in the general population.[13–15] What is not known is whether athletes have more or less risk of recurrent and potentially chronic LBP after these episodes.

ANATOMY

There are multiple pain generators in the human spine. This anatomy is important to bear in mind when evaluating an athlete with back pain. The lumbar spine is largely made up of the five vertebral bodies, which have a major weight-bearing function. Caudal to the spine is the sacrum, which has a synovial and partially ligamentous articulation with the iliac crests on either side. The SIJ is the largest axial joint in the body and is primarily a stabilizing joint, whose exact innervation remains unclear.[16,17] The pedicles of the lumbar vertebral bodies connect the posterior elements to the vertebral bodies. The posterior spine consists of the laminae, articular processes, and spinous processes. The superior and inferior articular processes of adjacent vertebrae create the zygapophyseal or facet joints. The pars interarticularis is part of the lamina between the articular processes[18] (**Fig. 1**). A defect in this area is called **spondylolysis**,[19] which is covered at length in another article elsewhere in this issue.

The intervertebral disc has three structural components: the nucleus pulposus, which comprises the central core; the annulus fibrosus, which forms the outer circumferential ring; and the cartilaginous vertebral endplates. The collagen layers of the annulus are arranged in a "criss-cross" type pattern, allowing it to resist axial, torsional, and tensile loads. The inner nucleus pulposus, which is composed of approximately 70% water, determines the disc height and also provides resistance to axial compression.[20] The proteoglycan and water content decreases with age, as do the number of viable cells in the nucleus.[21] The intervertebral disc is largely avascular and receives its nutrition from diffusion through the endplates and connective tissue transport. It has been suggested that this diminished blood supply leads to the

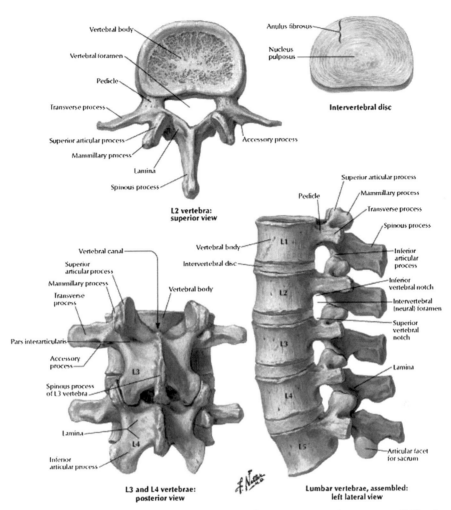

Fig. 1. Lumbar spine anatomy. (*Netter illustration from* www.netterimages.com. © Elsevier Inc. All Rights Reserved; Used with permission.)

beginning of degenerative breakdown of the disc in the second decade of life.[22] Both the inner portion of the annulus and the nucleus have no innervation, while the outer third of the annulus has small penetrating branches from the sinuvertebral nerve.[20] Interestingly, degenerated discs and adjacent endplates have more extensive innervation with nociceptive properties when compared with asymptomatic discs.[23,24]

Any of the three components of the disc can be involved in a disc herniation. These can be classified further: a **protrusion** occurs when nuclear material bulges but remains contained by the annulus. An **extrusion** is nuclear material that has migrated behind the vertebral body either superior or inferior to the annulus, which remains intact. A **herniation** occurs when fragments have ruptured through the annulus (**Fig. 2**).

Interestingly, mechanical compression of a nerve root may not be responsible for radicular pain. Biochemical, inflammatory processes are thought to contribute to pain

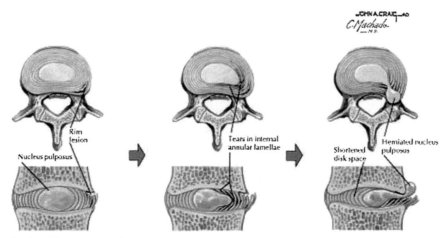

Fig. 2. Disk rupture and disc herniation. Peripheral tear of annulus fibrosus and cartilage endplate (rim lesion) initiates sequence of events that weaken and tear internal annular lamellae, allowing extrusion and herniation of nucleus pulposus. (*Netter illustration from www.netterimages.com.* © Elsevier Inc. All Rights Reserved; Used with permission.)

caused by a herniated disc.[20] Specifically, high levels of phospholipase A_2 and prostaglandin E_2, potent proinflammatory enzymes, have been found in human lumbar disc herniations and extrusions, respectively.[25,26] However, this condition typically has a favorable natural history. Multiple studies have shown clinical improvement and/or resorption of herniated materials in up to 90% of individuals without surgical intervention.[27–30] This is important to remember when considering a treatment plan for young adult athletes with radicular pain from a herniated disc.

While disc herniation can contribute to radicular discomfort, IDD without herniation is a very common source of back pain. Disrupted intervertebral discs have been shown to have higher concentrations of sensory fibers.[23] Also, levels of inflammatory mediators are elevated in both herniated discs[31] and degenerated discs[32]; in fact, one study showed a higher elevation of inflammatory markers in both the annulus and nucleus of degenerated discs than in the discs of patients with sciatica.[33] It is presumed that nociceptors within fissures in the annulus or adjacent to endplates are the source of this pain.[34]

A widely accepted theory exists regarding the sequence of events in the degeneration of the intervertebral disc, which was first described by Kirkaldy-Willis and colleagues in 1978. These events occur in individuals with or without significant back pain. First, repetitive microtrauma from shearing forces causes small, circumferential tears in the annulus. These tears can coalesce into larger radial tears, which may or may not lead to herniation. Over time, the disc becomes more disrupted and loses its height and its connection to the vertebral endplates. This segmental dysfunction results in instability, which can then lead to lateral recess and foraminal narrowing with subsequent nerve root impingement. It also results in muscular weakness and instability of the posterior elements, leading to degenerative changes over time. These mechanical changes affect the levels above and below this segmental degeneration, resulting in multilevel degenerative changes and stenosis. Eventually, the formation of scar tissue, osteophytes, and joint surface irregularities result in loss of motion, restabilization, and often a decrease in pain.[35,36]

EVALUATION

Evaluation of the athlete with LBP should begin with a thorough history of the injury or onset of back pain. This should include mechanism of injury (if any); location, character, and radiation of pain; exacerbating activities; and positions that alleviate the pain. For example, discogenic pain is usually made worse with prolonged periods of sitting or twisting activities.[37] The history should also include details pertinent to the particular sport, such as the athlete's position, training regimen, and injury history. A history of low back injury is a significant predictor for a subsequent back injury in varsity athletes.[38] The examiner should also be aware of previous treatments or modalities being used for the current injury. If there are radicular symptoms, the athlete should be asked to trace the pattern in the extremity for the examiner. The pattern and specific location of LBP can help determine the etiology of pain. Those who describe midline LBP are more likely to have discogenic pain (IDD), as opposed to those who report paramidline LBP, which is more likely to be caused by SI or facet joints.[39,40] However, when treating the young adult athletic population, the examiner should bear in mind the possibility of inflammatory spondyloarthropathy. Complaints of LBP and morning stiffness that improves with exercise are consistent with this diagnosis. Of course, past medical history and review of systems, including "red flag" signs and symptoms (**Table 2**), are also critical. These findings should prompt further evaluation or urgent surgical referral in the case of cauda equina syndrome.

The next step in evaluation is the physical exam, which should always include inspection of the back and limbs, palpation of the spine (standing and prone), and evaluation of gait and range of motion. The neurologic exam then follows, which includes testing of strength, sensation, and reflexes in both lower extremities. The combination of weakness, sensory loss, and diminished or absent reflexes may indicate nerve root impingement.[18] Special tests are also helpful, such as straight leg raise (SLR), crossed SLR, the slump test, and ankle dorsiflexion with SLR (Braggard's test).[37] The SLR test is fairly sensitive (0.91) but less specific (0.29), whereas the opposite is true for the crossed SLR (0.29 and 0.88).[41] The sensitivity for the slump test was recently shown to be 0.84 and its specificity is 0.83.[42]

It should be noted that this article does not discuss signs or symptoms of psychosocial factors, such as inappropriate behaviors and nonorganic physical signs, which are commonly referred to as Waddell's signs. It is thought that these factors can be predictors of poor patient outcomes and the likelihood of more chronic complaints.[37] Although the examiner may expect a high level of motivation for an

Table 2 Red flag signs and symptoms	
Sign/Symptom	**Possible Cause**
Bowel and/or bladder dysfunction Sexual dysfunction Saddle anesthesia	Cauda equina syndrome[a]
Night or rest pain Unexplained weight loss History of cancer	Cancer
Fever/chills Recent infection Intravenous drug use	Infection

[a] True surgical emergency.

athlete to return to sports, this cannot be assumed as psychosocial influences on injuries in athletes has been documented.[43,44] Attention to these signs and symptoms during the evaluation is critical when evaluating young adult athletes with LBP.

In addition, this article does not discuss spondylolysis and spondylolisthesis. These are two issues that certainly can present as pain in young adult athletes but they are extensively covered in the pediatric and older adult articles in this issue as they are more prevalent in these populations.

IMAGING

Once the history and physical examination have been performed, and a differential diagnosis formulated ruling out serious etiologies, it is completely acceptable to begin treatment of the athlete without obtaining imaging. Routine imaging for those with nonspecific acute LBP is not recommended.[45] Although lumbar radiographs have been shown to increase patient satisfaction,[46] and most patients believe they are important,[47] they are often unnecessary[48] and have not been shown to lead to better outcomes.[46,49] It is also important to avoid unnecessary radiation exposure, especially in the female population. Gonadal radiation from one set of AP and lateral films of the lumbar spine is equivalent to a year's worth of daily chest radiographs.[50] Obtaining plain films would be appropriate if there is a history of trauma, chronic steroid use, possible instability, or spondylolysis. It may also be considered if LBP persists beyond 6 weeks despite conservative treatment.[37]

Advanced imaging such as magnetic resonance imaging (MRI) is indicated if there is a history of "red flag" signs and symptoms or findings of neurologic compromise, as it is the test of choice for infection and metastases. Plain radiography is not highly sensitive for these etiologies. MRI is also the test of choice to evaluate disc morphology,[51] but because of the favorable natural history of herniated discs, MRI is not necessary in those with isolated radicular symptoms and a stable examination. MRI is, however, commonly utilized in planning interventional procedures such as epidural steroid injections.[45]

Although MRI is a useful diagnostic tool, it should be ordered with care. Boden and colleagues first described the prevalence of a degenerated or bulging in 35% of a group of asymptomatic patients younger than the age of 60 years who had never experienced back or radicular pain.[52] Others have reported similar findings, including Jensen, who reported abnormal findings in 64% of asymptomatic individuals. The incidence of these disc bulges has also been shown to increase with age.[53,54] This indicates the need to carefully correlate an MRI with a patient's clinical findings, as the MRI findings may not be responsible for the pain. In fact, Modic and colleagues noted that although the level of disc herniation on MRI correlated with patient symptoms, there was no correlation between size or number of herniations and patient symptoms or examination.[55] When looking specifically at an athletic population, the recommendations are the same. An evaluation of lumbar MRI scans of 19 asymptomatic males who were highly active for at least 10 years resulted in only 3 normal scans.[56] Another study involving college athletes showed a 29% incidence of disc degeneration in athletes without back pain. However, this study did find a correlation between athletes with history of LBP and disc degeneration.[4]

There is debate regarding which imaging modality is better for evaluating the source of discogenic pain. Discography, which involves fluoroscopically guided injection into the intervertebral disc in the hopes of reproducing the patient's pain, simply helps determine whether a disc is painful. In other words, it can help rule out a disc as a source of pain if the procedure does not reproduce the patient's pain. Discography has been even more scrutinized recently owing to increased risks associated with the procedure. Known complications of discography include increased pain, nausea, headache, and discitis.[57] In one study, 40% of individuals who were asymptomatic before discography reported new LBP afterwards. It should be noted that all of these patients had abnormal psychometrics.[58] In animal models, intentional injury to the intervertebral discs has been correlated with subsequent degenerative changes on MRI similar to IDD.[59,60] Recently, more degenerative changes and herniations in the discs of patients who had previously undergone discography were seen on MRI when compared with controls,[61] suggesting that intradiscal procedures result in accelerated degeneration. Because of these risks, at this time discography is recommended only when there is high suspicion for discogenic pain after unequivocal imaging, failure of nonoperative treatment, and surgery is being considered.[57,62]

In lieu of discography, MRI is being utilized more to help diagnose discogenic pain. The finding of a "high-intensity zone" (HIZ) within the posterior annulus on T2 sequences is thought by some to be a reliable marker of painful annular disruption in those with low back pain (**Fig. 3**). Histologic studies of the HIZs reveal inflammatory cell infiltration and remodeling of the tissue.[63] Multiple studies have supported correlation between the HIZ and a concordant response on discography, with positive predictive values being reported as high as 88%.[63–67] However, other studies have either not found the same correlation,[68,69] or have concluded that the HIZ is not a reliable indicator because up to 25% of asymptomatic individuals also have HIZs on MRI.[53,70] Lei and colleagues found a sensitivity of 94% and specificity of 77% of all MRI findings predicting a painful disc, but they concluded that HIZs themselves have low predictive value.[62]

DISCOGENIC PAIN

Discogenic pain is the most common source of LBP in the young to middle-aged adult, with a prevalence rate near 40%.[12,71] It differs from nerve root pain secondary to chemical irritation or compression from a disc; it is mechanical and usually

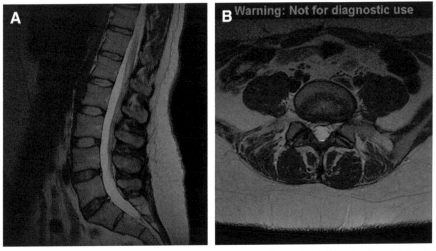

Fig. 3. High-intensity zones seen in the posterior annulus on T2 (*A*) sagittal and (*B*) axial images.

nonradicular with a somatic pattern.[62] IDD was first described in 1986 as a painful syndrome that results from chemical irritation from substances released from a damaged disc.[72] The culprit is a disc that exhibits a normal external contour but has changes in the internal structure. Many sports place significant, repetitive forces through the intervertebral disc, putting athletes at high risk for IDD.[73,74]

It was previously thought that no clinical features existed to identify IDD in a patient with LBP.[71] However, some history and exam findings can support the diagnosis. As mentioned previously, a complaint of midline pain in a young adult is most likely to be discogenic in nature.[12,39] Also, athletes with IDD typically complain of pain with periods of unsupported sitting, especially while leaning forward,[75] which correlates with the finding that intradiscal pressure is greater in a forward flexed, sitting position.[18] Back pain during class or with prolonged sitting at work is a common complaint. Pain with rising from sitting can also be reported with discogenic pain, but it is not specific.[40] Contrary to popular belief, posterior annular tears without nerve root compression can also cause radicular type buttock, groin, and leg pain.[75–77]

On examination, palpation of the lumbar spine may reveal midline tenderness. There should be no neurologic deficits. SLR and neural tension testing should also be negative. It has recently been suggested that reproduction of LBP with sustained hip flexion (**Fig. 4**) or pelvic rock is associated with an increased probability of IDD.[78] To perform the sustained hip flexion test, flex the hips to 70° while the patient is supine

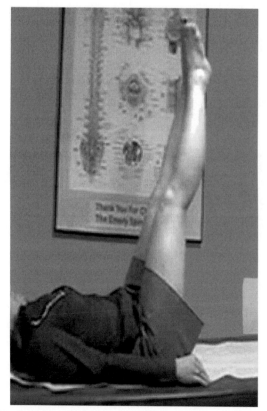

Fig. 4. Sustained hip flexion.

and ask the patient to slowly lower the legs, looking for reproduction of a patient's typical LBP.

Because the natural history of acute LBP is generally favorable, athletes should be educated on the prognosis and be encouraged to remain active. Activity modification has been shown to lead to quicker recovery when compared to bed rest.[37,45] Unfortunately, the recurrence rate for LBP can be quite high, up to 84% in one study.[79] Studies aimed at preventing recurrence of LBP have focused on specific control of core muscles. As mentioned previously, muscular weakness is a component of segmental instability and degenerative changes in the spine. Biomechanical studies have shown that effective muscle control, specifically that of the lumbar multifidus and transversus abdominus, can provide segmental stability by controlling motion of the spine.[80,81] Also, although an acute episode of LBP pain may resolve after 2 to 4 weeks, multifidus function does not recover spontaneously.[82] Therapy that targets retraining of the stabilizing spinal musculature has been shown to result in less LBP recurrence compared to those who do not undergo specific exercise training.[83,84] This type of therapy, called motor control, has been shown to be more effective than medical management and education in chronic, nonspecific LBP.[85]

In addition to the core muscles discussed in the preceding text, hip extensors and abductors are also important, as they function as stabilizers of the pelvis and transmit forces from the lower extremities to the spine. Nadler and colleagues demonstrated that athletes with LBP had a greater gluteus medius imbalance when compared to those without LBP, although this did not reach significance ($P = .07$).[86] An association has also been found between hip abductor imbalance in females and future occurrence of LBP.[87] Greater fatigability of gluteus maximus muscles has also been demonstrated in patients with chronic LBP.[88] Therefore, physical therapy should include an evaluation of and directed treatment toward strengthening gluteal muscle weakness and imbalances.

First-line medications for acute LBP include nonsteroidal anti-inflammatory drugs (NSAIDs) and acetaminophen. Athletes should be cautioned about possible side effects, such as gastrointestinal and renovascular risks with NSAIDs and asymptomatic aminotransferase elevations with acetaminophen. Skeletal muscle relaxants have been shown to be beneficial for short-term (2–4 days) relief only. Sedation and dizziness are common side effects. Opioid medications, although effective for pain relief, should be used with caution secondary to side effect profiles and risk for dependency or addiction. Oral corticosteroids have not been proven effective for axial LBP and are generally not recommended.[45,89]

Caudal epidural steroid injections (ESIs) have been suggested to provide positive short-term clinical outcomes for patients with ongoing discogenic pain,[90,91] but no study has been done with a placebo control. A recent review of studies evaluating caudal epidural injections for various etiologies of LBP suggested Level 1 evidence for this treatment method for chronic (not acute) discogenic back pain. It did note, however, a paucity of the literature for this diagnosis; only three trials were reviewed.[92] Recently, good outcomes were reported in one study after interlaminar ESI for discogenic pain.

Other experimental treatments have been reported, but more research is necessary before they can be recommended. Peng and colleagues reported significant decrease or complete alleviation of pain in 87% of patients with discogenic back pain who received intradiscal injection of methylene blue.[93] However, this was a small study and needs replication with bigger numbers. Platelet-rich plasma (PRP) has also been studied as an intradiscal injection. It has been shown to stimulate proteoglycan and collagen production in animal intervertebral discs,[94,95] as well as induce nucleus pulposus proliferation and collagen synthesis in human disc tissues in vivo.[96] Again, more studies in humans are needed before these procedures should be considered for treatment.

RADICULAR PAIN

Radicular symptoms are commonly caused by a herniated disc, which may cause mechanical compression or chemical irritation of the nerve root. Symptoms include numbness, tingling, and sharp radiating pain in the lower extremity. Ninety percent of symptomatic disc herniations occur at L4–L5 and L5–S1.[97] Patients may complain of concomitant LBP or no LBP at all. The pain can be made worse by coughing, sneezing, or Valsalva maneuver.

As with all lumbar spine examinations, the spine should be inspected and palpated. Range of motion should be documented, including flexion, extension, and lateral flexion. The neurologic examination must be performed carefully, as deficits may be subtle. Examination should include thorough strength testing of the bilateral lower extremities. It is important to document any focal weakness as well as diminished sensation or reflexes. Evaluation of the athlete's gait, which includes walking on the heels and toes, can be helpful. Special tests, such as SLR, can also be helpful. This involves passive flexion of the leg at the hip with the patient in the supine or sitting position. Classically, a positive test reproduces pain that travels beyond the popliteal fossa when the hip is flexed between 30° and 60°. It has been suggested that distribution of pain on SLR can predict location of the herniation in 88.5% of patients.[98] A crossed SLR sign occurs when the unaffected limb is flexed at the hip, causing reproduction of the radicular pain in the affected limb. This is less sensitive, but more specific, than the SLR.[99] The slump test, which is also more specific than the SLR, is performed with the patient seated at the edge of the table with knees flexed. The test is positive if the leg pain is reproduced with the thoracic and cervical spines flexed and the knee extended.[42]

As previously mentioned, the natural course of disc herniation with radiculopathy is favorable. If there is no evidence of progressing neurologic deficit or cauda equina syndrome, imaging is not necessary. The first step in management should include physical therapy and medications, such as NSAIDs. Although not Food and Drug Administration (FDA) approved for this diagnosis, gabapentin has been shown to provide relief for radicular pain when compared to placebo.[100] Systemic steroids, on the other hand, despite anecdotal success, have demonstrated no benefit over placebo.[45,89]

Athletes should be encouraged to remain active with relative rest from sporting activities, as bed rest is not beneficial.[37] Physical therapy should also be encouraged. A recent systematic review of randomized, controlled trials reported that there is moderate evidence for stabilization exercises versus no intervention for treatment of radicular pain. It was noted, however, that there were no trials comparing stabilization exercises to other treatments. It was also suggested that manipulation is more beneficial than sham manipulation for acute radicular pain with disc protrusion (extrusions were excluded).[101] One review of 100 high-level young adult athletes with radicular pain reported that 79 were able to return to their sport after relative rest and an individualized training program.[102] The use of lumbar corsets and braces is not supported by the literature.[20] There is also not enough evidence to recommend traction for LBP with or without leg pain.[103]

A common approach to LBP is the McKenzie method, or mechanical diagnosis and treatment. This begins with assessment of pain patterns to determine a classification. The objective is to look for "centralization" of the pain in response to sustained postures or repeated movements of the lumbar spine in a single direction. Centralization occurs when distal referred pain progressively retreats back toward the lumbar spine with these repeated movements. A patient's "directional preference" (DP) is identified as the direction (ie, flexion or extension) that leads to centralization. The subsequent intervention relies heavily on repeated lumbar exercises that match the patient's DP.[104,105] Long and colleagues found that patients who underwent directional preference-based exercises fared significantly better in all measured outcomes at short-term follow-up than those who were given nonspecific exercises or exercises opposite of their directional preference.[105] Other results suggest that outcomes with the McKenzie method to be equal to or superior to those from stabilization exercises. It has also been shown that centralization predicts an excellent prognosis if directed by DP.[104]

If there is no improvement in the athlete's condition in 4 to 6 weeks despite conservative management and intervention is necessary, a lumbar spine MRI is indicated.[50] This can help the interventionalist decide at which level an epidural steroid injection may be beneficial. Epidural corticosteroid injections are commonly used in the treatment of radicular pain, with the goal of decreasing the inflammation surrounding the nerve root. It is critical that these be performed with fluoroscopic guidance; if not, the target may be missed 30% to 40% of the time.[106] Riew and colleagues conducted a prospective, randomized, controlled study of subjects appropriate for surgery who instead underwent transforaminal nerve root block with bupivacaine plus betamethasone or bupivacaine alone. Results indicated that the ESI was more effective than anesthetic alone. Also, 29 of 51 patients avoided surgery in the first 2 years, and 21 of those 29 had still avoided surgery with good outcomes at 5-year follow-up.[107] Another prospective study randomized patients with radicular pain and a large disc herniation who had failed 6 weeks of conservative treatment into either discectomy or epidural injection treatment groups. Almost all patients who underwent surgery were satisfied with their results and had quicker resolution of symptoms. Although approximately only 50% of the injection patients reported relief at 3 years, it still suggests a positive role of epidural steroid injection in the noninvasive treatment of pain from a herniated lumbar disc. This study also showed no detrimental effects on neurologic recovery if surgery was delayed.[108]

When ESI is compared with placebo, results are conflicting. Transforaminal ESI was shown to provide superior outcomes at 1 year when compared to placebo trigger point injections in a small study,[109] but a large, multicenter, randomized, placebo-controlled trial evaluating the effects of ESI for sciatica showed no medium or long-term difference between the two treatment groups. There was a greater improvement in function at 3 weeks in the ESI group.[110] This suggests that ESIs are reasonable for acute radicular pain when other conservative measures have failed and while waiting for the natural healing process to take effect.

Although surgical management is discussed in a separate article in this issue, it is worth mentioning outcomes of surgical versus nonoperative treatment of lumbar radicular pain. The Spine Patient Outcomes Research Trial (SPORT), which was a large, randomized trial performed at 13 institutions, aimed to evaluate outcomes after open discectomy versus nonoperative treatment for radiculopathy with disc herniation. However, "because of the large numbers of patients who crossed over in both directions, conclusions about the superiority or equivalence of the treatments are not warranted based on the intent-to-treat analysis." Patients in both groups showed improvement over a 2-year period.[111] However, results from the observational cohort group in this study showed those who received surgery had significant improvements in primary outcome measures at 4 years when compared with the nonoperative group. Forty-four percent of the initial nonoperative group had surgery by the end of 4 years.[112] In addition, a large Cochrane review reported that discectomy provides a more rapid improvement in acute radicular leg pain compared with conservative treatment.[113]

SACROILIAC JOINT PAIN

The SIJ is also a common cause of LBP in athletes. It presents as pain in the area of the SIJ and it can radiate into the lower limb with variable pain patterns. Unilateral pain is more common than bilateral pain.[17] SIJ pain is commonly seen in cross-country skiers and rowers, thought to be secondary to biomechanical issues.[114] It is also commonly seen in athletes performing single-leg stance activities, such as skating, gymnastics, and bowling.[115] It can also be caused by ligamentous injury, enthesopathy, shearing forces, and capsular disruption, among others. Injury can result from a combination of axial loading and rotation, as well as direct trauma. It is thought that anatomic abnormalities, such as scoliosis and leg length discrepancy, can put one at risk for developing SIJ pain. Pregnancy is also a known risk factor.[16] It has been established that there are no definitive aggravating or relieving movements or postures that are specific to the SIJ.[116] Some suggest that the "Fortin finger sign," which is demonstrated by the patient putting his or her finger on the exact location of pain, can be a helpful diagnostic tool.[117] It was more recently suggested that there is a 96% chance that the patient will report paramidline LBP if SIJ is involved.[39]

Although sacroiliitis can be a cause of LBP, the term should not be used synonymously with SIJ pain. Sacroiliitis is a true inflammation of the joint that is typically associated with seronegative spondyloarthropathies, such as ankylosing spondylitis. The resulting inflammatory and destructive changes can be detected early on MRI.[118] Some authors suggest that SIJ pain should also be differentiated from SIJ dysfunction, which is a perceivable anterior rotary subluxation of the ilium and has a suggested prevalence of 20% in college students.[119] However, asymmetric SIJ movement and/or hypomobility has been seen in up to 20% of asymptomatic individuals with flexion and Gillett tests.[120] Although some suggest that SIJ pain can be treated by correcting this abnormal movement at the joint, there is no solid evidence to suggest that SIJ pain results directly from dysfunction.[119]

The examination targeting the SIJ is difficult because clinical stress testing in the area can load other nearby structures. Radiologic testing is also not reliable for diagnosis, and there is no gold standard for imaging.[16,114,115] Double comparative, intra-articular blocks using fluoroscopic guidance are considered the current standard for diagnosis of SIJ pain.[116,121] While others have been unable to correlate physical exam findings or clinical features to the diagnosis of SIJ pain,[116,122] Laslett and colleagues have shown that a combination of provocative SIJ maneuvers, including compression, distraction, sacral thrust, and thigh thrust testing (**Fig. 5**A–D, respectively), can help identify the SIJ as the pain generator. They report a sensitivity of 93.8% if three or more tests are positive and suggest that if all of these tests are negative, the SIJ can be ruled out as an etiology of pain. They also suggested that Gaenslen's test lacks diagnostic value.[121]

Treatment should begin with relative rest, NSAIDs as needed, and physical therapy. Osteopathic techniques, such as manipulation and soft tissue release, can also be helpful. Muscle imbalances should be addressed, as well as shoe modifications if a leg length discrepancy is present.[115,123] Although it is generally recommended that rehabilitation should focus on the whole lumbosacral–pelvic–glute region with core strengthening,[114,115] it has been suggested that contraction of the transversus abdominis decreases laxity in the SIJ, suggesting a role for more targeted strengthening.[124] In

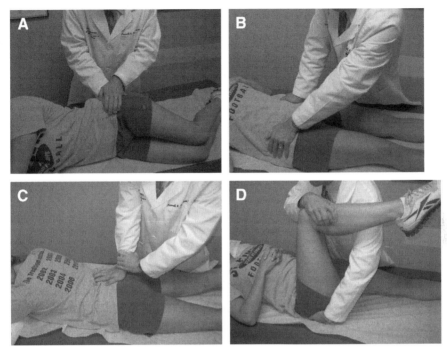

Fig. 5. SIJ provocation tests. (*A*) compression, (*B*) distraction, (*C*) sacral thrust, (*D*) thigh thrust.

addition, the hamstrings are thought to play a role in SIJ stability.[114] In fact, activation of the obterator internus, multifidus, and gluteus maximus have been shown to be delayed, while biceps femoris activation was shown to be early in patients with SIJ pain when compared to asymptomatic individuals.[125] Although these studies may suggest benefit from stabilization-type exercises, there are no randomized trials to compare conservative treatments for SIJ pain.[119]

Fluoroscopically guided SIJ injections have been shown to be beneficial and can be utilized if the athlete's progress plateaus or if pain is prohibiting progress of therapy. Multiple studies have evaluated the effectiveness of SIJ injections, but many involve only patients with inflammatory spondyloarthropathies. One study included patients with degenerative joint disease, as well as those with normal radiographs, and reported 50% relief or more in 64% of the patients. Another study showed two thirds of patients with SIJ pain received at least 50% relief at 6 weeks.[126] Another small, retrospective study reported significant decreases in disability and pain scores after treatment with both SIJ injections and physical therapy, although there was no control group.[123]

SUMMARY

In summary, LBP is a common problem for the young adult athlete, with discogenic pain being the most common of all etiologies. Although rare, more serious etiologies such as tumor or infection should be included in the differential diagnosis until effectively ruled out. Regardless of the cause, nonoperative and conservative strategies should be the cornerstone of treatment, owing to the favorable natural history of most LBP etiologies. Short-term non-narcotic medications are helpful, and avoidance of bed rest is critical for the athletic population. Rehabilitation should focus on stabilization and strengthening of the core and pelvic muscle groups, and biomechanical imbalances should be addressed. Surgical intervention ought to be utilized as a last resort in this population. Return to play should be considered only when the athlete is pain free with full range of motion and daily medications have been discontinued. Careful monitoring of the training regimen should always be undertaken, especially with chronic pain or recurrent injuries.

REFERENCES

1. Decade USBaJ. Spine: low back and neck pain. In: Surgeons AAoO, editor. The burden of musculoskeletal disease in the United States. Rosemont (IL): American Academy of Orthopaedic Surgeons; 2008. Available at: http://www.boneandjointburden.org/. Accessed March 2, 2012.
2. Dreisinger TE, Nelson B. Management of back pain in athletes. Sports Med 1996; 21(4):313–20.
3. Hosea T, Hannafin J, Bran J, et al. Aetiology of low back pain in young athletes: role of sport type. Br J Sports Med 2011;45:352.
4. Hangai M, Kaneoka K, Hinotsu S, et al. Lumbar intervertebral disk degeneration in athletes. Am J Sports Med 2009;37(1):149–55.
5. Sward L, Hellstrom M, Jacobssen B, et al. Disc degeneration and associated abnormalities of the spine in elite gymnasts: a magnetic resonance imaging study. Spine (Phila Pa 1976) 1991;16(4):437–43.
6. Videman T, Sarna S, Battie MC, et al. The long-term effects of physical loading and exercise lifestyles on back-related symptoms, disability, and spinal pathology among men. Spine 1995;20(6):699–709.
7. Weistroffer JK, Wellington KH. Return-to-play rates in National Football League linemen after treatment for lumbar disk herniation. Am J Sports Med 2011;39(3): 632–6.
8. Shaffer B, Wiesel S, Lauerman W. Spondylolisthesis in the elite football player: an epidemiologic study in the NCAA and NFL. J Spinal Disord 1997;10(5):365–70.
9. Standaert CJ, Herring SA. Expert opinion and controversies in sports and musculoskeletal medicine: the diagnosis and treatment of spondylolysis in adolescent athletes. Arch Phys Med Rehabil 2007;88:537–40.
10. Deyo RA, Weinstein JN. Low back pain. N Engl J Med 2001;344(5):363–70.
11. Micheli LJ, Wood R. Back pain in young athletes: significant differences from adults in causes and patterns. Arch Pediatr Adolesc Med 1995;149:15–8.
12. DePalma MJ, Ketchum JM, Saullo T. What is the source of chronic low back pain and does age play a role? Pain Med 2011;12:224–33.
13. Von Korff M, Deyo RA, Cherkin D, et al. Back pain in primary care: outcomes at 1 year. Spine 1993;18(7):855–62.
14. Troup J, Martin J, Lloyd D. Back pain in industry: a prospective survey. Spine 1981;6(1):61–9.
15. Pengel LH, Herbert RD, Maher CG, et al. Acute low back pain: systematic review of its prognosis. BMJ 2003;327:1–5.
16. Cohen SP. Sacroiliac joint pain: a comprehensive review of anatomy, diagnosis, and treatment. Anesth Analg 2005;101:1440–53.
17. Foley BS, Buschbacher RM. Sacroiliac joint pain: anatomy, biomechanics, diagnosis, and treatment. Am J Phys Med Rehabil 2006;85:997–1006.
18. Barr KP, Harrast MA. Low back pain. In: Braddom RL, editor. Physical medicine and rehabilitation. 3rd edition. Philadelphia: Saunders/Elsevier; 2007. p. 883–927.

19. Standaert CJ, Herring SA. Spondylolysis: a critical review. Br J Sports Med 2000; 34:415–22.
20. Rhee JM, Schaufele M, Abdu W. Radiculopathy and the herniated lumbar disc. J Bone Joint Surg [Am] 2006;88A(9):2070–80.
21. Intervertebral disc aging, degeneration, and herniation. In: Buckwalter JA, editor. Orthopaedic basic science: biology and biomechanics of the musculoskeletal system. 2nd edition. Rosemont (IL): American Academy of Orthopaedic Surgeons; 2000.
22. Boos N, Weissbach S, Rohrbach H, et al. Classification of age-related changes in lumbar intervertebral discs: 2002 Volvo Award in Basic Science. Spine 2022;27(23): 2631–44.
23. Coppes MH, Marani E, Thomeer RT, et al. Innervation of "painful" lumbar discs. Spine 1997;22(20):2342–9.
24. Brown M, Hukkanen M, McCarthy I, et al. Sensory and sympathetic innervation of the vertebral endplate in patients with degenerative disc disease. J Bone Joint Surg [Am] 1997;79-B:147–53.
25. Saal J, Franson RC, Dobrow R, et al. High levels of inflammatory phospholipase A2 activity in lumbar disc herniations. Spine 1990;15(7):674–8.
26. O'Donnell J, O'Donnell A. Prostaglandin E2 content in herniated lumbar disc disease. Spine 1996;21(14):1653–5.
27. Saal JA, Saal JS, Herzog RA. The natural history of lumbar intervertebral disc extrusions treated non-operatively. Spine 1990;15(7):683–6.
28. Hakelius A. Prognosis in sciatica: a clinical folow-up of surgical and non-surgical treatment. Acta Orthop Scand (Suppl) 1970;129:1–76.
29. Weber H. Spine update: the natural history of disc herniation and influence of intervention. Spine 1994;19(19):2234–8.
30. Hiromichi K, Kenichi S, Osamu N, et al. The natural history of herniated nucleus pulposus with radiculopathy. Spine 1996;21(2):1877–83.
31. Saal JS, Franson RC, Dobrow R, et al. High levels of inflammatory phospholipase A$_2$ activity in lumbar disc herniations. Spine 1990;15(7):674–8.
32. Weiler C, Nerlich AG, Bachmeier BE, et al. Expression and distribution of tumor necrosis factor alpha in human lumbar intervertebral discs: a study in surgical specimen and autopsy controls. Spine 2004;30(1):44–54.
33. Burke J, Watson R, McCormack D, et al. Intervertebral discs which cause low back pain secrete high levels of proinflammatory mediators. J Bone Joint Surg [Br] 2002;84-B:196–201.
34. DePalma MJ, Lee J-E, Peterson L, et al. Are outer annular fissures stimulated during diskography the source of diskogenic low back pain? An analysis of analgesic diskography data. Pain Med 2009;10(3):488–94.
35. Kirkaldy-Willis W, Wedge J, Yong-Hing M, et al. Pathophysiology and pathogenesis of lumbar spondylosis and stenosis. Spine 1978;3(4):319–28.
36. Panjabi M. The stabilizing system of the spine. Part I: function, dysfunction, adaptation and enhancement. J Spinal Disord 1992;5:383–9.
37. Gaunt AM. Caring for patients who have acute and subacute low back pain. CME Bull 2008;7:1–8.
38. Greene HS, Cholewicki J, Galloway MT, et al. A history of low back injury is a risk factor for recurrent back injuries in varsity athletes. Am J Sports Med 2001;29(6): 795–800.
39. DePalma MJ, Ketchum JM, Trussell BS, et al. Does the location of low back pain predict its source? PM R 2011;3(1):33–9.

40. Young S, Aprill CN, Laslett M. Correlation of clinical examination characteristics with three sources of chronic low back pain. Spine J 2003;3(6):460–5.

41. Devillé WL, Van der Windt DA, Dzaferagić A, et al. The test of Lasègue: systematic review of the accuracy in diagnosing herniated discs. Spine 2000;25(9):1140–7.

42. Majlesi J, Togay H, Un'alan H, et al. The sensitivity and specificity of the slump and the straight leg raising tests in patients with lumbar disc herniation. J Clin Rheumatol 2008;14:87–91.

43. Hanson SJ, McCullagh P, Tonymon P. The relationship of personality characteristics, life stress, and coping resources to athletic injury. J Sport Exerc Psychol 1993;14(3):262–72.

44. Ahern DK, Lohr BA. Psychosocial factors in sports injury rehabilitation. Clin Sports Med 1997;16(4):755–68.

45. Chou R, Qaseem A, Snow V, et al. Diagnosis and treatment of low back pain: a joint clinical practice guideline from the American College of Physicians and the American Pain Society. Ann Intern Med 2007;147:478–91.

46. Chou R, Fu R, Carrino JA, et al. Imaging strategies for low-back pain: systematic review and meta-analysis. Lancet 2009;373(9662):463–72.

47. Espeland A, Baerheim A, Albrektsen G, et al. Patients' views on importance and usefulness of plain radiography for low back pain. Spine 2001;26(12):1356–63.

48. Atlas SJ, Deyo RA. Evaluating and managing acute low back pain in the primary care setting. J Gen Intern Med 2001;16:120–31.

49. Kendrick D, Fielding K, Bentley E, et al. Radiography of the lumbar spine in primary care patients with low back pain: randomised controlled trial. BMJ 2001;322:400–5.

50. Jarvik J. Imaging of adults with low back pain in the primary care setting. Neuroimaging Clin N Am 2003;13:293–305.

51. Roudsari B, Jarvik JG. Lumbar spine MRI for low back pain: indications and yield. AJR Am J Radiol 2010;195:550–9.

52. Boden SD, Davis DO, Dina TS, et al. Abnormal magnetic resonance scans of the lumbar spine in asymptomatic subjects. J Bone Joint Surg [Am] 1990;72-A(3):403–8.

53. Jensen MC, Brant-Zawadski MN, Obuchowski N, et al. Magnetic resonance imaging of the lumbar spine in people without back pain. N Engl J Med 1994;331(2):69–73.

54. Weishaupt D, Zanetti M, Hodler J, et al. MR imaging of the lumbar spine: prevalence of intervertebral disk extrusion and sequestration, nerve root compression, end plate abnormalities, and osteoarthritis of the facet joints in asymptomatic volunteers. Radiology 1998;209:661–6.

55. Modic MT, Obuchowski NA, Ross JS, et al. Acute low back pain and radiculopathy: MR imaging findings and their prognostic role and effect on outcome. Radiology 2005;237:597–604.

56. Healy JF, Healy BB, Wong WH, et al. Cervical and lumbar MRI in asymptomatic older male lifelong athletes: frequency of degenerative findings. J Comput Assist Tomogr 1996;20(1):107–12.

57. Guyer RD, Ohnmeiss DD. Lumbar discography. Position statement from the North American Spine: Society Diagnostic and Therapeutic Committee. Spine 1995;20(18):2048–59.

58. Carragee EJ, Chen Y, Tanner CM, et al. Can discography cause long-term back symptoms in previously asymptomatic subjects? Spine (Phila Pa 1976) 2000;25(14):1803–8.

59. Sobajima S, Kompel JF, Kim JS, et al. A slowly progressive and reproducible animal model of intervertebral disc degeneration characterized by MRI, X-ray, and histology. Spine 2004;30(1):15–24.

60. Kim KS, Yoon ST, Li J, et al. Disc degeneration in the rabbit: a biochemical and radiological comparison between four disc injury models. Spine 2004;30(1):33–7.
61. Carragee EJ, Don AS, Hurwitz EL, et al. 2009 ISSLS Prize winner: does discography cause accelerated progression of degeneration changes in the lumbar disc? A 10 year study. Spine 2009;34(21):2338–45.
62. Lei D, Rege A, Koti M, et al. Painful disc lesion: can modern biplanar magnetic resonance imaging replace discography? J Spinal Disord Tech 2008;21:430–5.
63. Peng B, Hou S, Wu W, et al. The pathogenesis and clinical significance of a high-intensity zone (HIZ) of lumbar intervertebral disc on MR imaging in the patient with discogenic low back pain. Eur Spine J 2006;15:583–7.
64. Aprill CN, Bogduk N. A diagnostic sign of painful lumbar disc on magnetic resonance imaging. Br J Radiol 1992;65:361–9.
65. Schellhas KP, Pollei SR, Gundry CR, et al. Lumbar disc high-intensity zone: correlation of magnetic resonance imaging and discography. Spine 1996;21(1):79–86.
66. Lam K, Carlin D, Mulholland R. Lumbar disc high-intensity zone: the value and significance of provocative discography in the determination of the discogenic pain source. Eur Spine J 2000;9:36–41.
67. Saifuddin A, Braithwaite I, White J, et al. The value of lumbar spine magnetic resonance imaging in the demonstration of anular tears. Spine 1998;23(4):453–7.
68. Ricketson R, Simmons JW, Hauser BO. The prolapsed intervertebral disc: the high-intensity zone with discography correlation. Spine 1996;21(23):2758–62.
69. Buirski G, Silberstein M. The symptomatic lumbar disc in patients with low back pain: magnetic resonance imaging appearances in both a symptomatic and control population. Spine 1993;18(13):1808–11.
70. Carragee EJ, Paragioudakis SJ, Khurana S. Lumbar high-intensity zone and discography in subjects without low back problems. Spine 2000;25(23):2987–92.
71. Schwarzer AC, Aprill CN, Derby R, et al. The prevalence and clinical features of internal disc disruption in patients with chronic low back pain. Spine 1995;20(17): 1878–83.
72. Crock H. Internal disc disruption: a challenge to disc prolapse 50 years on. Spine 1986;11:650–3.
73. Bono CM. Low back pain in athletes. J Bone Joint Surg [Am] 2004;86-A(2):382–96.
74. Cooke P, Lutz G. Internal disc disruption and axial back pain in the athlete. Phys Med Rehabil Clin North Am 2000;11:837–65.
75. Zhou Y, Abdi S. Diagnosis and minimally invasive treatment of lumbar discogenic pain – a review of the literature. Clin J Pain 2006;22:468–81.
76. Saifuddin A, Emanuel R, White J, et al. An analysis of radiating pain at lumbar discography. Eur Spine J 998;7:358–62.
77. Ohnmeiss D, Vanharanta H, Ekholm J. Relationship of pain drawings to invasive tests assessing intervertebral disc pathology. Eur Spine J 1999;8:126–31.
78. DePalma MJ, Ketchum JM, Queler E, et al. Does sustained hip flexion, pelvic rock, or location of low back pain predict the etiology of low back pain? An interim analysis of 170 consecutive low back pain cases. Pain Med 2009;10(5):948.
79. Valkenburg H, Haanen H. The epidemiology of low back pain. In: White AA, Gordon SL, editors. Symposium on idiopathic low back pain. St. Louis: Mosby; 1982. p. 9–22.
80. Goel V, Kong W, Han J. A combined finite element and optimization investigation of lumbar spine mechanics with and without muscles. Spine 1993;18:1531–41.
81. Wilke H-J, Wolf S, Claes LE, et al. Stability increase of the lumbar spine with different muscle groups. Spine 1995;20(2):192–8.

82. Hides JA, Richardson CA, Jull GA. Multifidus muscle recovery is not automatic after resolution of acute, first-episode low back pain. Spine 1996;21(23):2763–9.

83. Hides JA, Jull GA, Richardson CA. Long-term effects of specific stabilizing exercises for first-episode low back pain. Spine 2001;26(11):E243–E8.

84. Hides JA, Richardson CA, Jull GA. Multifidus muscle rehabilitation decreases recurrence of symptoms following first episode low back pain. Paper presented at National Congress of the Australian Physiotherapy Association. Brisbane, July 14–19, 1996.

85. Ferreira P, Ferreira M, Maher C, et al. Specific stabilisation exercise for spinal and pelvic pain: a systematic review. Aust J Physiother 2006;52:79–88.

86. Nadler SF, Malanga GA, DePrince M, et al. The relationship between lower extremity injury, low back pain, and hip muscle strength in male and female collegiate athletes. Clin J Sport Med 2000;10:89–97.

87. Nadler SF, Malanga GA, Bartoli LA, et al. Hip muscle imbalance and low back pain in athletes: influence of core strengthening. Med Sci Sports Exerc 2002;34(1):9–16.

88. Kankaanpää M, Taimela T, Laaksonen D, et al. Back and hip extensor fatigability in chronic low back pain patients and controls. Arch Phys Med Rehabil 1998;79(4): 412–7.

89. Chou R, Huffman LH. Medications for acute and chronic low back pain: a review of the evidence for an American Pain Society/American College of Physicians Clinical Practice Guideline. Ann Intern Med 2007;147:505–14.

90. Manchikanti L, Cash KA, McManus CD, et al. Preliminary results of a randomized, equivalence trial of fluoroscopic caudal epidural injections in managing chronic low back pain. Part 1: discogenic pain without disc herniation or radiculitis. Pain Phys 2008;11:785–800.

91. Butterman G. The effect of spinal steroid injections for degenerative disc disease. Spine J 2003;4:495–505.

92. Conn A, Buenaventura RM, Datta S, et al. Systematic review of caudal epidural injections in the management of chronic low back pain. Pain Phys 2009;12:109–35.

93. Peng B, Zhang Y, Hou S, et al. Intradiscal methylene blue injection for the treatment of chronic discogenic low back pain. Eur Spine J 2007;16:33–8.

94. Akeda K, An HS, Pichika R, et al. Platelet-rich plasma (PRP) stimulates the extracellular matrix metabolism of porcine nucleus pulposus and anulus fibrosus cells cultured in alginate beads. Spine 2006;31(9):959–66.

95. Nagae M, Ikeda T, Mikami Y, et al. Intervertebral disc regeneration using platelet-rich plasma and biodegradable gelatin hydrogel microspheres. Tissue Engin 2007;13(1): 147–58.

96. Chen W-H, Lo W-C, Lee J-J, et al. Tissue-engineered intervertebral disc and chondrogenesis using human nucleus pulposus regulated through TGF-b1 in platelet-rich plasma. J Cell Physiol 2006;209:744–54.

97. Lawrence JP, Greene HS, Grauer JN. Back pain in athletes. J Am Acad Orthop Surg 2006;14(13):726–35.

98. Qin S, Zhang Q, Fan D. Significance of the straight-leg raising test in the diagnosis and clinical evaluation of lower lumbar intervetebral disc protrusion. J Bone Joint Surg [Am] 1987;69:517–22.

99. Deyo RA, Rainville J, Kent DL. What can the history and physical examination tell us about low back pain? JAMA 1992;268(6):760–5.

100. Yildirim K, Sışeciogˇlu M, Karatay S, et al. The effectiveness of gabapentin in patients with chronic radiculopathy. Pain Clin 2003;15(3):213–8.

101. Hahne AJ, Ford JJ, McMeeken JM. Conservative management of lumbar disc herniation with associated radiculopathy. Spine 2010;35(11):E488–E504.

102. Iwamoto J, Sato Y, Takeda T, et al. Return to play after conservative treatment in athletes with symptomatic lumbar disc herniation: a practice-based observational study. J Sports Med 2011;2:25–31.

103. Gay RE, Brault JS. Evidence-informed management of chronic low back pain with traction therapy. Spine J 2008;8:234–42.

104. May S, Donelson R. Evidence-informed management of chronic low back pain with the McKenzie method. Spine J 2008;8:134–41.

105. Long A, Donelson R, Fung T. Does it matter which exercise? A randomized control trial of exercise for low back pain. Spine 2004;29(23):2593–602.

106. Weinstein SM, Herring SA, Derby R. Contemporary concepts in spine care: epidural steroid injections. Spine 1995;20:1842–6.

107. Riew KD, Park J-B, Cho Y-S, et al. Nerve root blocks in the treatment of lumbar radicular pain: a minimum five-year follow-up. J Bone Joint Surg [Am] 2006;88-A(8): 1722–5.

108. Buttermann GR. Treatment of lumbar disc herniation: epidural steroid injection compared with discectomy. J Bone Joint Surg [Am] 2004;86-A(4):670–80.

109. Vad VB, Bhat AL, Lutz GE, et al. Transforaminal epidural steroid injections in lumbosacral radiculopathy. Spine 2002;27(1):11–6.

110. Arden N, Price C, Reading I, et al. A multicentre randomized controlled trial of epidural corticosteroid injections for sciatica: the WEST study. Rheumatology 2005; 44:1399–406.

111. Weinstein JN, Tosteson TD, Lurie J, et al. Surgical vs nonoperative treatment for lumbar disk herniation: the Spine Patient Outcomes Research Trial (SPORT): a randomized trial. JAMA 2006;296(20):2441–50.

112. Weinstein JN, Lurie J, Tosteson TD, et al. Surgical versus non-operative treatment for lumbar disc herniation: four-year results for the Spine Patient Outcomes Research Trial (SPORT). Spine (Phila Pa 1976) 2008;33(25):2789–800.

113. Gibson JA, Waddell G. Surgical interventions for lumbar disc prolapse: updated Cochrane Review. Spine 2007;32(16):1737–45.

114. Brolinson PG, Kozar AJ, Cibor G. Sacroiliac joint dysfunction in athletes. Curr Sports Med Rep 2003;2(1):47–56.

115. Prather H. Sacroiliac joint pain: practical management. Clin J Sport Med 2003;13: 252–5.

116. Dreyfuss P, Michaelsen M, Pauza K, et al. The value of medical history and physical examination in diagnosing sacroiliac joint pain. Spine 1996;21(22):2594–602.

117. Fortin JD, Falco FJ. The Fortin finger test: an indicator of sacroiliac pain. Am J Orthop 1997;26(7):477–80.

118. Puhakka K, Jurik A, Schiottz-Christensen B, et al. Magnetic resonance imaging of sacroiliitis in early seronegative spondylarthropathy: abnormalities correlated to clinical and laboratory findings. Rheumatology 2004;43:234–7.

119. Laslett M. Evidence-based diagnosis and treatment of the painful sacroiliac joint. J Man Manip Ther 2008;16(3):142–52.

120. Dreyfuss P, Dreyer S, Griffin J, et al. Positive sacroiliac screening tests in asymptomatic adults. Spine 1994;19(10):1138–43.

121. Laslett M, Aprill CN, McDonald B, et al. Diagnosis of sacroiliac joint pain: validity of individual provocation tests and composites of tests. J Man Manip Ther 2005;10: 207–18.

122. Schwarzer AC, Aprill CN, Bogduk N. The sacroiliac joint in chronic low back pain. Spine 1995;20(1):31–7.

123. Slipman CW, Lipetz JS, Plastaras CT, et al. Fluoroscopically guided therapeutic sacroiliac joint injections for sacroiliac joint syndrome. Am J Phys Med Rehabil 2001;80:425–32.

124. Richardson CA, Snijders CJ, Hides JA, et al. The relation between the transversus abdominis muscles, sacroiliac joint mechanics, and low back pain. Spine 2002; 27(4):399–405.

125. Hungerford B, Gilleard W, Hodges P. Evidence of altered lumbopelvic muscle recruitment in the presence of sacroiliac joint pain. Spine 2003;28(14):1593–600.

126. Liliang P-C, Lu K, Weng H-C, et al. The therapeutic efficacy of sacroiliac joint blocks with triamcinolone acetonide in the treatment of sacroiliac joint dysfunction without spondyloarthropathy. Spine 2009;34(9):896–900.

The Aging Spine in Sports

Joanne Borg-Stein, MD*, Lauren Elson, MD, Erik Brand, MD, MSc

KEYWORDS

- Aging • Lumbar spine • Disc • Arthritis • Stenosis

KEY POINTS

- Masters athletes may experience low back pain from multiple sources. Masters athletes with discogenic back pain should avoid or modify sports with combined rotational and compressive forces; individuals with facet-mediated pain should avoid or modify sports with excessive extension and rotation.
- Optimization of flexibility, strength, endurance, and core control is critical. Sports-specific training, realistic goal setting, and counseling are of maximal importance.
- Overall, the health benefits of continued sports and athletic participation outweigh the potential risks of spinal degeneration in middle-aged athletes. There is little correlation between radiographic appearance of the spine and symptoms; therefore, symptoms should serve as the primary guide when determining activity modifications. Overall, masters athletes should be encouraged to remain active and fit to enhance their quality of life and reduce the risk of cardiovascular disease.

Team physicians and sports medicine physicians in general often treat active patients age 50 years and older. *Masters* is the term used to designate individuals or events that are based on age groups, generally older than 35 years and typically older than 50 years. The United States Senior Games begin at age 50. The Senior Olympics sponsors games in 50 states and involves 250,000 older adults in training, competition, and education.[1,2]

EPIDEMIOLOGY/ETIOLOGY OF LOW BACK PAIN AND THE MASTERS ATHLETE

Low back pain will affect approximately 65% of the US population during their lifetime, with 26% having low back pain at least 1 day in the last 3 months.[3,4] Muscle mass declines with age; approximately 1.25% per year after age 35 with accelerated decline after age 70. This is attributed to decreased cross-sectional area as well as sarcopenia, characterized by the replacement of muscle fibers with fat and fibrosis. Musculoskeletal reaction time, muscle endurance, tendon and cartilage structure,

Department of PM&R, Harvard Medical School, Spaulding Rehabilitation Hospital, 125 Nashua Street, Boston, MA 02114, USA
* Corresponding author.
E-mail address: jborgstein@partners.org

Clin Sports Med 31 (2012) 473–486
doi:10.1016/j.csm.2012.03.002
0278-5919/12/$ – see front matter © 2012 Elsevier Inc. All rights reserved.

flexibility, and balance all decrease with aging and will effect the lumbar spine.[1] The aging spine itself is characterized by 2 parallel but independent processes: development of degenerative discogenic changes and bone mass reduction. The etiology of low back pain in the masters athlete includes degenerative disc disease with or without radiculopathy, lumbar facet osteoarthropathy, lumbar stenosis with neurogenic claudication, and osteoporosis complicated by compression fracture, deformity, and kyphosis. These topics will be covered in this review.

DEGENERATIVE DISC DISEASE IN THE MASTERS ATHLETE
Anatomy and Physiology

The lumbar disc is composed of a gel substance (nucleus pulposus) surrounded by outer collagen fibers, which are arranged in a crossed manner (annulus fibrosis). These discs are further supported by the anterior and posterior longitudinal ligaments. Together, the vertebral disc complex resists spinal compression. During axial rotation and flexion of the spine, the annular fibers are placed at a mechanical disadvantage. A common mechanism of lumbar disc herniation in athletes is combined flexion, rotation, and compression of the spine. Football, wrestling, hockey, dance, gymnastics, tennis, and golf are some of the sports in which this injury mechanism commonly occurs.[5]

Clinical Presentation

The clinical presentation of disc-related back pain is primarily divided into 3 subtypes: axial pain (back pain alone), radicular pain (leg pain alone), or axial and radicular pain. Axial discogenic low back pain often presents as severe episodes of acute pain, muscle spasm, and lost time from sport. The symptoms are exacerbated by prolonged sitting, standing, or axial loading. There are no neurologic deficits or referred pain. Athletes may also present with radicular pain without back pain. Pain is most often in the L5 or S1 distribution beginning in the buttock, thigh, or hip girdle with radiation into the lateral or posterior leg and foot. In the acute phase, the athlete may have a lumbar shift away from the side of radicular pain. This represents an involuntary reactive muscle spasm. In addition, neural tension signs, such as straight leg raising, cross straight leg raising, or slump test will reproduce leg pain. There may be associated motor or sensory deficits. Last, the athlete may have a combination of axial and radicular pain with an overlap in clinical presentation.[6]

Management

Management begins with a careful physical examination to confirm the diagnosis clinically and rule out other sources of back and leg pain, such as vascular, infectious, neoplastic, or hip. If the clinician has medical concerns in the presence of a "red flag" (fever, weight loss, history of cancer), then appropriate laboratory or radiographic evaluation is performed (refer to the article by Mautner and Huggins elsewhere in this issue). Initial management emphasizes[6–8] pain reduction with judicious use of nonsteroidal anti-inflammatory drugs or opiates and gabapentin considered for neuropathic pain and sleep. Physical therapy may include manual treatments and modalities with graded exercise and sports-specific training program. Lumbar epidural steroid injections are indicated for radicular pain that is not responding to the above measures.[9] In the case of intractable radicular pain or progressive neurologic deficit, lumbar discectomy is offered. Most younger athletes will return to sport on average 5 months after operation. No data are specifically available on masters athletes. Lumbar functional stabilization and rehabilitation will be critical[10] (refer to articles Donatelli and colleagues and d'Hemecourt and Luke elsewhere in this issue).

LUMBAR FACET OSTEOARTHROPATHY
Epidemiology in the Masters Athlete

The effect of participation in sports on arthropathy of the spine in unclear. It has been shown that there are an increased number of anatomic changes of the spine in adolescent athletes compared with sedentary controls; however, there is no correlation between these findings and symptoms. The occurrence of radiographic changes of the lumbar spine in track and field athletes showed a higher prevalence of osteophytes in shot putters, discus throwers, and high jumpers when compared with runners in the study by Schmitt and colleagues.[11] The increased loading conditions of the spine in sports involving extension and rotation has been presumed to increase the risk for facet arthropathy. Because most master athletes have spent decades mastering their respective sports, it is impossible to determine if symptoms that they develop are a result of degenerative changes that appeared while they were younger or are newer findings. A study by Lundin and coworkers[12] evaluated radiologic changes and back pain in the thoraco-lumbar spine of 134 former elite wrestlers, gymnasts, and soccer and tennis players and compared the results with 28 controls. There was no difference in the incidence of back pain between the 2 groups, but there were more radiographic abnormalities in the athletes.[13]

Pain appeared independent of radiographic changes in athletes versus controls. Low back pain is less in athletes than in control subjects. Soccer players have a greater incidence of degeneration in the lower lumbar region, and weight lifting is associated with greater degeneration throughout the lumbar spine.[5] Lumbar mobility in former elite male athletes from soccer, long-distance running, weight-lifting, and shooting is not significantly different when compared with controls.[13]

Anatomy and Neurophysiology of Pain

The facet joints are the articulations between consecutive vertebrae. They are synovial-lined joints with hyaline cartilage. Repetitive hyperextension and rotation can lead to inflammation and synovitis. Eventually, tropism may develop in response. In the elderly patient, other degenerative changes, including loss of disc height, can lead to a great load through the facets.[14–17]

Common Sports Involved

Sports with some of the highest torsional loads include baseball, golf, javelin, and tennis.[18] In baseball, irregular and uncoordinated motion of arm and upper torso puts undue rotational strain on the lumbar spine. Ball players with low back pain show loss of spine extension, loss of rotation (often) unilaterally, poor rotational mechanics, and weak abdominals. Pitchers may develop irritation of the lower lumbar facets from increased torsional strain, usually when restarting training after a break. Golfers tend to bend to left, loading the spine asymmetrically. Lumbar pain involving rotary motion is incapacitating in a javelin thrower.[18] Tennis involves extremes of lumbar flexion, extension, and lateral bending.[15] Thirty-eight percent of professional tennis players have missed games because of back pain.

Clinical Presentation: Axial Pain, Stiffness, Decreased Motion

Controversy exists over the specific elements of history and physical that is diagnostic of facet arthropathy.[14] Patients with facet-mediated pain often have reproduction of pain with extension with rotation. Avoidance of this motion often leads to stiffness and impaired motion. Presentation may involve pain with rising from flexion or with a lateral shift in the extension motion. There may be point tenderness to palpation in the paraspinal region over the corresponding facet joint. Associated radicular pain may also occur from the proximity of the inflammatory mediators to the exiting nerve root. Facet referral patterns are nonspecific and levels may overlap. Low-volume intra-articular anesthetic injection and medial branch blocks are the most accepted method for diagnosing facet-mediated pain.[14]

Management

Pharmacologic
Short-term nonsteroidal anti-inflammatory drugs can be used to reduce acute symptoms; however, in the elderly population, there is greater risk for gastrointestinal, renal, and hepatic side effects. In cases of severe pain, methylprednisolone may be indicated; however, there is the potential for many systemic side effects.

Bracing
Corsets and braces do not produce any long-term improvements and may lead to deconditioning of the core musculature.[18,19]

Exercise
Bed rest for more than 3 to 5 days is not beneficial to the natural history of disease. It also produces profound weakness, loss of biomechanical function, and increased weakness and stiffness requiring a longer rehabilitation course. Rapid mobilization with nonexacerbatory exercise is important. A neutral-based isometric trunk-strengthening program is progressed as tolerated to resistive strengthening, motion, and aerobic conditioning. For athletes involved in high-torque sports, progression with a trainer or physical therapist through exercises with resisted rotation in supine, then sitting, then standing is key for improving thoraco-lumbar control.[18]

Injections (steroid, radiofrequency, prolotherapy)
Well-controlled trials demonstrate mixed results in the treatment of facet arthropathy with intra-articular corticosteroid injections, with normal saline producing similar effects. Diagnostic medial branch blocks are predictive of the efficacy or radiofrequency ablation of these nerves. Aspiration and corticosteroid injection is helpful in the treatment of synovial cysts in the facet. There is no conclusive evidence supporting the use of prolotherapy for the treatment of generalized low back pain. None of the prolotherapy studies specifically address its use in the treatment of facet arthropathy.[14]

Acupuncture, manipulation, massage
Although there are no conclusive studies in the specific treatment of facet arthropathy, the mentioned modalities may modulate the pain response by providing nonnoxious mechanical and chemical stimulation that decrease the transduction of nociception.

Surgery
The facet joints are important for the structural stability of the spine. Removal of more than 50% of the facet joint led to unacceptable movement of the segment in cadaver studies. Arthrodesis is unsupported in the literature for improving facet-related symptoms.[14,19] Minimally invasive surgical excision of facet cysts reduces related symptoms.[20]

Sports-Specific Training
Return to sport requires a trunk stabilization program, sport-specific strengthening exercises, adequate sport-specific aerobic conditioning, full ability to participate in

the sport, graded return to activity, and maintenance of a strengthening program. In golfers, prevention of lumbar spine pain is obtained by minimizing the torsion stress by absorbing the rotation in the hips, knees, and shoulders. Improvement of muscle strength in golfers improves the coordination, firing sequence of the muscles, and balance, which enhances neuromuscular control. Tennis requires the quadriceps strength to allow the player to play with a knee and hip flexed position to protect the back. Strengthening of the latissimus dorsi, abdominal obliques, rectus abdominus, and gluteal musculature help to control the rotator forces and leg-trunk-arm coordination.[18]

LUMBAR STENOSIS
Epidemiology in the Masters Athlete

The incidence of acquired lumbar stenosis is known to increase with age. There are no studies that compare the rates of symptomatic stenosis of the athletic versus the nonathletic population. Healy and coworkers,[21] however, examined the incidence of degenerative changes of the cervical and lumbar spine in the magnetic resonance images of asymptomatic high-level triathletes and handball players. Compared with the study by Jensen[22] which examined lumbar magnetic resonance images in 100 asymptomatic elderly patients, 15% of whom had stenosis, Healy and colleagues[21] also found a 15% incidence rate, albeit in a much smaller sample size. The incidence of other degenerative changes that may lead to acquired stenosis, including disc degeneration and facet arthropathy, were also equal.

Anatomy and Neurophysiology of Pain

The lumbar spinal canal is surrounded anteriorly by the vertebral bodies, the disc, and the posterior longitudinal ligament. The lateral margin is comprised of the pedicles and the lateral extension of the ligamentum flavum. Posteriorly, the border is lined by the ligamentum flavum, facet joints, and laminae. As the spinal nerves exit at each level, the neuroforamina are surrounded by the discs and vertebral bodies anteriorly, by the facets joints posteriorly, and by the pedicles superior and inferiorly,[19] Degenerative changes of any of these components can lead to compression of the neural elements. Interestingly, most individuals who have evidence of mechanical compression of the nerve roots do not have pain. Symptoms develop in the lower extremities when there is inflammation and irritation of the nerve root. Normally, with the straight-leg-raise maneuver, the nerve moves up to 5 mm within the neural foramen. An inflammatory reaction may occur if the normal motion is obstructed, leading to tension and disruptions of the neural architecture.[19]

Compression of the neural elements can lead to electrophysiologic changes. This may result in the stimulation of pain fibers, a decrease in blood flow and thus nutritional support of the neural elements.

Common Sports Involved

Athletes involved in sports that require prolonged extension are more likely to be symptomatic if they have an underlying stenosis. Masters athletes are unlikely to be involved with sports with extreme lumbar hyperextension loads, specifically gymnastics, ballet, and pole vaulting. There are, however, masters-level competitions in weight lifting and swimming. Weight lifting causes large extension forces of the lumbar spine. The breast stroke requires large flexion/extension movements.[18]

Clinical Presentation: Axial Pain, Radicular Pain, Polyradiculopathy, Neurogenic Claudication

Initially, lumbar stenosis presents as vague low back pain and stiffness, relieved with rest and exacerbated with activity. Depending on the location of the stenosis, the pain typically begins in the low back and radiates caudally. Symptoms include numbness, tingling, and pain and may be present in a single dermatome or myotome in the setting of focal neuroforaminal stenosis. With central stenosis, the symptoms often are less specific or may present as a polyradiculopathy. Ninety percent of patients with spinal stenosis will experience unilateral or bilateral radicular pain.[23] Often, patients will complain of a feeling of weakness and giving way, cramping, diffuse paresthesis, and a dull, aching pain. Classically, these symptoms are exacerbated with spinal extension and are rapidly improved with flexion.

On physical examination, specific motor deficits are uncommon, especially if the patient has been resting immediately before the examination. Brief exercise to reproduce symptoms may bring out claudicatory functional deficits. Diminished or absent reflexes corresponding to the suspected nerve root levels are common. Reflexes to test for the presence of upper motor neuron disease should be negative or absent. Nerve conduction studies may be helpful in excluding other causes of similar symptoms, including peripheral neuropathies and focal nerve entrapments.

Radiologic evaluation should start with anteroposterior and lateral x-rays with flexion and extension views to examine for any deformities or functional instability. Magnetic resonance imaging has become the imaging study of choice in the diagnosis and surgical planning of lumbar stenosis.[19]

Management

Pharmacologic

Analgesics, anti-inflammatories, and neurogenic-acting agents are useful in reducing the symptoms. In the older patient, extra care needs to be used in the prescribing of such agents. Acetaminophen can affect hepatic and renal function. Nonsteroidal anti-inflammatories can affect hepatic and renal function, leading to hypertension, and affect the gastrointestinal system, leading to ulcers. The dose of opioids and agents such as gabapentin and pregabalin need to be adjusted for cognitive side effects in the elderly population.

Exercise and education

Education and reassurance are components of every rehabilitation program. Nonexacerbatory exercise is important. Physical therapists can provide education and instructions on a safe, individualized exercise program. The program should include aerobic conditioning as well as spinal stabilization and strengthening exercises. Stationary bike riding is generally well tolerated and is accessible to many patients. There is no evidence for the use of physical modalities in patients with lumbar stenosis; however, they may decrease the symptoms of certain individuals. Long-term use of corsets should be avoided, as it leads to additional muscle deconditioning.[19] Exercise and physical therapy may potentially lead to a flare of symptoms; however, with careful monitoring, education, and planning, this may be avoided.[18,19] Even if exercise does not diminish the symptoms, it will improve the individual condition, allowing for more definitive procedures to be better tolerated.

Injection

Epidural administration of steroids may provide relief of radicular symptoms associated with spinal stenosis. Although there are relatively few side effects associated with image-guided delivery of these agents, the difficulty of the procedure increases in patients with severe degenerative changes.[19]

Surgery

Severe debilitating deterioration in patients who have been treated conservatively is rare; however, surgery may decrease the neurologic signs and improve the quality of life. Surgery does not usually reverse all of the neurologic symptoms; however, it does improve them, leading to a higher level of function. Surgery is indicated for patients whose pain, numbness, or weakness in the lower extremities severely restricts their activities of daily living. The most common procedures done are decompressive laminectomy with nerve-root decompression and limited laminotomy with foraminotomy.

Sports-Specific Training

Appropriate cross training and conditioning can help decrease the hyperextension loads and mechanics that exacerbate the symptoms of lumbar stenosis. Weight lifting training now emphasizes the role of general body conditioning flexibility, aerobic conditioning, speed, and cross-training. Dancers are educated to achieve the desired aesthetic positions by using hip extension, improving core strength, and obtaining lumbar extension throughout the spine. Although runners are not necessarily predisposed to lumbar stenosis, those with the underlying condition can mitigate symptoms by improving flexibility and strengthening the abdominal and spinal stabilizing musculature. Maintaining balance between lower extremity and the trunk flexors and extensors is also important in all athletes.[18]

Prognosis

Most people who are older than 60 years have degenerative changes that lead to chemical, mechanical, and anatomic processes that lead to nerve-root compression. The majority of these individuals, however, do not have pain. Because the signs and symptoms of neurogenic claudication are not solely dependent on the underlying compressive changes, symptoms may decrease, remain stable, or progress without regard to the specific anatomy.[19]

OSTEOPOROSIS AND COMPRESSION FRACTURE
Epidemiology in the Master Athlete

Spinal osteoporosis is an important consideration in the aging athlete. This condition can put the athlete at risk for spinal compression fracture, resultant kyphotic deformity, and associated comorbidities, such as gait and balance dysfunction and chronic pain. Participation in sports in the second and third decade of life may help develop higher peak bone mass and improved architecture via changes in geometric properties and density in a pattern specific to the load. Such appears to be the case for sports that involve odd impact loading (ie, basketball, soccer, step aerobics, racquet sports, and speed skating, which deliver blows in a variety of directions, affecting the entire bone circumference, for instance, by moving forward, backward and sideways) or high impact loading (ie, volleyball, gymnastics, jumping sports, karate). Repetitive low-to-moderate sports (ie, running) may also improve bone geometry. In contrast, nonimpact sports (ie, cycling, swimming) are not associated with better bone mineral density (BMD) or mineral composition.[24] Improvements in peak bone mass obtained during youth may carry a benefit of decreased fracture risk in the older ex-athlete, even if resistance training is not maintained. Continued loading exercise in the older-age masters groups, however, appears to help maintain BMD better than that in nonathletic controls.[25] Standard recommendations for osteoporosis prevention in the elderly include resistance training and weight-bearing exercise 30 to 60 minutes per day, 3 to 5 days per week and avoidance of tobacco and excessive alcohol.[26] Additionally, nutrition, hormones, and genetics can also play a role in osteoporosis in the masters athlete. The benefits of low-to-moderate impact activity, such as running, in the maintenance of BMD remain unclear.[27] In the 2005 National Senior Olympic Games, runners greater than 65 years old had total body BMD significantly higher than that of sedentary controls and marginally higher than that of swimmers. However, this advantage was not demonstrated in the female subset, and spine BMD of either sex demonstrated no significant difference among runners, swimmers, and controls.[27] Even 1 hour per week of weight-bearing physical activity has been found to improve regional BMD compared with sedentary control females.[28] Diet, exercise, menstrual history, and heredity may all play a role.

Anatomy and Neurophysiology of Pain

The spinal vertebrae consist mainly of trabecular bone, which has a high rate of turnover and may not respond with as much osteogenesis as cortical bone when stressed with low-to-moderate impact activities such as running.[27] Although vertebrae fractures can cause significant pain, there is scarce evidence of innervation of the vertebral bodies themselves. Only 35% of cadaver vertebrae stained positive for nerve fibers, 95% of which were perivascular.[29] Osteoporosis without fracture can cause vague low back pain of unknown origin.[30] In vitro, risedronate decreased neuron calcitonin gene-related peptide immunoreactive (CGRP-ir) activity. In vivo, Risedronate decreased CGRP expression and increased BMD, especially in combination with exercise. Some CGRP-ir or transient receptor potential vanilloid 1 immunoreactive nerve fibers were found in the bone marrow.[30]

Common Sports Involved

Any sport that exceeds the flexion, compression, and sheer force tolerance of the vertebrae may predispose to fracture. For instance, acute osteoporotic vertebral compression fractures have been reported during midswing in healthy, active postmenopausal long-term golfers with BMD of L2-5 vertebrae in the first through third percentiles for age.[31] Low-impact sports such as cycling may predispose to osteoporosis. In women age 55 to 75 years initiating regular exercise (mainly tennis but also swimming, weight lifting, golf, and aerobic exercise) as late at 50 years, BMD was significantly higher than that in age-matched controls and in the same range as intercollegiate athletes.[32] Spine vertebral BMD was higher in intercollegiate female tennis players versus swimmers, which was attributed to gravitational stress on weight-bearing bones.[32] Over a 7-year period, competitive male master cyclists had lower BMD than nonathletes at all measured body sites. Complementary resistance and plyometric and other high-impact training was associated with less spine BMD loss and was recommended because of high fracture risk from falls in cycling.[33] Over an 18-month period, female masters cyclists and controls have been found to lose spine BMD, whereas runners maintained it.[28] Over a 4.6-year average period, male masters runners age 40 to 80 years did not have lower spine BMD.[34]

Clinical Presentation

Axial pain
The usual mechanism of compression fracture is an elderly or osteoporotic individual bending forward, who experiences acute onset of severe back pain in the thoracic or

lumbar region. As many as one-third of patients with vertebral compression fractures may progress to chronic pain.[35,36]

Muscular pain

Spinal compression fracture in the aging athlete may masquerade as muscle strain or other soft tissue injury; therefore, approximately 500,000, or two-thirds, of vertebral fracture each year in the United States go undiagnosed.[37] In addition, because of changes in posture or kinetic chain kinematics, a spinal compression fracture may result in reactive myofascial pain.

Gait and balance impairment

Spinal compression fractures can result in deformity such as excessive thoracic kyphosis and pelvic obliquity in addition to pain and stiffness, which can also impair gait and balance, partly by shifting the center of gravity relative to the base of support. Fall prevention, bracing, and gait training may help address these issues.

Management

Acute management of vertebral fractures may include initial bed rest (24–48 hours usually, with mobilization as soon as possible). One-third of fractures may cause pain,[36] and analgesic medications may be useful in treating this. Osteoporosis medications may be initiated but can take 6 months to 1 year to achieve efficacy, and up to 19% of patients have a been found to have an additional fracture within a year of initiating osteoporosis medication treatment.[36] Acute management may also include consideration of bracing and progression to physical therapy.[36]

Pharmacologic

Opioids may be necessary acutely. Nonsteroidal anti-inflammatory drugs may delay fracture healing and should ideally be avoided in the elderly with acute vertebral compression fracture.[26] Other pain medications risk sedation, which may affect fall risk or training ability in the masters athlete. Bisphosphonate medications can increase density of vertebral bone by inhibiting osteoclast activity. Newer nitrogen-containing bisphosphonates are significantly more effective than the first-generation etidronate. Treatment can be initiated in women with dual energy x-ray absorptiometry of the hip with (1) Less than equal to 2.0 and no risk factors, (2) Less than equal to 1.5 and greater than 1 risk factor, or (3) a prior vertebral or hip fracture.[26] Dosage for treatment or prevention varies but may be daily to yearly, oral, or intravenous. Formulations may include calcium or vitamin D. Newer bisphosphonates can reduce spine fractures approximately 40% to 70%.[26] Side effects may include gastrointestinal, atypical femur fracture, and jaw osteonecrosis. Recombinant parathormone may reduce vertebral fracture risk 65% but may cause leg cramps or dizziness.[26] Calcitonin intranasal spray is approved for osteoporosis treatment. Estrogen hormone replacement therapy is approved for osteoporosis prevention but should be used for the shortest duration necessary because of cardiovascular risks. Selective estrogen receptor modulators prevent and treat osteoporosis in postmenopausal women. Over 3 years, selective estrogen receptor modulators may reduce vertebrae fracture risk 30% to 55% and are an alternative if bisphosphonates are not tolerated.[26] Regardless of the medication regimen used, the care provider must be cognizant of the risks of polypharmacy in the elderly athlete and respect changes in drug metabolism pathway that accompany aging (see the article by Mautner and Huggins elsewhere in this issue for more information).

Nonpharmacologic

Exercise Weight-bearing exercise such as walking, jogging, or stair climbing 50 to 60 minutes 3 times weekly at 70% to 90% of maximal oxygen uptake (with 90% compliance) with calcium supplementation of 1500 mg daily resulted in increase lumbar bone mineral content 5.2% at 9 months and 6.1% at 22 months in postmenopausal women age 55 to 70 years. After 13 months of reduced weight-bearing exercise, bone mineral content returned to baseline.[38] The greatest stimulus for bone formation includes high strain rates, high strain magnitudes, uneven distribution across the bone, and high magnitude of ground reaction force.[33] Systematic back muscle exercise regimens after percutaneous vertebroplasty for spinal osteoporotic compression fracture resulted in significantly improved scores on Oswestry Disability Index and visual analogue scale as far out as 2 years out.[36] Although it is generally agreed that prolonged low-to-moderate-intensity physical activity in postmenopausal women is associated with higher L1–4 BMD,[39] it remains controversial whether higher-intensity training for competitive events is less benefi-cial.[40] Although exercise in the elderly can increase bone density, as of 2002 it had not been definitively documented to decrease fracture rate.[36] Particular sports may affect site-specific BMD. For instance, in female masters athletes (average age 50 years) cyclists and controls had decreased lumbar BMD over 18 months, whereas runners maintained BMD.[36] Impact exercise for 24 weeks can increase L2–4 BMD in osteopenic postmenopausal individuals age 48 to 65 years compared with a decline in controls. Exercise can also increase lumbar BMD in osteoporotic women age 60 to 68 years, in addition to reduced fracture risk. Physical therapy can play a role in the standard nonmedical management.[36] Extension exercises, including isometrics, should be emphasized and may decrease pain. Flexion should be minimized.[26] Fall prevention, balance, posture support training, spine neutral body mechanics, and muscle strengthening should be emphasized. Precautions include no lifting and avoidance of spinal flexion. Resistance training should be avoided for 2 months.[26] In women athletes age 23 to 75 years, exercising more than 3 times per week, greater than 8 or more months per year, for greater than 3 years may reduce the normal rate of lumbar bone mass loss.

Nutrition Calcium is the most important mineral for osteoporosis prevention. Vitamin D increases intestinal absorption of phosphate and calcium. Serum level quantifica-tion and supplementation should be considered, especially in northern climates or for indoor athletes. Other factors in bone health include magnesium; vitamins C, K, A, and B12; folate; and protein balance.[26] The recommended calcium intake for women and men 51 to 70 years is 1000 and 1200 mg/d, respectively, and 1200 mg/d for everyone 71 years and older.[41] Recommended serum (25)-OH Vitamin D concentra-tions are 20 to 50 ng/mL.[41] Vitamin K supplementation of 10 mg/d, and calcium intake have been found to not influence the rate of bone loss in elite female runners aged 15 to 50 years.[42] Refer to the article by Anderson elsewhere in this issue for more information.

Endocrine Amenorrhea was the only significant factor predisposing to bone loss in elite female runners aged 15 to 50 years. Age of menarche was not significantly related to bone loss.[42]

Bracing Bracing the spine for postural training and support after vertebral compres-sion fractures is an option. For instance, some feel that rigid back support for golfers with osteoporosis may be helpful.[31] However, compliance in proper tightening and use is poor, and patients with osteoporosis often find a brace constraining.[36] Bracing after acute vertebral compression fracture can reduce pain and improve posture and load on fracture site. Current recommendations are for a neutral thoraco lumbo sacral orthosis or lumbar corset for comfort.[26]

Modalities Moist heat, ice/cold packs, and massage may be beneficial in pain control for osteoporotic vertebral compression fracture.

Gait and balance Balance training programs such as tai chi chuan improve balance and can reduce fall risk by 40%, possibly via improved knee extensor strength and endurance associated with improved gait stability.[36] Rolling walker may be necessary.

Comorbid condition management Constipation should be managed to avoid excess valsalva, which may put undue pressure on vertebrae. Costal iliac impingement syndrome may occur when spinal deformity causes lower ribs to abut the iliac crest. Lateral bending and rotation may exacerbate this condition. This can be treated with a soft wide belt or rib resection.[26]

Injection Vertebroplasty and kyphoplasty are reasonably safe and effective in osteoporotic fractures with worsening collapse and persistent pain.[36] Both involve percutaneous injection of cement into a vertebral body fracture using local or general anesthesia and fluoroscopic guidance. Vertebroplasty uses pressurized cement. The most common complication is cement leakage into epidural space, which can rarely cause neural compromise.[36] One or more spine levels can be treated at 1 session. Positive bone scans may increase likelihood of pain relief with vertebroplasty.[36] Kyphoplasty uses a pressurized balloon to re-expand the vertebral body and instill cement at low pressure, which can reduce the risk of cement extravasation.[36]

Surgery There are no specific surgical options for management of osteoporotic compression fracture in the aging athlete at this time.

Sports-Specific Training

Impact loading sports provide the most protection to the lumbar spine, whereas nonimpact sports (cycling) do not.[28] Female masters cyclists and controls (average age approximately 50 years) decreased L1–4 BMD over 18 months, whereas runners did not.[28] Female ex-elite runners have demonstrated greater spine BMD than nonathletes years after cessation of training.[28] It is also higher in high peak stress sports such as weightlifting compared with lower-force repetitive sports, such as cycling or cross-country skiing.[28] Women with a lifetime history of impact loading sports (tennis, running) had greater lumbar BMD than sedentary controls.[28]

Prognosis

Determination of prognosis should include quantification of bone mass. Site-specific measurements improve prognostication. The approximate risk of fracture doubles for every 1 point decrease in T-score. However, after 65 years of age, the bone mass measurements of the lumbar spine may be inaccurate because of osteoarthritis or fractures. Bone loss rate can by quantified by at least 2 measurements of bone mass over a 2- to 4-year interval or predicted by serum/urine markers of bone turnover, such as serum bone-derived fraction of alkaline phosphatase and osteocalcin or fasting urine calcium/creatinine ratio or urine hydroxyproline. High rates of bone resorption are associated with twice the risk of vertebrae fracture independent of BMD. The provider may also evaluate risk factors aside from bone mass, such as immobilization, comorbid diseases, or medications that increase fall risk, and environmental factors (slippery surfaces and inadequate lighting).[43] Prior vertebral compression fracture may predispose the patient to subsequent fracture.

SUMMARY

1. Masters athletes may experience low back pain from multiple sources. Masters athletes with discogenic back pain should avoid or modify sports with combined rotational and compressive forces; individuals with facet-mediated pain should avoid or modify sports with excessive extension and rotation.
2. Optimization of flexibility, strength, endurance, and core control is critical. Sports-specific training, realistic goal setting, and counseling are of maximal importance.
3. Overall, the health benefits of continued sports and athletic participation outweigh the potential risks of spinal degeneration in middle-aged athletes. There is little correlation between radiographic appearance of the spine and symptoms; therefore, symptoms should serve as the primary guide when determining activity modifications. Overall, masters athletes should be encouraged to remain active and fit to enhance their quality of life and reduce the risk of cardiovascular disease.

REFERENCES

1. American Academy of Family Physicians; American Academy of Orthopaedic Surgeons; American College of Sports Medicine; American Medical Society for Sports Medicine; American Orthopaedic Society for Sports Medicine; American Osteopathic Academy of Sports Medicine, Kibler WB, Putukian M. Selected issues for the master athlete and the team physician: a consensus statement. Med Sci Sports Exerc 2010;42(4):820–33.
2. Masters athletes pursue many sports. International Council on Active Aging. Available at: http://www.icaa.cc. Accessed April 3, 2012.
3. Deyo RA, Tsui-Wu YJ. Descriptive epidemiology of low back pain and its related medical care in the United States. Spine 1987;12(3):264–8.
4. Deyo RA, Mirza SK, Martin BI. Back pain prevalence and visit rates: estimates from US national surveys 2002. Spine 2006;31(23):2724–7.
5. Videman T, Sarna S, Battié MC, et al. The long-term effects of physical loading and exercise lifestyles on back-related symptoms, disability, and spinal pathology among men. Spine 1995;20(6):699–709.
6. Hackley DR, Wiesel SW. The lumbar spine in the aging athlete. Clin Sports Med 1993;12(3):465–85.
7. Patel AT, Ogel AA. Diagnosis and management of acute low back pain. Am Fam Physician 2000;61(6):1779–86.
8. Vuori IM. Dose-response of physical activity and low back pain, osteoarthritis, and osteoporosis. Med Sci Sports Exerc 2001;33(6 Suppl):S551–86.
9. Gharibo CG, Varlotta GP, Rhame EE, et al. Interlaminar versus transforaminal epidural steroids for the treatment of subacute radicular pain: a randomized, blinded, prospective outcome study. Pain Physician 2011;14(6):499–511.
10. Lennard TA, Crabtree HM, editors. Spine in sports. Philadelphia: Elsevier Mosby; 2005.
11. Schmitt H, Dubljanin E, Schneider S, et al. Radiographic changes in the lumbar spine in former elite athletes. Spine 2004;29(22):2554–9.

12. Lundin O, Hellström M, Nilsson I, et al. Back pain and radiological changes in the thoraco-lumbar spine of athletes. A long-term follow-up. Scand J Med Sci Sports 2001;11(2):103–9.

13. Friery K. Incidence of injury and disease among former athletes: a review. J Exer Physiol-online 2008:11(2)26–45.

14. Cohen SP, Raja SN. Pathogenesis, diagnosis, and treatment of lumbar zygapophysial (facet) joint pain. Anesthesiology 2007;106(3):591–614.

15. Mayle R, Ellenbecker T, Safran M. Tennis. In: Madden C, Putukian M, McCarthy E, et al, editors. Netter's sports medicine. Philadelphia: Saunders; 2009. p. 592–9.

16. Anish E. The senior athlete. In: Madden C, Putukian M, McCarthy E, et al, editors. Netter's sports medicine. Philadelphia: Saunders; 2009. p. 86–100.

17. Schnebel B. Thoracic and lumbar spine injuries. In: Madden C, Putukian M, McCarthy E, et al, editors. Netter's sports medicine. Philadelphia: Saunders; 2009. p. 393–403.

18. Watkins RLumbar spine. editors. Clinical sports medicine. In: Frontera WRMicheli LJHerring SA, et al, editors. Philadelphia: Saunders; 2006. p. 433–47.

19. Garfin SR, Herkowitz HN, Mirkovic S. Spinal stenosis. J Bone Joint Surg Am 1999;81(4):572–86.

20. Sandhu FA, Santiago P, Fessler RG, et al. Minimally invasive surgical treatment of lumbar synovial cysts. Neurosurgery 2004;54(1):107–11.

21. Healy JF, Healy BB, Wong WH, et al. Cervical and lumbar MRI in asymptomatic older male lifelong athletes: frequency of degenerative findings. J Comput Assist Tomogr 1996;20(1):107–12.

22. Jensen MC, Brant-Zawadzki MN, Obuchowski N, et al. Magnetic resonance imaging of the lumbar spine in people without back pain. N Engl J Med 1994;331(2):69–73.

23. Rohrer S. Spinal stenosis. In: Bracker MD, editor. The 5-minute sports medicine consult. 2nd edition. Philadelphia: Lippincott Williams & Wilkins; 2011.

24. Tenforde AS, Fredericson M. Influence of sports participation on bone health in the young athlete: a review of the literature. PM R 2011;3(9):861–7.

25. Nordström A, Karlsson C, Nyquist F, et al. Bone loss and fracture risk after reduced physical activity. J Bone Miner Res 2005;20(2):202–7.

26. Heckert K, Anan E. Osteoporosis. Kessler PM&R Review Course. March 1, 2011.

27. Velez NF, Zhang A, Stone B, et al. The effect of moderate impact exercise on skeletal integrity in master athletes. Osteoporos Int 2008;19(10):1457–64.

28. Beshgetoor D, Nichols JF, Rego I. Effect of training mode and calcium intake on bone mineral density in female master cyclist, runners, and non-athletes. Int J Sport Nutr Exerc Metab 2000;10(3):290–301.

29. Buonocore M, Aloisi AM, Barbieri M, et al. Vertebral body innervation: implications for pain. J Cell Physiol 2010;222(3):488–91.

30. Orita S, Ohtori S, Koshi T, et al. The effects of risedronate and exercise on osteoporotic lumbar rat vertebrae and their sensory innervation. Spine 2010;35(22):1974–82.

31. Ekin JA, Sinaki M. Vertebral compression fractures sustained during golfing: report of three cases. Mayo Clin Proc 1993;68(6):566–70.

32. Jacobson PC, Beaver W, Grubb SA, et al. Bone density in women: college athletes and older athletic women. J Orthop Res 1984;2(4):328–32.

33. Nichols JF, Rauh MJ. Longitudinal changes in bone mineral density in male master cyclists and nonathletes. J Strength Cond Res 2011;25(3):727–34.

34. Wiswell RA, Hawkins SA, Dreyer HC, et al. Maintenance of BMD in older male runners is independent of changes in training volume or VO(2)peak. J Gerontol A Biol Sci Med Sci 2002;57(4):M203–8.

35. Chen BL, Huang YL, Zeng LW, et al. Systematic back muscle exercise after percutaneous vertebroplasty for spinal osteoporotic compression fracture patients: a randomized controlled trial. Clin Rehabil 2011. [Epub ahead of print].

36. Lin JT, Lane JM. Nonmedical management of osteoporosis. Curr Opin Rheumatol 2002;14(4):441–6.

37. Dalsky GP, Stocke KS, Ehsani AA, et al. Weight-bearing exercise training and lumbar bone mineral content in postmenopausal women. Ann Intern Med 1988;108(6): 824–8.

38. Boden S. When back pain is a spine compression fracture. Available at: http://www.spine-health.com/conditions/osteoporosis/when-back-pain-a-spine-compression-fracture. Accessed November 23, 2011.

39. Hagberg JM, Zmuda JM, McCole SD, et al. Moderate physical activity is associated with higher bone mineral density in postmenopausal women. J Am Geriatr Soc 2001;49(11):1411–7.

40. Kohrt WM. Osteoprotective benefits of exercise: more pain, less gain? J Am Geriatr Soc 2001;49(11):1565–7.

41. National Institute of Health. Dietary Supplement Fact Sheet. Available at: http://ods.od.nih.gov/factsheets/. Accessed November 17, 2011.

42. Braam LA, Knapen MH, Geusens P, et al. Factors affecting bone loss in female endurance athletes: a two-year follow-up study. Am J Sports Med 2003;31(6): 889–95.

43. Kanis JA, Delmas P, Burckhardt P, et al. on behalf of the European Foundation for Osteoporosis and Bone Disease. Position paper: guidelines for diagnosis and management of osteoporosis. Osteoporos Int 1997;7:390–406.

Lumbar Spine Surgery in Athletes:
Outcomes and Return-to-Play Criteria

Ying Li, MD[a], M. Timothy Hresko, MD[b],*

KEYWORDS

- Lumbar spine surgery • Athlete • Outcome • Return-to-play

KEY POINTS

- Surgical treatment of lumbar spine conditions in athletes can produce excellent outcomes.
- Professional and competitive athletes participating in both noncontact and contact sports can return to their preinjury level of performance and have successful careers after discectomy for lumbar disc herniation.
- Athletes who undergo direct pars repair for spondylolysis may be able to return to sports, but their participation level may vary.
- There is great variability in published return-to-play criteria, which are based primarily on expert opinion.
- Physicians must ultimately base their decision to release athletes back to sport on each individual's condition and on the chosen sport.

Low back pain affects up to 80% of the general population. Nearly 30% of athletes will experience acute low back pain during their careers.[1] Athletes who participate in sports that involve repetitive hyperextension, twisting, axial loading, and direct contact are at higher risk of lumbar spine injuries. A study of 4790 college athletes competing in 17 varsity sports over a 10-year period found significantly higher back injury rates in football and gymnastics.[2] Lumbar disc herniation (LDH) is a common problem among football players, especially in offensive and defensive linemen.[3–5] Spondylolysis and spondylolisthesis can be diagnosed in 15% to 50% of college football players[6–8] and in 6% to 11% of gymnasts.[9] Sward and colleagues reported that 75% of elite gymnasts had evidence of disc degeneration compared to 31% of nonathletes.[10] Wrestling, rowing, weightlifting, hockey, ballet, diving, swimming,

The authors have nothing to disclose.

[a] Division of Pediatric Orthopaedic Surgery, University of Michigan, 2912 Taubman Center, 1500 East Medical Center Drive, Ann Arbor, MI 48109-5328, USA; [b] Harvard Medical School, Children's Hospital Boston, 300 Longwood Avenue, Boston, MA 02115, USA
* Corresponding author.
E-mail address: timothy.hresko@childrens.harvard.edu

running, golf, and baseball are other sports that demonstrate a higher incidence of lumbar spine injuries.[11-13]

Lumbar spine injuries in athletes can result in poor performance or inability to perform, which can lead to a shortened career and financial loss. McCarroll and colleagues found that low back pain was the reason for lost playing time in 30% of college football players.[6] Hainline reported that 38% of professional tennis players missed at least one tournament secondary to low back pain.[14]

Treatment of lumbar spine injuries begins with conservative management. A brief period of rest of 1 to 2 days provides initial pain relief without leading to muscle atrophy. Medications include nonsteroidal anti-inflammatory drugs with or without a short course of muscle relaxants if the athlete is experiencing muscle spasms. Physical therapy modalities, including ice, heat, and massage, and local anesthetic or epidural steroid injections can help with pain relief. Once the athlete's pain is under control, a regimen of stretching and strengthening exercises is started. Return to sports activity is gradual as the athlete's symptoms improve.[15,16] Cooke and Lutz recommended that athletes may return to play when they have full painless range of motion; the ability to maintain a neutral spine position during sport-specific exercises; and return of muscle strength, endurance, and control.[15]

Surgery may be necessary if conservative management fails. LDH can be treated with lumbar discectomy. Spondylolysis and spondylolisthesis may require repair of the pars defect or fusion. Degenerative disc disease (DDD) can be treated with fusion or total disc replacement (TDR). Studies report excellent outcomes with these procedures in the general population.[17-23] Traditional outcome measures used to evaluate the efficacy of treatment of lumbar spine conditions, such as visual analog scales (VASs), the Oswestry Disability Index (ODI), and the Short Form-36 (SF-36), are self-reporting questionnaires that primarily assess a patient's ability to perform activities of daily living without pain. Many patients now lead an active lifestyle and desire to return to sports after treatment of lumbar spine conditions. In addition, patients who are competitive and professional athletes are interested in returning to their preinjury level of performance and career longevity after treatment of a lumbar spine injury. There is a paucity of evidence on outcomes after lumbar spine surgery in athletes and return-to-play (RTP) criteria. This article summarizes the current literature.

OUTCOMES OF SURGICAL TREATMENT OF LUMBAR DISC HERNIATION

The Spine Patient Outcomes Research Trial (SPORT) observational cohort demonstrated that patients with LDH who underwent standard open discectomy had significant improvement in the bodily pain and physical function scales of the SF-36 and ODI compared to patients who were treated nonoperatively at 3 months, 1 year, and 2 years. The differences between the two groups narrowed between 3 months and 2 years but remained significant. The authors also looked at work status as a secondary outcome. They found that work status was worse in the surgically treated group at 6 weeks but there was no difference at 3 and 6 months. Work status then showed a small benefit for surgery at 1 year but this equalized at 2 years.[17] These results were not reproduced in the SPORT randomized trial. The randomized trial demonstrated that both the nonoperative and surgically treated groups had substantial improvements for all primary and secondary outcomes. There was a considerable amount of crossover between treatment groups. Intent-to-treat analysis showed that although there was a trend toward larger improvements in the surgically treated group, the differences were not statistically significant.[18]

The SPORT studies reported on outcomes of patients from the general population who were treated for LDH. These results cannot necessarily be applied to the athletic population. Competitive and professional athletes are interested in different outcomes, such as performance, RTP rates, and career length. Hsu and coworkers looked at performance-based outcomes after nonoperative and surgical management of LDH in 342 athletes in the National Football League (NFL), National Hockey League (NHL), Major League Baseball (MLB), and National Basketball Association (NBA). The authors examined RTP rates, number of games played after treatment, and number of years played before official retirement. Successful RTP was defined as return to the active roster for at least one professional regular season game after treatment. Overall, 82% of the athletes successfully returned to play regardless of treatment, with an average career length of 3.4 years after injury. RTP rates and career length were equal between treatment groups. There was significant variation in RTP rates depending on the sport. MLB athletes had the highest rate of RTP and NFL athletes had the lowest rate of RTP. A player's professional experience before injury was found to be a positive predictor for RTP rate and career length, whereas increased age was a negative predictor. Subgroup analysis demonstrated that NFL athletes who underwent lumbar discectomy had significantly longer careers compared to those who underwent nonoperative treatment.[4]

Hsu and colleagues[4] further examined performance-based outcomes in NFL athletes after treatment of LDH. He found that RTP rates for the nonoperative and surgical groups were equal. Seventy-eight percent of the athletes who underwent LDH returned to play, which is comparable to return-to-work rates in the general population.[17,18] However, career length after treatment was significantly greater for the athletes who had undergone lumbar discectomy. The author noted that a potential confounding factor for these results is that the nonoperative group was significantly older. Surgeons may be more likely to recommend nonoperative treatment for older athletes. In spite of this, subgroup analysis did not reveal any significant difference in RTP rates between athletes younger and older than the age of 30, suggesting that older athletes can return to a successful career after lumbar discectomy. Hsu also calculated a performance score for each individual player's position. No difference in performance scores was found between treatment groups. Further, performance scores within each treatment group were equal before and after treatment, demonstrating that players in all positions may be able to return to their preinjury level of performance after either nonoperative or surgical treatment of LDH. Eight percent of athletes in the surgical group experienced recurrent LDH requiring revision discectomy. This recurrence rate is comparable to reported rates in the general population.[24]

Offensive and defensive football linemen may be at even higher risk of lumbar disc problems secondary to their high body mass indices (BMIs), consistent play in squatting and crouching positions, frequent high-velocity trauma, and intense weight-training.[5] Weistroffer and Hsu reported on RTP rates in 66 NFL linemen after nonoperative or surgical treatment of LDH. They observed that a significantly greater number of linemen successfully returned to play after operative treatment (80.8% vs 28.6%). Linemen treated with lumbar discectomy played an average of 33 games over a 3.0-year period, whereas those treated nonoperatively played an average of 5.1 games over a 0.8-year period. Seven linemen in the operative group underwent revision discectomy for recurrent symptoms. Six of these athletes successfully returned to play.[5]

Anakwenze and colleagues compared RTP rates and performance outcomes in 24 NBA players who had undergone lumbar discectomy for LDH to a control group matched for experience, position, age, and BMI. Performance outcome measures included number of games played; number of minutes per game; shooting percentage; and rebounds, assists, steals, and blocks per 40 minutes. The authors found that

RTP rates were equal between the two groups. There was a trend toward the surgically treated group playing fewer games one season after surgery but this difference was not significant. The only significant differences were a greater increase in blocked shots and a smaller decrease in rebounds in the surgically treated group. The clinical significance of these differences is unknown. However, the results suggest that NBA athletes who undergo lumbar discectomy are able to achieve the same level of performance as NBA athletes who did not require surgery.[25]

Watkins and colleagues reviewed RTP rates in 59 professional and Olympic athletes who had undergone microscopic lumbar discectomy for LDH. Eighty-eight percent of athletes returned to active participation in their sport at an average of 5.2 months after surgery. No performance-based outcomes were assessed. The authors emphasized the importance of an intense postoperative rehabilitation program that focuses on trunk stabilization and strengthening to return athletes back to their sport.[26]

Although these studies demonstrate that outcomes of single-level discectomy are excellent in athletes, results of multilevel discectomy may be suboptimal. Wang and colleagues reported on 14 athletes from schools in the National Collegiate Athletic Association who had been treated with lumbar discectomy for LDH. Ninety percent of the athletes who underwent single-level open discectomy returned to play at the varsity level, whereas none of the athletes who had a 2-level discectomy returned to sports secondary to continued symptoms.[27]

RTP CRITERIA AFTER SURGICAL TREATMENT OF LUMBAR DISC HERNIATION

Very few evidence-based RTP criteria for postsurgical treatment of LDH are available. The recommendations published in the literature are based on authors' opinions and experience (**Table 1**). All authors emphasize the importance of postoperative physical therapy and rehabilitation. Neither single-level nor multilevel discectomy appears to be a contraindication to return to contact sports.[16,26,28,29] Watkins and coworkers permit athletes to return to sport once they demonstrate completion of a trunk stabilization program, achievement of excellent aerobic condition, return to a satisfactory skill level in the sport, and ability to perform sport-specific stretching and strengthening exercises.[26] Eck and Riley allow their patients to return to sport once they have sufficient pain relief and range of motion. Typically, athletes who have undergone microdiscectomy return to noncontact sports at 6 to 8 weeks and contact sports at 4 to 6 months postoperatively. The authors delay RTP for athletes who have had a percutaneous discectomy until 2 to 3 months after surgery.[16] Abla and colleagues conducted a survey of 523 members of the North American Spine Society (NASS) to assess return to golf after lumbar spine surgery. The majority of respondents allowed

Table 1	
Summary of recommendations for RTP after treatment of LDH	
Treatment	**RTP**
Percutaneous discectomy	2–3 months for all sports (Eck & Riley[16])
Microdiscectomy	6–8 weeks for noncontact sports
	4–6 months for contact sports (Abla et al[30])
Microdiscectomy	4–8 weeks for golf (Cahill et al[29])
Microdiscectomy	8–12 weeks for all sports

return to golf 4 to 8 weeks after microdiscectomy. Surgeons were significantly more likely to recommend a shorter time to return to play for professional and competitive golfers compared to noncompetitive golfers.[30] Cahill and coworkers reviewed 87 pediatric patients who had undergone lumbar microdiscectomy. Sixty-four percent of the patients were athletes. The authors released the athletes back to full sports participation at 8 to 12 weeks postoperatively.[29]

OUTCOMES OF SURGICAL TREATMENT OF SPONDYLOLYSIS AND SPONDYLOLISTHESIS

Spondylolysis and spondylolisthesis are responsible for up to 47% of low back pain in adolescent athletes.[31] Athletes who participate in sports that involve repetitive lumbar hyperextension, such as football and gymnastics, are at higher risk of developing these conditions.[6–9] Rossi and Dragoni examined 3132 competitive athletes and found spondylolysis in 43% of divers, 30% of wrestlers, and 23% of weightlifters.[32] Soler and Calderon reviewed 3152 elite athletes and reported spondylolysis in 27% of throwing athletes, 17% of gymnasts, and 17% of rowers.[33]

Posterolateral fusion with or without instrumentation is an effective treatment for spondylolysis and spondylolisthesis that is refractory to conservative management. Helenius and colleagues reported satisfactory long-term outcomes in 108 young patients treated with in situ fusion for low-grade spondylolisthesis at an average follow-up of 20.8 years.[19] The authors used the ODI and Scoliosis Research Society (SRS) questionnaire to measure outcomes. Lamberg and colleagues reviewed 69 young patients with high-grade spondylolisthesis who had undergone posterolateral, anterior, or circumferential in situ fusion. All groups had good ODI scores at an average follow-up of 17.2 years, with the circumferential fusion group demonstrating slightly better outcomes.[20]

There are no dedicated series in the English-language literature examining the outcomes of posterolateral fusion for spondylolysis or spondylolisthesis in athletes. However, there are several reports of outcomes of direct pars repair in athletes. Direct pars repair may be advantageous in athletes because spinal motion is preserved. Several techniques have been described, including the Buck screw, the Morscher hook screw, and the Scott wiring technique. A biomechanical study demonstrated that the Buck screw provided the stiffest and strongest repair, whereas wiring was the least stable construct.[34] Debnath and coworkers studied 22 competitive athletes with spondylolysis who had undergone pars repair. Nineteen athletes were treated with the Buck screw technique and three athletes were treated with the Scott wiring technique. Ninety-five percent of the athletes who underwent Buck repair returned to play at an average of 7 months postoperatively, whereas none of the athletes who underwent wiring returned to play.[35] Reitman and Esses published comparable results with the Buck screw technique. They reported on four young athletes who began returning to sport within 6 months after Buck repair for spondylolysis. By 1 year, all of the athletes had returned to their preinjury level of performance.[36]

Nozawa and colleagues described better outcomes of the wiring technique in 20 competitive athletes with spondylolysis or grade I spondylolisthesis. All of the athletes returned to sports postoperatively, although not all returned to their previous level of participation. The authors categorized various sports into different levels of intensity by modifying a classification devised by the American Academy of Pediatrics. Ninety percent of the athletes returned to sports at the same intensity level, but not all athletes returned to their preinjury sport.[37]

RTP CRITERIA AFTER SURGICAL TREATMENT OF SPONDYLOLYSIS AND SPONDYLOLISTHESIS

Evidence-based RTP criteria after surgical treatment of spondylolysis and spondy-lolisthesis is scarce. Similarly to lumbar discectomy, a structured postoperative physical therapy and rehabilitation program are critical to return an athlete back to sport. Radcliff and colleagues describe their rehabilitation protocol, which begins with core strengthening and nonimpact aerobic activity at 2 weeks postoperatively. All exercises are performed with a neutral spine during the first 3 months. Higher impact activity may start at 3 months, and sport-specific training can be introduced at 4 to 6 months. Athletes may return to play when they demonstrate normal strength, normal range of motion, and no pain with sport-specific activity. This typically occurs between 6 to 12 months after surgery. Although solid radiographic fusion is preferred, the authors believe this to be the least important determinant for RTP.[38]

There is no information on RTP criteria after direct pars repair. Published recom-mendations for return to noncontact sports after fusion for spondylolisthesis are controversial (**Table 2**). Rubery and Bradford conducted a survey of 261 members of the SRS who commonly treat spondylolisthesis. They found that 62% to 66% of surgeons allowed return to low-impact, noncontact sports by 6 months postopera-tively for both low-grade and high-grade slips.[39] The survey of Abla and colleagues of NASS demonstrated comparable results. The majority of respondents permitted return to golf at 6 months after fusion for spondylolisthesis. Surgeons were signifi-cantly more likely to allow professional and competitive golfers to return to play sooner, such as at 2 to 3 months or 4 to 8 weeks.[30] Eck and Riley disagree and suggest delaying return to noncontact sports for 1 year.[16]

RTP criteria for contact sports are even more controversial. Eck and Riley do not recommend returning to full-contact sports.[16] Burnett and Sonntag allow return to contact sports but do not specify a timeframe.[28] Rubery and Bradford's survey of the SRS demonstrated that 51% to 56% of surgeons permitted return to contact sports, such as basketball and soccer, at 1 year after surgery regardless of slip grade. The most important factors that influenced decision making on RTP were radiographic appearance and time from surgery. The authors placed football and hockey into a separate category defined as collision sports. Only 27% to 36% of surgeons allowed return to collision sports at 1 year postoperatively. Forty-nine percent and 58% of surgeons recommended against or forbade collision sports for low-grade and

Table 2
Summary of recommendations for RTP after treatment of spondylolysis and spondylolisthesis with fusion

	Type of Sport	RTP
Abla et al[30]	Golf	6 mo
Rubery and Bradford[39]	Non-contact	6 mo
	Contact	1 y
	Collision	Not recommended
Eck and Riley[16]	Non-contact	1 y
	Contact	Not recommended
Burnett and Sonntag[28]	Contact	Allowed but no defined time-frame
Radcliff et al[38]	All	6–12 mo
Herman et al[40]	All	1 y

high-grade slips, respectively. The most common sports that surgeons forbade patients to resume after spondylolisthesis fusion were gymnastics, football, rugby, wrestling, weightlifting, skydiving, and bungee jumping.[39]

Although some authors do not restrict return to contact sports after fusion for spondylolisthesis, they advise that athletes participating in activities that require extreme mobility or involve heavy loads may be limited after surgery. Herman and coworkers allow unrestricted RTP in athletes who are asymptomatic, have achieved stable fusion, and are fully rehabilitated to their previous playing capacity. This typically occurs within 1 year after surgery. The authors believe that a single-level lumbosacral fusion has minimal impact on spine function, whereas a multilevel fusion may impair mobility and performance.[40] Radcliff and coworkers caution that fusion may be a career-ending surgery for activities that require extreme lumbar hyperextension, such as gymnastics and dance. They also state that athletes participating in sports that involve heavy loads may be reduced from highly competitive to recreational.[38]

OUTCOMES OF SURGICAL TREATMENT OF DEGENERATIVE DISC DISEASE

Outcomes of lumbar fusion and lumbar TDR for the treatment of DDD in the general population are satisfactory. Blumenthal and colleagues conducted a prospective, randomized, multicenter trial comparing lumbar TDR to lumbar fusion. Primary outcome measures were a VAS and the ODI and SF-36 questionnaires. Both treatment groups improved significantly after surgery. However, the TDR group showed significantly greater improvement in pain and disability scores during the early postoperative period. At 2-year follow-up, the differences between the groups equalized. The authors also reported a significantly higher rate of patient satisfaction in the TDR group at 2-year follow-up.[22] These results suggest that lumbar TDR is at least equivalent to lumbar fusion, although no long-term results of TDR are available. Siepe and coworkers reviewed 92 patients who had undergone lumbar TDR with a minimum follow-up of 2 years. VAS and ODI scores showed significant and lasting improvement throughout the postoperative course. At final follow-up, 56% of patients had returned to work without restrictions in full-time labor, 4.4% had some restrictions, and 7.7% were employed in new positions.[23]

There are no published series that describe outcomes of lumbar fusion for treatment of DDD in athletes. However, there are reports on outcomes of lumbar TDR in athletes and the military.[41,42] Siepe and colleagues reviewed 39 professional, competitive, and recreational athletes who had undergone lumbar TDR for DDD with an average follow-up of 26.3 months. VAS and ODI scores were significantly improved after surgery, and these results were maintained until final follow-up. RTP rate was 94.9%. Overall, 9 of 12 professional or elite athletes returned to play at a competitive level after TDR. Return to competitive contact sports, including parachute jumping, diving, soccer, cross-country motor biking, wild water rafting, and kayaking, was possible with no or only minor restrictions. Athletes reported that they achieved full recovery and peak fitness at an average of 5.2 months postoperatively.[41]

Military personnel, especially the Marines and special operations communities, experience extraordinary daily forces on the lumbar spine. Frequent activities include parachute jumps, diving, high-impact water entries, and prolonged runs bearing heavy loads. Tumialan and coworkers compared 12 military patients who had undergone lumbar TDR to an age-matched and level-matched cohort who had undergone lumbar fusion. Average follow-up was 10.7 months. Eighty-three percent of the TDR group returned to unrestricted full duty at an average of 22.6 weeks, compared to 67% of the fusion group returning at an average of 32.4 weeks. The

Table 3	
Summary of recommendations for RTP after treatment of DDD	
Treatment	RTP
Lumbar fusion/lumbar TDR	Allow contact sports but no defined (Burnett & Sonntag[28]) timeframe
Lumbar TDR	3 months for noncontact sports (Siepe et al[41])
	4–6 months for contact sports
Lumbar TDR	3 months for nonimpact training (Tumialan et al[42])
	4–5 months for light impact and weight-training
	6 months for unrestricted full military duty

results were not statistically significant, likely because the study was underpowered. Although these data suggest that TDR has a better outcome than fusion, the authors describe some potential confounding factors. Military surgeons may be more likely to permit a service member who works in a sedentary environment to return to full duty sooner. Surgeons also typically wait for evidence of radiographic fusion before releasing patients back to full duty, even if all symptoms have resolved. There are no radiographic criteria for TDR that can indicate a safe return to full duty. These patients are allowed to return when they are asymptomatic, which can be relatively early in the postoperative period. Nevertheless, these results confirm that individuals who undergo lumbar TDR are able to return to a high level of rigorous training and physical performance.[42]

RTP CRITERIA AFTER SURGICAL TREATMENT OF DEGENERATIVE DISC DISEASE

There is little evidence in the literature on RTP criteria after treatment of DDD (**Table 3**). Bono permits athletes who have undergone lumbar fusion to return to play when there is radiographic evidence of a solid fusion; resolution of pain; and restoration of strength, flexibility, and endurance.[43] Burnett and Sonntag state that neither lumbar fusion nor lumbar TDR is a contraindication to resuming contact sports but they do not specify a timeframe for return.[28] Siepe and colleagues recommend participating in noncontact sports within the first 3 months after lumbar TDR and returning to preoperative sports at 3 to 6 months. These authors believe that even contact sports and extreme sports can be safely resumed at 4 to 6 months after TDR.[41] Tumialan and colleagues have published an algorithm for return to active duty for military personnel after lumbar TDR. They allow nonimpact training at 3 months, light-impact training and weight-training at 4 to 5 months, and a fitness test at 6 months. Service members may return to unrestricted full duty at 6 months if they demonstrate preservation of motion, absence of hardware complications, and resolution of preoperative symptoms.[42]

RTP CRITERIA AFTER SURGICAL TREATMENT OF SPINAL STENOSIS AND SCOLIOSIS

Spinal stenosis and scoliosis are other lumbar spine conditions that may require treatment in athletes. There are no studies that examine outcomes of treatment in athletes. Similarly to treatment of LDH, spondylolysis and spondylolisthesis, and DDD, published RTP recommendations are based on expert opinion (**Table 4**). The survey of Abla and colleagues of survey of NASS found that the majority of surgeons permitted return to golf at 4 to 8 weeks after laminectomy for spinal stenosis.[30] Eck

Table 4
Summary of recommendations for RTP after treatment of spinal stenosis and scoliosis

Condition	Treatment	RTP
Spinal stenosis	Laminectomy	4–8 weeks for golf (Abla et al[30])
Spinal stenosis	Laminectomy	4–6 months (Eck & Riley[16])
	Fusion	1 y for noncontact sports
	Contact sports	Not recommended
Spinal stenosis	Laminectomy	Allow contact sports but no defined timeframe (Burnett & Sonntag[28])
Fusion		Allow contact sports but no defined timeframe
Scoliosis fusion		6 months for noncontact sports (Rubery & Bradford[39])
		1 y for contact sports
		Collision sports not recommended

and Riley recommend RTP at 4 to 6 months postoperatively if athletes demonstrate lack of neurologic symptoms or instability and full range of motion. If a fusion is also performed, the authors allow noncontact sports at 1 year but forbid contact sports.[16] Burnett and Sonntag believe that contact sports are safe after single-level and multilevel laminectomy, as well as single-level and multilevel fusion.[28]

Fabricant and colleagues recently performed an analysis of independent predictors of RTP in 42 athletes who had undergone posterior spinal fusion for adolescent idiopathic scoliosis. Patients were allowed to return to full activity at a minimum of 4 months postoperatively if they had resolution of pain, and radiographs did not demonstrate any change in curve correction or implant position. Average time to return to play was 7.4 months. At an average follow-up of 5.5 years, 59.5% of patients returned to athletics at an equal or higher level of participation. The most common reasons for a decline in activity level were loss of flexibility, back pain, and deconditioning. Distal fusion level was found to be a significant predictor of successful RTP. A stepwise decline in activity level was seen with more distal fusion levels, with 73% of patients with a T12 distal fusion level returning to their previous activity compared to 20% of patients with a L4 distal fusion level. The authors emphasize that these findings should not be used as a guideline for releasing patients back to sport, but should be used when counseling patients and families about the likelihood of RTP after posterior spinal fusion for adolescent idiopathic scoliosis.[44]

Rubery and Bradford's survey of SRS is the only available source of RTP criteria after fusion for scoliosis. Forty-three percent of surgeons recommended low-impact, noncontact sports at 6 months and 61% allowed contact sports at 1 year postoperatively. The factors that most influenced RTP were time from surgery, use of instrumentation, and chosen sport. Collision sports, including wrestling, football, hockey, and gymnastics, were permitted only by 32% of respondents at 1 year. Sixty percent of surgeons recommended against or forbade return to collision sports after scoliosis fusion. The most common sports forbidden after surgery were football, gymnastics, collision, skydiving, and trampoline. Distal fusion level did not influence decision making on return to sports for the majority of surgeons.[39]

SUMMARY

Surgical treatment of lumbar spine conditions in athletes can produce excellent outcomes. Professional and competitive athletes participating in both noncontact and contact sports can return to their preinjury level of performance and have successful careers after lumbar discectomy for LDH. NFL players, especially offensive and defensive linemen, may experience greater improvement with lumbar discectomy than nonoperative treatment. Athletes who undergo direct pars repair for spondylolysis or grade I spondylolisthesis may be able to return to sports but their participation level may vary. Athletes and military personnel who undergo lumbar TDR are capable of returning to rigorous activities, including contact and extreme sports and unrestricted full-service military duty. Distal fusion level may be an independent negative predictor of successful RTP after posterior spinal fusion for adolescent idiopathic scoliosis. There is great variability in published RTP criteria, which are based primarily on authors' opinions and experience. Athletes must demonstrate resolution of preoperative symptoms, full range of motion, and successful completion of a structured rehabilitation program before returning to play. Physicians must ultimately base their decision to release an athlete back to sport on each individual's condition and on the chosen sport.

REFERENCES

1. Dreisinger TE, Nelson B. Management of back pain in athletes. Sports Med 1996; 21(4):313–20.
2. Keene JS, Albert MJ, Springer SI, et al. Back injuries in college athletes. J Spinal Disord 1989;2(3):190–5.
3. Hsu WK. Performance-based outcomes following lumbar discectomy in professional athletes in the National Football League. Spine (Phila Pa 1976) 2010;35(12):1247–51.
4. Hsu WK, McCarthy KJ, Savage JW, et al. The Professional Athlete Spine Initiative: outcomes after lumbar disc herniation in 342 elite professional athletes. Spine J 2011;11(3):180–6.
5. Weistroffer JK, Hsu WK. Return-to-play rates in National Football League linemen after treatment for lumbar disk herniation. Am J Sports Med 2011;39(3):632–6.
6. McCarroll JR, Miller JM, Ritter MA. Lumbar spondylolysis and spondylolisthesis in college football players: a prospective study. Am J Sports Med 1986;14(5):404–6.
7. Ferguson RJ, McMaster JH, Stanitski CL. Low back pain in college football linemen. J Sports Med 1974;2(2):63–9.
8. Semon RL, Spengler D. Significance of lumbar spondylolysis in college football players. Spine (Phila Pa 1976) 1981;6(2):172–4.
9. Jackson DW, Wiltse LL, Cirincoine RJ. Spondylolysis in the female gymnast. Clin Orthop Relat Res 1976(117):68–73.
10. Sward L, Hellstrom M, Jacobsson B, et al. Disc degeneration and associated abnormalities of the spine in elite gymnasts: a magnetic resonance imaging study. Spine (Phila Pa 1976) 1991;16(4):437–43.
11. Dunn IF, Proctor MR, Day AL. Lumbar spine injuries in athletes. Neurosurg Focus 2006;21(4):E4.
12. Lawrence JP, Greene HS, Grauer JN. Back pain in athletes. J Am Acad Orthop Surg 2006;14(13):726–35.
13. Watkins RG. Lumbar disc injury in the athlete. Clin Sports Med 2002;21(1):147–65, viii.
14. Hainline B. Low back injury. Clin Sports Med 1995;14(1):241–65.

15. Cooke PM, Lutz GE. Internal disc disruption and axial back pain in the athlete. Phys Med Rehabil Clin North Am 2000;11(4):837–65.

16. Eck JC, Riley LH 3rd. Return to play after lumbar spine conditions and surgeries. Clin Sports Med 2004;23(3):367–79, viii.

17. Weinstein JN, Lurie JD, Tosteson TD, et al. Surgical vs nonoperative treatment for lumbar disk herniation: the Spine Patient Outcomes Research Trial (SPORT) observational cohort. JAMA 2006;296(20):2451–9.

18. Weinstein JN, Tosteson TD, Lurie JD, et al. Surgical vs nonoperative treatment for lumbar disk herniation: the Spine Patient Outcomes Research Trial (SPORT): a randomized trial. JAMA 2006;296(20):2441–50.

19. Helenius I, Lamberg T, Osterman K, et al. Scoliosis research society outcome instrument in evaluation of long-term surgical results in spondylolysis and low-grade isthmic spondylolisthesis in young patients. Spine (Phila Pa 1976) 2005; 30(3):336–41.

20. Lamberg T, Remes V, Helenius I, et al. Uninstrumented in situ fusion for high-grade childhood and adolescent isthmic spondylolisthesis: long-term outcome. J Bone Joint Surg Am 2007;89(3):512–8.

21. Pizzutillo PD, Mirenda W, MacEwen GD. Posterolateral fusion for spondylolisthesis in adolescence. J Pediatr Orthop 1986;6(3):311–6.

22. Blumenthal S, McAfee PC, Guyer RD, et al. A prospective, randomized, multicenter Food and Drug Administration investigational device exemptions study of lumbar total disc replacement with the CHARITE artificial disc versus lumbar fusion: part I: evaluation of clinical outcomes. Spine (Phila Pa 1976) 2005;30(14):1565–75 [discussion: E1587–91].

23. Siepe CJ, Mayer HM, Wiechert K, et al. Clinical results of total lumbar disc replacement with ProDisc II: three-year results for different indications. Spine (Phila Pa 1976) 2006;31(17):1923–32.

24. Barth M, Weiss C, Thome C. Two-year outcome after lumbar microdiscectomy versus microscopic sequestrectomy. Part 1: evaluation of clinical outcome. Spine (Phila Pa 1976) 2008;33(3):265–72.

25. Anakwenze OA, Namdari S, Auerbach JD, et al. Athletic performance outcomes following lumbar discectomy in professional basketball players. Spine (Phila Pa 1976) 2010;35(7):825–8.

26. Watkins RG 4th, Williams LA, Watkins RG 3rd. Microscopic lumbar discectomy results for 60 cases in professional and Olympic athletes. Spine J 2003;3(2):100–5.

27. Wang JC, Shapiro MS, Hatch JD, et al. The outcome of lumbar discectomy in elite athletes. Spine (Phila Pa 1976) 1999;24(6):570–3.

28. Burnett MG, Sonntag VK. Return to contact sports after spinal surgery. Neurosurg Focus 2006;21(4):E5.

29. Cahill KS, Dunn I, Gunnarsson T, et al. Lumbar microdiscectomy in pediatric patients: a large single-institution series. J Neurosurg Spine 2010;12(2):165–70.

30. Abla AA, Maroon JC, Lochhead R, et al. Return to golf after spine surgery. J Neurosurg Spine 2011;14(1):23–30.

31. Micheli LJ, Wood R. Back pain in young athletes: significant differences from adults in causes and patterns. Arch Pediatr Adolesc Med 1995;149(1):15–8.

32. Rossi F, Dragoni S. Lumbar spondylolysis: occurrence in competitive athletes. Updated achievements in a series of 390 cases. J Sports Med Phys Fitness 1990;30(4): 450–2.

33. Soler T, Calderon C. The prevalence of spondylolysis in the Spanish elite athlete. Am J Sports Med 2000;28(1):57–62.

34. Kip PC, Esses SI, Doherty BI, et al. Biomechanical testing of pars defect repairs. Spine (Phila Pa 1976) 1994;19(23):2692–7.
35. Debnath UK, Freeman BJ, Gregory P, et al. Clinical outcome and return to sport after the surgical treatment of spondylolysis in young athletes. J Bone Joint Surg Br 2003;85(2):244–9.
36. Reitman CA, Esses SI. Direct repair of spondylolytic defects in young competitive athletes. Spine J 2002;2(2):142–4.
37. Nozawa S, Shimizu K, Miyamoto K, et al. Repair of pars interarticularis defect by segmental wire fixation in young athletes with spondylolysis. Am J Sports Med 2003;31(3):359–64.
38. Radcliff KE, Kalantar SB, Reitman CA. Surgical management of spondylolysis and spondylolisthesis in athletes: indications and return to play. Curr Sports Med Rep 2009;8(1):35–40.
39. Rubery PT, Bradford DS. Athletic activity after spine surgery in children and adolescents: results of a survey. Spine (Phila Pa 1976) 2002;27(4):423–7.
40. Herman MJ, Pizzutillo PD, Cavalier R. Spondylolysis and spondylolisthesis in the child and adolescent athlete. Orthop Clin North Am 2003;34(3):461–7, vii.
41. Siepe CJ, Wiechert K, Khattab MF, et al. Total lumbar disc replacement in athletes: clinical results, return to sport and athletic performance. Eur Spine J 2007;16(7): 1001–13.
42. Tumialan LM, Ponton RP, Garvin A, et al. Arthroplasty in the military: a preliminary experience with ProDisc-C and ProDisc-L. Neurosurg Focus 2010;28(5):E18.
43. Bono CM. Low-back pain in athletes. J Bone Joint Surg Am 2004;86–A(2):382–96.
44. Fabricant PD, Admoni SH, Green DW, et al. Return to athletic activity after posterior spinal fusion for adolescent idiopathic scoliosis: analysis of independent predictors. J Pediatr Orthop 2012;32(3):259–65.

Injuries and Abnormalities of the Cervical Spine and Return to Play Criteria

Christopher K. Kepler, MD, MBA[a,b,]*,
Alexander R. Vaccaro, MD, PhD[a,b]

KEYWORDS

- Cervical spine injury • Spinal cord injury • Sports-associated injury
- Sideline physician • Return to play

KEY POINTS

- Sports-associated injuries are the second most common of spinal cord injury in the United States in the first 30 years of life.
- Benign injury types such as isolated spinous process fractures or compression fractures can be treated with immobilization and typically do not preclude return to play once healed.
- More complex injuries must be evaluated based on spinal stability, need for fusion, and the number of levels fused if necessary; fusion of 3 or more cervical levels is a contraindication to return to play.
- Players with a third stinger in a single season or a recurrent transient quadriparesis must undergo imaging to rule out stenosis and parenchymal injury; return to play is dependent on resolution of symptoms and severity of episode.
- Players with symptomatic disk herniation(s) who undergo successful cervical fusion may return to play after fusion of 1 or 2 segments.

Sporting injuries are a common cause of accidental injury in the United States, resulting in approximately 5.3 million visits to health care providers in 2009.[1] Although not as common as extremity fractures and ligament injuries, sports-related cervical spine and spinal cord injury rates are capable of producing catastrophic disability when they do occur. In particular, American football,[2-4] hockey,[5,6] and wrestling[7] are the commonly played sports with high incidence of cervical spine and spinal cord

[a] Thomas Jefferson University, 1015 Walnut Street, Curtis Building, Room 801, Philadelphia, PA 19107, USA; [b] Rothman Institute, 925 Chesnut Street, 5th Floor, Philadelphia, PA 19107, USA
* Corresponding author. Thomas Jefferson University, 1015 Walnut Street, Curtis Building, Room 801, Philadelphia, PA 19107.
E-mail address: chris.kepler@gmail.com

Clin Sports Med 31 (2012) 499–508
doi:10.1016/j.csm.2012.03.005
0278-5919/12/$ – see front matter © 2012 Elsevier Inc. All rights reserved.

injury (SCI), although SCI has also been described during skiing/snowboarding,[8] mountain biking,[9] diving,[10,11] and horseback riding.[12,13] Internationally, rugby has also been identified as having a relatively high incidence of cervical spine injury.[14,15] Several relevant databases are maintained by various organizations to help track the incidence, severity, and circumstances of injuries sustained during sports.

Epidemiology of Cervical Injury in Sports

Sports injuries were the fourth most common cause of SCI in the United States between 2005 and 2010 after motor vehicle accidents, violence, and falls and the second most common cause of SCI in the first 30 years of life. Sports injuries accounted for 7.9% of SCI between 2005 and 2010.[16] Although cervical injury has been described in many sports, these injuries occur predominantly in contact sports, and football in particular, in the United States. A study spanning 12 years at 2 SCI centers in the United States reported that approximately 60% of patients injured during sports were football players, followed by wrestlers (21%).[17] Diving accidents have made up 11% of admissions to SCI centers in some series,[18] but these are typically recreational, not competitive, diving injuries. Cervical vertebral fracture or dislocation is the most common cause of catastrophic neurologic injury in sports, causing approximately 75% of catastrophic cervical spine injuries, as shown in 1 large study of football cervical injuries spanning the introduction of guidelines, which demonstrated effectiveness in reducing cervical fracture rate. Despite several recent, high-profile catastrophic injuries resulting in quadriplegia, it is exceedingly rare across all commonly played sports.

Transient episodes of cervical neuropraxia commonly known as *stingers* or *burners* affect 1 upper extremity and are common, occurring in 50% or more of college football players,[19,20] and are likely underreported because of the rapid resolution of symptoms and desire of players to avoid missing playing time. Cervical cord neuropraxia, also referred to as *transient quadriplegia*, results in a neurologic deficit in more than 1 extremity that resolves completely within 2 days, often within 10 to 15 minutes. This condition is relatively rare, occurring in approximately 2 per 100,000 football players at the collegiate level.[3]

INJURY PATHOPHYSIOLOGY AND MECHANISM OF INJURY

Cervical spine fractures take a variety of forms and may be relatively benign, such as in spinous process fractures, or result in catastrophic injury, such as after cervical fracture/dislocation. Isolated spinous process fractures are most often the result of strong contraction of the trapezius and rhomboid muscles or hyperflexion injury leading to an avulsion of the spinous process.[21] Similarly benign in isolation, compression fractures are the result of hyperflexion and may share a mechanism with more severe cervical fracture but may occur in lower-energy mechanisms. By definition, compression fractures have an intact posterior vertebral body that prevents injury to the spinal cord in most cases.

The most common type of sport-related cervical spine fractures, however, are flexion-distraction injuries, which result in considerably higher rates of spinal instability and resulting SCI. Forced cervical flexion after axial loading of a flexed neck results more commonly in tensile failure of the posterior spinal elements followed by failure of the vertebral body, often with the production of a stereotypic anteroinferior fragmentation of the cranial vertebral body known as the "teardrop fragment." A variety of combinations of ligamentous and bony injuries are possible in both-column injuries of the cervical spine; facet dislocations in the setting of a both-column injury carry high rates of SCI likely because the intact articular processes prevent spontaneous reduction and canal decompression, which may occur after both-column injuries with fracture of the articular process. Slightly less cervical spine flexion at the moment of impact will instead produce concentric compression of the vertebral body, resulting in a burst fracture. Burst fractures differ from compression fractures by involvement of the posterior wall of the vertebral body, which may result in an SCI through bony retropulsion into the spinal canal.

Finally, the term *spear-tackler's spine* refers to radiographic findings of the reversal of normal cervical lordosis, evidence of previous vertebral injury, and cervical stenosis in a football player who has been confirmed to use a tackling technique of leading with the head, or "spearing." This constellation of findings and tackling technique carries a very high risk of neurologic injury.

Stingers result in weakness, pain, and paresthesias in a multidermatomal distribution in a single upper extremity; athletes commonly endorse symptoms of burning and tingling radiating from the neck to the shoulder, arm, or hand along with transient weakness. The mechanism of injury may involve ipsilateral shoulder depression with side bending of the neck to the contralateral side, which results in a traction injury to the brachial plexus. Alternately, similar symptoms can be the result of direct nerve root compression either through neck extension and contralateral rotation or ipsilateral neck side bending. Either mechanism can narrow the neural foramen and mechanically compress the exiting nerves, although it has been suggested that the foraminal narrowing mechanism is most common and results in more severe symptoms.[22]

Cervical cord neuropraxia or transient quadriparesis differs from stingers in the involvement of more than 1 extremity, and symptoms can range from temporary mild paresthesias to transient quadriplegia. Forced hyperflexion or hyperextension in a stenotic canal causes superimposition of compression secondary to the apposition of the posteroinferior margin of the cranial vertebral body and the anterosuperior lamina of the caudal vertebral body, resulting in temporary neurologic symptoms.

Along with players with spear-tackler's spine, players who experience transient cervical cord neuropraxia have been repeatedly identified as commonly showing findings of congenital spinal stenosis in the cervical spine. As defined by Pavlov and colleagues,[23] the ratio of the width of the vertebral body to the width of the central canal as demonstrated on a lateral cervical radiograph can be used to assess for spinal stenosis—ratios of less than 0.8 are routinely used to define stenosis and identify players with the associated increased risk of neurologic injury.

Klippel-Feil anomalies are characterized by congenital fusion of adjacent vertebrae. These anomalies may involve only 2 vertebral bodies or may be more complex with fusion of multiple contiguous or noncontiguous vertebral bodies. Congenital cervical fusions may be associated with pulmonary, cardiac, and urologic malformations, which may present additional considerations.

RETURN TO PLAY CRITERIA

Many investigators have proposed criteria to guide team or treating physicians in allowing return to play for athletes after cervical spine fracture,[17,21,24,25,26,27] stingers,[20,25,28,29] transient quadriplegia,[24,25,28,30] and other related conditions, such as congenital stenosis and disk herniation.[24,31] The relative rarity of these injuries is reflected in the literature composed of retrospective case series, which limits the ability to provide recommendations based on high-level evidence. Return-to-play guidelines are ultimately based largely on the judgment of experts who use the relatively sparse published literature as well as clinical acumen and experience to guide recommendations. The recommendations that follow here represent a combination of the accumulated experience and advice of experts in the field.

Cervical Fracture

No patient should return to play after a cervical spine fracture until 8 to 10 weeks after the injury to allow for bony healing. Because of the risk of additional injury to the cervical spine or physical limitations after surgery that will limit athletic performance and possibly increase the risk of repeated injury, the following are permanent contraindications to return to play after cervical fracture: atlanto-occipital fusion, atlantoaxial rotatory fixation or instability, spear tackler's spine, subaxial instability on dynamic radiographs (>3.5 mm translation, >11° angulation), trauma-induced sagittal malalignment, residual canal compromise from retropulsed bone or disk herniation, persistent neurologic findings, limitation in range of motion, or 3 or more level anterior or posterior fusion.

Relative contraindications to return to play include healed upper cervical spine fractures (healed nondisplaced Jefferson fracture, a healed type 1 or type 2 odontoid fracture, or a healed lateral mass fracture of C2), healed minimally displaced compression fracture, healed posterior element fracture excluding spinous process fracture, or a successful 1 or 2 level anterior or posterior fusion. Criteria that must be satisfied before patients with relative contraindications may return to play include painless, full range of motion; radiographic evidence of fracture healing or fusion union; and return of muscle strength after immobilization associated with the injury. Patients with healed spinous process (clay shoveler's) fractures or nondisplaced subaxial fractures have no contraindication to returning to contact sports once they regain motion and are no longer tender at the fracture site.

Stingers

Decisions about return to play after stingers should consider the number of episodes a player has suffered, the timing of these episodes, and the duration of the symptoms. After a first stinger or second stinger in a different season from the first stinger, the athlete may return to play immediately, once symptoms have resolved completely and he or she regains full, painless range of neck motion. If symptoms do not completely resolve, the player should undergo radiographs and advanced imaging as necessary; the player can return to contact sports when all symptoms have resolved and full range of motion is restored provided radiographs are not concerning for fracture or other destabilizing injury. If a patient experiences a second stinger in the same season as the first stinger, they may return the following game if symptoms resolve completely and they regain full range of motion. If these criteria are not satisfied, the player must wait for symptoms to resolve before returning. If the severity of lingering symptoms is severe, the physician should consider terminating the player's season, even if the symptoms eventually resolve before the season's end. A player who suffers a third stinger in the same season should sit out the remainder of the game even if symptoms resolve completely. Radiographs are warranted for all players with a third stinger and advanced imaging should be obtained for severe or persistent symptoms to rule out contributing anatomic factors such as congenital or foraminal stenosis. Physicians should strongly consider terminating a patient's season if symptoms are severe or persistent; persistent symptoms may permanently preclude a return to contact sports, even if they eventually resolve.

Transient Quadriparesis

Players who experience an episode of transient quadriparesis with rapid and complete resolution of symptoms must at least have plain radiographs and magnetic resonance imaging to screen for injury and evaluate the player's spinal cord dimensions and any evidence of intrinsic cord abnormality or neural compression. If there is no evidence of stenosis or spinal cord parenchymal injury, a player may return to play when asymptomatic and full range of motion of the neck is regained. Some physicians reserve advanced imaging studies such as computed tomography and magnetic resonance imaging in this setting only if there is evidence of stenosis on screening radiographs. Patients with mild or moderate stenosis and no evidence or spinal cord parenchymal injury who quickly regain full range of motion of the neck and who have no residual symptoms are considered to have a relative contraindication to returning to contact sports; decisions regarding return to play should be made based on the degree of stenosis, the propensity for injury during the sport in question, and the severity of symptoms in the initial episode of transient quadriparesis. Players who have a single episode of transient quadriparesis with evidence of severe stenosis or who experience more than 1 occurrence should not be allowed to return to contact sports, regardless of the degree or speed of postinjury recovery.

Spinal Stenosis

Players may be discovered to have spinal stenosis through radiographs or advanced imaging obtained after an episode of transient quadriparesis, persistent symptoms related to a stinger, or a traumatic/sporting injury to the cervical spine possibly unrelated to the presence of stenosis. Regardless of what prompts the initial radiographs, the presence of stenosis in a contact athlete must be considered carefully with the best interests of the player in mind, as stenosis predisposes that player to a neurologic injury after cervical trauma, which may not cause any injury in a player who does not have cervical stenosis. Players who have no history of cervical injury in whom spinal stenosis is diagnosed incidentally have no contraindication to return to play. If a player suffers an injury in the setting of spinal stenosis (stinger with persistent symptoms, neck pain, limited neck range of motion), the algorithm described above for transient quadriparesis should be followed.

Disk Herniation

Although disk herniations often are degenerative in nature, sporting activity that results in frequent, significant axial load on the head and neck may contribute to the high rates of cervical disk herniation seen in some athletes, such as front-row rugby players.[32] In this sense, such conditions can be considered chronic athletic injuries. Patients with a symptomatic disk herniation should be considered to have an absolute contraindication to return to play because of the increased risk of spinal cord injury due to relative spinal stenosis caused by the herniated disk, and because the pain and limited range of motion of the neck and upper extremities may endanger protective responses to prevent further injury. Patients with asymptomatic herniated disks noted incidentally on imaging must be questioned and examined carefully for insidious signs of radiculopathy or myelopathy and should demonstrate full range of motion of the neck before they are cleared to play. As described above for cervical fracture, patients who undergo 1 or 2 level cervical instrumented or noninstrumented fusion for symptomatic disk herniation and who demonstrate evidence of successful union have a relative contraindication to return to play and must demonstrate full, painless range of motion before return. Players with multilevel disease who undergo 3 or more level fusion should not return to contact sports. Minimally invasive techniques to resect herniated disk material without destabilization of the spine or the need for concomitant fusion are increasingly performed—patients may return to play without limitations once they regain full, painless range of motion and symptoms prompting the surgery have resolved completely.

Klippel-Feil Anomalies

There are no limitations to return to play for players with Klippel-Feil anomalies, which only affect 1 or 2 motion segments; biomechanically, short-segment Klippel-Feil anomalies are no different from 1 or 2 level fusions. Consistent with guidelines for players who undergo fusion of more than 2 motion segments, players with evidence of congenital fusion of 3 or more levels or malformation involving the occipitocervical or atlantoaxial regions should not be allowed to return to play.

Formal Return to Play Guidelines

No major sporting organizations (eg, National Collegiate Athletic Association, National Football League) have endorsed any particular algorithm or policy regarding return to play after cervical spine injuries, likely for a variety of reasons. In contrast to injuries that have received significant attention in the popular press, such as anterior cruciate ligament injuries in female collegiate athletes and concussions, the incidence of cervical spine injuries does not appear to be increasing, possibly because of rule changes specifically instituted to minimize the risk of these injuries. Secondly, as is evident from the return-to-play discussion, cervical spine injuries as a whole have complex, heterogeneous pathoanatomy, which precludes adoption of a single, simple algorithm. Because of these factors, decisions about when and if athletes may return to play after cervical spine injury must be made by the treating physician in consultation with the player, coaches, and training staff to serve the best interests of the player's off-field future well-being. The team physician must develop an accurate understanding of the natural history of the injury, posttreatment recovery process, and the risks specific to the sport in consideration.

ROLE OF SIDELINE PHYSICIAN

One of the most critical responsibilities of the sideline physician does not occur during a game but well in advance—a comprehensive series of algorithms must be established to facilitate optimal on-the-field treatment of an injured player and transfer to a hospital when necessary. Contingency plans must ensure availability of proper equipment necessary for early stabilization of an injured player: a spine board and stretcher, immobilizing cervical collars, tools to remove protective gear such as a facemask, airway management devices, and cardiopulmonary resuscitation equipment. Additionally, it is important that the physician have several individuals who are familiar with the techniques used to immobilize and transfer patients without causing secondary injury who can assist the physician during an emergency.

A player who walks off the field before notifying the coaches or physician of a potential cervical spine injury should be questioned and examined on the sideline in a seated position. In contrast, when a player is unable or unwilling to leave the field and communicates a potential injury while still on the field, that player should be questioned and, to the degree possible based on the player's positioning, examined on the field without moving the player. If necessary, the player can be log-rolled into a supine position with cervical spine precautions, and any helmet or pads should be left in place as they provide some measure of protection by promoting relative immobility and neutral alignment.[33]

Assessment should begin with the standard ABCD protocol, assessing airway, breathing, and circulation first. Next, disability is assessed through questioning about symptoms, such as the presence of neck or extremity pain including laterality, weakness, paralysis, and paraesthesias. Patients presenting prone with evidence of airway compromise will have to be carefully log-rolled into a supine position where the face mask can be removed with shears or bolt cutters, if present. Patients with neck pain, bilateral extremity pain, weakness, paralysis, or paraesthesias should be treated as though they have a potentially unstable cervical fracture or spinal cord injury and transferred to a medical facility for imaging and further workup. A complete secondary survey will typically be conducted at the medical facility for patients with severe injuries. Patients who have symptoms suggesting a relatively minor injury such as a stinger can be monitored according to the return to play criteria outlined above.

HOW LIKELY IS RETURN TO PLAY AFTER CERVICAL INJURY IN ATHLETES?

Many types of cervical spine injury preclude return to play, such as an episode of neuropraxia in the setting of severe congenital stenosis or unstable fractures requiring multilevel fusion. For less-severe injuries that do not present a contraindication to contact sports or are considered a relative contraindication, knowledge of the rate at which athletes return to competition at the same performance level is useful for physicians to provide guidance to athletes after injury. Unfortunately, the literature is relatively sparse, likely because of the relative rarity of these injuries and small number of elite athletes for which return to play is sufficiently important to justify monitoring. No guidance on rate of return to competition in elite athletes is available for players who suffer minor cervical fractures, likely because of the clinical insignificance of the most common injury patterns such as spinous process fractures. Ironically, there is also little formal guidance about return to play for elite athletes after stingers but for the opposite reason. Stingers are extremely common and likely not reported by many athletes, either out of indifference to the transient nature of symptoms or fear of disclosing an injury that might result in being kept from play. Clancy and coworkers[19] reported a 4-year prevalence of recurrent stingers of approximately 50% in active college football players, and several series describing players with a history of stingers have been performed on active players indicating that many continue to play;[22,34] all indications suggest many players continue to play after suffering a stinger or recurrent stingers, although whether residual symptoms affect level of play has not been addressed.

As it often represents only a relative contraindication to return to play, the success of players continuing to compete after transient neuropraxia has been commented on in several series. Torg and colleagues[24] described a cohort of athletes with first episodes of neuropraxia, 70% of who were at the collegiate or professional level with another 26% at the high school level. Overall, 60% returned to their previous level of competition but at an average follow-up of 40 months, only 23% of the cohort continued to participate in contact sports without recurrent episodes of neuropraxia, 14% continued to play but with recurrent symptoms, and 5% continued to play at the same level after undergoing some type of surgical procedure. A smaller series of 10 athletes presenting with a first episode of transient neuropraxia in the setting of cervical stenosis was described by Bailes.[35] Six athletes retired as a result of the first episode, and 4 returned to play after conservative treatment an average of 36 months after injury. The follow-up of only 40 months was not long enough to accurately gauge the recurrence rate, but the long period of time before return to play should be a cautionary tale for physicians advising players after similar injury. Finally, a small series of 5 elite athletes with transient neuropraxia treated with anterior cervical diskectomy and fusion (ACDF) for disk herniation demonstrated that although all returned to play, 2 players were forced to retire after recurrent disk herniation 1 year and 2 years after the index surgery, respectively.[31]

In contact sports such as American football and rugby, which commonly result in axial loading of the head, symptomatic cervical disk herniation is relatively common and can be considered a chronic, sport-related injury. Andrews and coworkers[32] described a series of 19 professional rugby players who underwent ACDF for symptomatic cervical disk herniation over a 5-year period and had an average of 17 months of follow-up. Seventeen of the players underwent single-level surgery, whereas the remaining 2 players underwent 2 level surgery at an average age of 28 years. Thirteen players (68%) returned to play at the same level of competition with 12 of the 13 returning within a year of their surgery and 2 eventually experiencing recurrent symptoms. One additional player returned to competitive rugby but in a lower division. Similarly, a study of American football players conducted by Hsu[36] included 99 National Football League players confirmed through media reports and injury notifications to have undergone treatment for cervical disk herniation. Of this cohort, 38 of 53 players (72%) who underwent surgical treatment returned to play for an average of 2.8 years, echoing the results described in professional rugby players. Although this rate of return to play was higher than that in the nonoperative group, the lack of direct contact with players or access to medical records precluded any analysis of confounding factors that may have affected the rate of return to play between groups.

SUMMARY

Cervical spine injury has a wide spectrum of consequences for the contact athlete, ranging from minimal to catastrophic. Because of the potentially grave sequelae of cervical injury, it is incumbent on team physicians or treating spine surgeons to be knowledgeable of postinjury treatment and return-to-play algorithms. Sideline physicians must have a rehearsed, comprehensive protocol for ensuring rapid treatment should an on-field injury occur with contingency plans to transport an injured player to a medical facility if necessary. Likelihood of return to play is variable with the extent of injury, but high for stingers, relatively low for patients who suffer episodes of transient neuropraxia, and intermediate for players who undergo cervical fusion for disk herniation based on the best available evidence. However, patients must be evaluated carefully on a case-by-case basis because of the heterogeneity of injury severity and associated pathology.

REFERENCES

1. US Department of Health and Human Services. Summary Health Statistics for the U.S. Population: National Health Interview Survey 2009;2011(5/24).
2. Thomas BE, McCullen GM, Yuan HA. Cervical spine injuries in football players. J Am Acad Orthop Surg 1999;7(5):338–47.
3. Boden BP, Tacchetti RL, Cantu RC, et al. Catastrophic cervical spine injuries in high school and college football players. Am J Sports Med 2006;34(8):1223–32.
4. Rihn JA, Anderson DT, Lamb K, et al. Cervical spine injuries in American football. Sports Med 2009;39(9):697–708.
5. Wennberg RA, Cohen HB, Walker SR. Neurologic injuries in hockey. Neurol Clin 2008;26(1):243,55, xi.
6. Tator CH, Provvidenza C, Cassidy JD. Spinal injuries in Canadian ice hockey: an update to 2005. Clin J Sport Med 2009;19(6):451–6.

7. Boden BP, Lin W, Young M, et al. Catastrophic injuries in wrestlers. Am J Sports Med 2002;30(6):791–5.

8. Tarazi F, Dvorak MF, Wing PC. Spinal injuries in skiers and snowboarders. Am J Sports Med 1999;27(2):177–80.

9. Dodwell ER, Kwon BK, Hughes B, et al. Spinal column and spinal cord injuries in mountain bikers: a 13-year review. Am J Sports Med 2010;38(8):1647–52.

10. Aito S, D'Andrea M, Werhagen L. Spinal cord injuries due to diving accidents. Spinal Cord 2005;43(2):109–16.

11. Cusimano MD, Mascarenhas AM, Manoranjan B. Spinal cord injuries due to diving: a framework and call for prevention. J Trauma 2008;65(5):1180–5.

12. Hamilton MG, Tranmer BI. Nervous system injuries in horseback-riding accidents. J Trauma 1993;34(2):227–32.

13. Ball JE, Ball CG, Mulloy RH, et al. Ten years of major equestrian injury: are we addressing functional outcomes? J Trauma Manag Outcomes 2009;3:2.

14. Shelly MJ, Butler JS, Timlin M, et al. Spinal injuries in Irish rugby: a ten-year review. J Bone Joint Surg Br 2006;88(6):771–5.

15. Fuller CW, Brooks JH, Kemp SP. Spinal injuries in professional rugby union: a prospective cohort study. Clin J Sport Med 2007;17(1):10–6.

16. National Spinal Cord Injury Statistical Center. NSCISC Spinal Cord Injury Database; 2011(5/25).

17. Bailes JE, Hadley MN, Quigley MR, et al. Management of athletic injuries of the cervical spine and spinal cord. Neurosurgery 1991;29(4):491–7.

18. Tator CH, Edmonds VE, New ML. Diving: a frequent and potentially preventable cause of spinal cord injury. Can Med Assoc J 1981;124(10):1323–4.

19. Clancy WG Jr, Brand RL, Bergfeld JA. Upper trunk brachial plexus injuries in contact sports. Am J Sports Med 1977;5(5):209–16.

20. Shannon B, Klimkiewicz JJ. Cervical burners in the athlete. Clin Sports Med 2002; 21(1):29,35, vi.

21. Zmurko MG, Tannoury TY, Tannoury CA, et al. Cervical sprains, disc herniations, minor fractures, and other cervical injuries in the athlete. Clin Sports Med 2003;22(3): 513–21.

22. Meyer SA, Schulte KR, Callaghan JJ, et al. Cervical spinal stenosis and stingers in collegiate football players. Am J Sports Med 1994;22(2):158–66.

23. Pavlov H, Torg JS, Robie B, et al. Cervical spinal stenosis: determination with vertebral body ratio method. Radiology 1987;164(3):771–5.

24. Torg JS, Ramsey-Emrhein JA. Management guidelines for participation in collision activities with congenital, developmental, or postinjury lesions involving the cervical spine. Clin J Sport Med 1997;7(4):273–91.

25. Cantu RC, Bailes JE, Wilberger JE Jr. Guidelines for return to contact or collision sport after a cervical spine injury. Clin Sports Med 1998;17(1):137–46.

26. Vaccaro AR, Klein GR, Ciccoti M, et al. Return to play criteria for the athlete with cervical spine injuries resulting in stinger and transient quadriplegia/paresis. Spine J 2002;2(5):351–6.

27. Morganti C. Recommendations for return to sports following cervical spine injuries. Sports Med 2003;33(8):563–73.

28. Page S, Guy JA. Neurapraxia, "stingers," and spinal stenosis in athletes. South Med J 2004;97(8):766–9.

29. Standaert CJ, Herring SA. Expert opinion and controversies in musculoskeletal and sports medicine: stingers. Arch Phys Med Rehabil 2009;90(3):402–6.

30. Torg JS, Pavlov H, Genuario SE, et al. Neurapraxia of the cervical spinal cord with transient quadriplegia. J Bone Joint Surg Am 1986;68(9):1354–70.

31. Maroon JC, El-Kadi H, Abla AA, et al. Cervical neurapraxia in elite athletes: evaluation and surgical treatment. Report of five cases. J Neurosurg Spine 2007;6(4):356–63.
32. Andrews J, Jones A, Davies PR, et al. Is return to professional rugby union likely after anterior cervical spinal surgery? J Bone Joint Surg Br 2008;90(5):619–21.
33. Banerjee R, Palumbo MA, Fadale PD. Catastrophic cervical spine injuries in the collision sport athlete, part 2: principles of emergency care. Am J Sports Med 2004;32(7):1760–4.
34. Levitz CL, Reilly PJ, Torg JS. The pathomechanics of chronic, recurrent cervical nerve root neurapraxia. The chronic burner syndrome. Am J Sports Med 1997;25(1):73–6.
35. Bailes JE. Experience with cervical stenosis and temporary paralysis in athletes. J Neurosurg Spine 2005;2(1):11–6.
36. Hsu WK. Outcomes following nonoperative and operative treatment for cervical disc herniations in national football league athletes. Spine (Phila Pa 1976) 2011;36(10): 800–5.

Degenerative Disease of the Cervical Spine and Its Relationship to Athletes

Konstantinos M. Triantafillou, MD*, William Lauerman, MD,
S. Babak Kalantar, MD

KEYWORDS

- Degenerative • Cervical • Neck • Athlete • Neuropraxia • Spondylosis
- Stenosis

KEY POINTS

- Long-term participation in contact sports appears to increase the risk of radiographic evidence of cervical spine degeneration; however, the clinical relevance is unclear.
- Cervical spine stenosis is thought to be a risk factor for the severity of irreversible spinal cord injury and the frequency of transient neuropraxia.
- Athletes suspected of having a transient neuropraxia should be screened for cervical stenosis with magnetic resonance imaging (MRI) after appropriate cervical spine clearance protocols have been followed.
- High-risk athletes demonstrating functional cervical stenosis should be counseled against the return to contact sports.
- Prospective studies correlating MRI with clinical data are required to clarify the relationship of cervical spondylosis, acute neurologic injury, and chronic sequelae in athletes.

Although catastrophic and acute cervical spine injuries in sports have been the subject of great focus in orthopaedic literature, the possible long-term effects of the stresses and repetitive injuries sustained by athletes is less clear. One area of particular interest has been on the premature development of spondylosis, or degenerative disease, of the cervical spine. Cervical spondylosis consists of disk degeneration that may result in facet arthropathy, segmental instability, and/or spinal stenosis. Though typically asymptomatic, cervical spondylosis can result in a variety or combination of syndromes. Pain generators located in the capsules of degenerated

The authors have nothing to disclose.
Division of Spine Surgery, Department of Orthopaedic Surgery, Georgetown University Hospital, 3800 Reservoir Road, NW, Pasquerilla Healthcare Center (PHC) Ground Floor, Washington, DC 20007, USA
* Corresponding author.
E-mail address: triantafillou.md@gmail.com

facet joints may possibly be a source of axial neck pain. Impingement of the nerve roots from osteophytic spurs may result in signs and symptoms of radiculopathy. Osteophytes, disc bulges, and/or ligamentum flavum hypertrophy may result in canal stenosis that can clinically manifest as cervical myelopathy. The sequelae of cervical spondylosis are an exceedingly common cause of clinic visits, health care expenditures, and reduction in quality of life in the general population.

Fifty-five percent of high school students are reported to participate in competitive and contact sports.[1] Recent reports cited by the media have implicated long-term participation in contact sports in the development of premature osteoarthritis[2,3] and have renewed interest in exploring the effects of early and competitive competition poses on the musculoskeletal system. Of a sample of National Football League (NFL) retirees aged 30 to 49 years, 36.6% self-reported a diagnosis of arthritis and pain in the neck compared to 16.9% in the general population.[3] Identifying any potential risk factors for the development of early degenerative disease of the cervical spine in an athlete could have a large impact on the evolution of sports safety.

With these concerns in mind, three main questions need to be asked when examining the literature. First, does participation in certain sports increase the risk of premature cervical spine degeneration, and if so, what are the long-term clinical implications? Second, does evidence of degenerative disease increase the risk of acute cervical or neurologic injury during sports participation? Third, what are the return-to-play (RTP) guidelines if degenerative cervical spine disease is identified?

Many difficulties lie in interpreting the data that explores the relationship between athletes and cervical spondylosis. First, the majority of studies examining the natural history of sports participation and cervical spine degeneration use radiographic outcomes; therefore, conclusions about the long-term clinical sequelae are assumptive. Also, Dailey and colleagues recently reviewed the literature that examined the risk of cervical stenosis and acute neurologic injuries; notably, these studies are case series or retrospective and are therefore of low-quality evidence (Levels III and IV) based on the Grading of Recommendations Assessment, Development and Evaluation approach.[4] The basis of current guidelines for RTP are vulnerable to the bias and confounding variables inherent in these studies without the strength of prospective controlled studies.

Second, the radiologic criteria used to define cervical degeneration, and therefore the validity of the conclusions of studies that have used these definitions, has been called into question. Cervical spine radiographs are noted to have good interexaminer reliability for classifying degenerative disk disease,[5] and are useful as an initial screening tool for the presence of cervical stenosis.[6] Cervical stenosis, or narrowing of the spinal canal, has multiple etiologies, and in the context of degenerative disease is used as a marker of disease severity. Historically, the ratio of the sagittal diameter of the spinal column to that of the vertebral body (SC/VB) had been used to quantify the degree of cervical stenosis on radiographs, with a normal canal defined as a ratio 1.0 and a severely stenotic canal defined as 0.80.[7] This measurement, however, has been shown to have a high false-positive rate and a poor positive predictive value in the context of collision sport athletes who have larger vertebral bodies than the average person.[8,9] As a result, studies that have used the SC/VB ratio to improve our understanding of the relationship between cervical stenosis and acute neurologic injury in the athlete may have overcalled the incidence of stenosis by as much as 88%.[10] Unfortunately, this has confounded the results of a large volume of work and contributed to the poor consensus for RTP guidelines among experts. The use of magnetic resonance imaging (MRI), which incorporates the soft tissues and more accurately quantifies the amount of space available for the spinal cord, is more precise[11] and has supplanted radiographs as the standard for the evaluation of cervical stenosis in studies and RTP decision making.

Lastly, it is difficult to create guidelines for athletes when comparing studies between different sports, as there may be a large difference in mechanisms of injury and sustained stresses and loads both during training and game play. Others have noted the difficulty in establishing controls, especially given the often larger size and better fitness of the athlete compared to individuals in the general population.[12] Therefore, it is difficult to draw definitive conclusions without the strength of controlled longitudinal studies exploring patient-oriented outcomes. Despite these difficulties, clinical practitioners who care for the athlete will undoubtedly be presented with these questions in their practice, and therefore a basic understanding of the current beliefs and controversies exploring the relationship between degenerative conditions of the spine and its relationship to the athlete is imperative.

EPIDEMIOLOGY

Degenerative changes of the cervical spine increase with age in the general population. Studies of the cervical spine in asymptomatic individuals have shown that degenerative changes on MRI are present in 25% of persons younger than 40 years of age and in 60% of persons older than 40 years.[13] In persons older than the age of 60, degenerative changes on lateral cervical spine radiographs are present in more than 60% to 75% of persons, with MRI evidence in more than 85% of persons.[14,15] The prevalence of positive MRI findings in asymptomatic individuals "emphasizes the dangers of predicating operative decisions on diagnostic tests without precisely matching these findings with clinical signs and symptoms."[13(p408)] Similarly, given that the vast majority of patients in the general population with evidence of cervical degeneration will remain asymptomatic, how one defines degenerative disease in the spine is cited as a major difficulty in analyzing the data and comparing the literature.[16]

Sports participation exposes the cervical spine to theoretical risk factors not seen in the general population. Some of these risk factors, including body mechanics, repetitive loads, acute bony and ligamentous injuries, weightlifting, spondylolysis, and muscle imbalances, have been more extensively studied in the lumbar than in the cervical spine.[16–22] The incidence and risk factors for degenerative disease of the cervical spine in athletes, and more importantly, the clinical sequelae, are even less defined. Attention has focused mostly on the effect of acute injuries and chronic repetitive loads in contact and collision sports. Because of the high rates of acute cervical injury sustained by front-line players in a rugby scrum, these players have been a source of much of the literature regarding degenerative changes to the cervical spine (**Fig. 1**).[23–25]

To make comparisons between sports and elucidate the risk factors for degeneration, it may be helpful to categorize them into collision sports, noncollision contact sports, and noncontact sports. Although somewhat arbitrary, this may help interpret the mixed results shown in the literature and provide a framework for counseling parents and patients and highlight the importance of examining athletes on a case-by-case basis.

In collision sports, a recurrent observation is that athletes who have been observed to have higher rates of radiographic evidence of degeneration in the cervical spine are also the ones who incidentally have the highest rate of acute injuries or may experience the greatest frequency of repetitive loading.[26,27] Scher observed that rugby players presenting with radiculopathy had evidence of severe degenerative disease, prompting concerns that participating in rugby may be a risk factor for premature degenerative arthritis of the cervical spine in the young athlete.[28] To

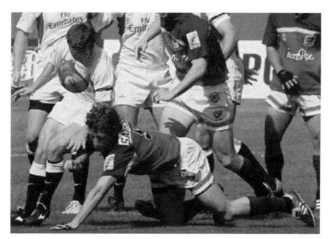

Fig. 1. A rugby player experiences a neck hyperextension injury.

explore this observation, Scher compared asymptomatic rugby players to a control, and noted that there appeared to be an increased incidence of early and severe degeneration seen on lateral cervical spine radiographs. Further, he noted that positions that sustain the largest loads and have higher rates of acute cervical spine injuries, namely the front-line players engaged in the scrum, also had the highest incidence of severe cervical degenerative changes.[29] Similar concerns have been noted in participation in American football, in which players presenting with chronic neck pain have had radiologic evidence of a previous acute cervical spine injury and undiagnosed fracture.[30] These early studies have raised the suspicion that long-term repetitive loads and/or acute cervical spine injuries may increase the risk for cervical disk degeneration.

The use of MRI as a modality for the evaluation of spine degeneration and a greater focus on the clinical implications of such findings has improved our understanding of the natural history of degeneration in collision sports. An MRI study of the cervical spine in asymptomatic competitive and professional front-line rugby players showed evidence that cervical disk disease was more severe in veteran rugby players compared to age-matched controls and to historical figures.[6] A recent study evaluated the symptoms of degenerative changes in professional rugby players averaging 23 years of competitive play as compared to a control. There was a significant increase in the radiographic evidence of C5/6 and C6/7 disk degeneration as well as apophyseal joint degeneration in the rugby group. Interestingly, there was **no** difference in the incidence of symptoms between rugby players and controls.[12] It was suggested that protective effects of muscle bulk and athleticism, a culture of toughness, or an unwillingness to admit symptoms for secondary gain may serve as confounders. Rugby players have been shown to have decreased range of motion of the neck, which may result in future functional disability.[31] The etiology is presumptively related to cervical degeneration, although this link has not been scientifically validated. These findings further highlight the difficulty in controlling variables and contribute to our lack of understanding of the natural history and long-term clinical implications of cervical degeneration in collision sport athletes.

Although collision sports have been the focus of most studies, other reports examining the incidence of degeneration from chronic repetitive loads in noncollision contact sports have shown mixed results. Schneider and colleagues studied a small group of high cliff divers in Acapulco compared to age-matched controls and concluded that evidence of spondylosis seen on lateral cervical radiographs may be related to the chronic repetitive forces to the cervical spine experienced during impact with water.[32] Indirect loads to the cervical spines in soccer players as a result of "heading" the ball has also been studied as a hypothetical risk factor for early degeneration. In one study published in 1982, cervical spine radiographs were taken from 43 retired members of the National Soccer Team of Norway and compared to an age-matched control. aqUsing an unvalidated novel scoring system, the authors concluded that these players exhibited degenerative changes "decades higher" than appropriate for their age, with no observed higher incidence of spondylosis in self-reported "headers."[33] The authors noted that the heavy all-leather soccer ball in use before the introduction of the modern lighter weight soccer ball may serve as a confounder when comparing to modern soccer players. A more recent study looked at radiographic and MRI findings of degenerative changes comparing young and veteran (>10 years) competitive soccer players versus age-matched and weight-matched controls. These players showed a tendency toward early degeneration on MRI and radiography, though not statistically significant, and exhibited a decreased cervical range of motion on cervical dynamometer,[34] similar to that of rugby players noted previously. These studies suggest that there is a risk of developing premature radiographic degeneration of the cervical spine in the noncollision contact athlete who sustains chronic repetitive loads to the head. However, the strength of these studies and lack of clinical outcome precludes making a definitive correlation.

Examining noncollision and noncontact activities may provide further insight into the risk that chronic indirect repetitive loads contribute to cervical degeneration. A prospective study comparing 32 jockeys without a history of acute cervical bony or ligamentous injury over 13 years with age-matched controls in the general population showed an increased incidence of cervical spine degeneration. The authors postulate that equestrians increase their risk of cervical degenerative arthritis from a repetitive loading force.[35] Scher reviewed the injury radiographs of a small group of adult African laborers who sustained acute neurologic injuries from accidents involving carrying loads of up to 200 pounds on their heads, a routine practiced since childhood.[36] Incidentally, he did not note any evidence of degenerative changes and suggested that chronic sustained loads to the cervical spine may not increase the risk of premature degeneration. Although not sports related, these findings suggest that repetitive chronic loads on the cervical spine that occur in sports, in distinction from sustained chronic loads to the cervical spine seen in this population of laborers, may increase the risk for premature degeneration.

Current epidemiologic studies suggest that athletes participating in collision sports, especially those in positions prone to acute bony and ligamentous injuries and high chronic repetitive loading of the cervical spine, appear to increase the risk of developing radiologic evidence of degenerative disease of the cervical spine. The risk of developing radiologic evidence of degenerative changes in noncollision sports, in which chronic repetitive loads predominate over acute injuries to the cervical spine, are even less defined. It has not yet been shown that these changes are clinically relevant. Prospective controlled studies with long-term follow-up of both radiologic and clinical outcomes are required to elucidate the incidence and natural history of premature spondylosis in athletes.

NATURAL HISTORY

Prudence suggests that it is best to assume that radiologic evidence of cervical premature degeneration will increase the incidence of the clinical syndromes of neck pain, radiculopathy, or myelopathy in the athlete until proven otherwise. The natural history of the clinical sequelae of asymptomatic degenerative cervical disease is not fully understood in the general population, let alone in the athlete. Similarly, the prognosis of patients who do become symptomatic is also unclear. There are currently no Level I/II/III studies that can reliably describe the expected natural history of cervical radiculopathy for degenerative disk disease.[37] Similarly, the natural history of myelopathy is unclear. A prospective cohort study was performed in patients who presented with radiculopathy or axial neck pain who had MRI evidence of cord compression without clinical signs or symptoms of myelopathy. It was estimated that symptomatic cord compression occurred at a rate of 5% per year.[38] A recent Cochrane review could not conclude definitively whether or not surgical treatment of either radiculopathy or myelopathy as a result of degenerative cervical spine is beneficial, although low-quality evidence does suggest that there are short-term but not long-term benefits over conservative therapies.[39]

CERVICAL SPONDYLOSIS AND ACUTE NEUROLOGIC INJURY

American football and wrestling high school athletes sustain the highest rates of head/neck/spine injuries in the United States.[40] The most feared neck injury is the irreversible spinal cord injury (SCI) and is typically caused by cervical spine fractures, fracture dislocations, and traumatic herniations. However, the two most common injuries are cervical cord neuropraxias and unilateral brachial plexus or cervical root neuropraxias, also known as "stingers" and "burners,"[41] which are generally self-limiting. Although cervical stenosis resulting from degenerative changes has not been studied in isolation, the relationship of these three entities and cervical stenosis as a whole has been the subject of much literature.

Cervical stenosis is thought to be a risk factor for catastrophic SCI in athletes and supported by the trauma literature. Eismont and colleagues reviewed the sagittal diameter of the spinal canal in patients sustaining a cervical fracture dislocation.[42] He noted that those sustaining a complete SCI had significantly narrower canals to those that did not. During neck hyperextension, the sagittal diameter of the spinal canal is narrowed by 30%, suggesting that athletes with preexisting cervical stenosis are predisposed to SCI if they sustain a fracture dislocation of the cervical spine. Similarly, a retrospective study by Matsuura and colleagues compared trauma patients sustaining SCI to a control group and demonstrated that those with injury had a smaller sagittal canal diameter per computed tomography (CT) measurements. This suggests that those patients with CT evidence of sagittal stenosis are at increased risk for acute SCI.[43] Kang and colleagues attempted to quantify this difference in a review of 288 patients with cervical fracture dislocations and noted that those with complete SCI had average canal diameter of 16.1 mm compared to 18.1 mm in those without SCI.[44] Drawing from results from the National Center for Catastrophic Sports Injury Research, Cantu anecdotally reported that of all athletes sustaining cervical spine fracture dislocations, 0% of players with MRI-documented stenosis versus 20% had full neurologic recovery after quadriplegia.[45] However, the validity of these results is unclear, as there is no documentation of the specific degree or neurologic deficit or spinal stenosis on which these findings were based.

Cervical cord neuropraxia results from a compression or concussive type injury to the cervical spinal cord in the absence of cervical fracture or fracture dislocation.

There is a transient complete or partial loss motor and/or sensation bilaterally that may last up to 36 hours. There are several suggested mechanisms; however, it is most commonly felt that compression occurs between the inferior posterior vertebral body and the sub-adjacent lamina during hyperflexion or hyperextension.[46] Therefore it is suggested that cervical stenosis increases the risk of neuropraxia.[46,47]

It is believed that there is an increased risk and recurrence of transient neuropraxia in athletes with cervical stenosis. An early retrospective study of competitive football players who had experience transient quadriplegia showed that all had evidence of congenital or acquired spinal stenosis as determined by the SC/VB ratio.[7] This has also been suggested in a retrospective study in rugby players,[48] and has been reported in patients with developmental or idiopathic stenosis.[49] A subsequent retrospective review comparing athletes experiencing recurrent transient neuropraxias to those without recurrence noted that a lower SC/VB ratio and narrower canal diameter correlated with risk of recurrence. Given the concern with the use of the SC/VB ratio,[8,11,49] MRI or CT myelography have been advocated to clarify the relationship between stenosis and neuropraxias in future studies.[10,45]

The risk that transient neuropraxia poses to SCI is still under debate. The previous studies had no reports of irreversible injury after athletes sustained initial or recurrent episodes of cervical cord neuropraxias; however, there have been some case series reporting permanent sequelae in patients with documented stenosis.[48,50]

The stinger and the burner are distinct from cervical neuropraxias because they involve lower motor neurons, namely the roots or brachial plexus, and therefore present with unilateral symptoms of weakness and sensory changes. The stinger and burner may result from a variety of mechanisms including a brachial plexus stretch from neck contralateral flexion and ipsilateral shoulder downward load, a direct blow to the plexus, or a neck extension compression injury of the roots as they exit the foramina.[4] This is supported by the work of Kelly and colleagues, who noted that football players without evidence of degenerative changes who experienced stingers and burners were measured to have smaller foramen compared to a control.[51] The authors therefore suggested that degenerative foraminal stenosis may exacerbate the normal physiologic stenosis during normal neck extension and rotation. However, the relationship between degenerative changes of the cervical spine and cervical burners or stingers has not been validated.

CLINICAL APPLICATION

Cervical stenosis presents a risk factor for irreversible SCI. Daily and colleagues have attempted to address the current debate regarding RTP criteria in a review of the literature examining the role of cervical stenosis, neuropraxias, and SCI in the athlete.[4] Importantly, he noted that of 16 relevant studies, the strength of the evidence was low to very low given their retrospective nature. However, given the serious consequences of ignoring this link, the evidence provides enough impetus to provide a rudimentary set of guidelines for the clinician presented with neuropraxia in the athlete.

Despite the multitude of low-quality evidence that implicates neuropraxia and cervical stenosis, currently it is recommended that a clinician who is presented an athlete with a transient neuropraxia should evaluate for cervical stenosis. The purpose of screening in this select population is based primarily on the potential risk of permanent neurologic sequelae if a catastrophic injury, such as a fracture or fracture dislocation of the cervical spine, were to occur, and on the potential for these sequelae to occur after transient neuropraxia. Routine screening for cervical stenosis

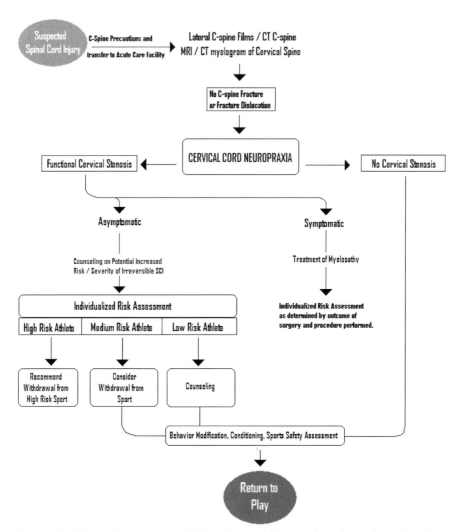

Fig. 2. Algorithm and treatment guidelines for cervical stenosis in the setting of transient cervical cord neuropraxia.

using radiographs or MRI, however, is not routinely recommended and not cost effective.[45,52]

When presented with an athlete sustaining a transient neuropraxia, the clinician should evaluate the patient for cervical stenosis (**Fig. 2**). The good sensitivity but poor predictive value of using SC/VB ratio alone to evaluate cervical stenosis has been previously discussed. Plain films may therefore be used for the initial screening of cervical stenosis if MRI has not already been performed to evaluate neurologic injury in the acute setting. This is rarely the case, however, as any player exhibiting spinal cord symptoms should be evaluated with an MRI. For RTP decisions, functional stenosis has been defined by a lack of cerebrospinal fluid around the cord on MRI.[4,11] This criterion has not yet been fully evaluated in the literature. It is generally agreed that the contact athlete return to contact sports if radiographic stenosis is not present, as permanent neurologic sequelae in this cohort have not been observed.[4]

When an athlete demonstrates canal compromise on MRI, the decision for return to contact sports may be approached on a case-by-case basis. To provide a framework for counseling patients, it may be practical for the practitioner to categorize risk of neurologic injury inherent in each sport, position, and level of competition into high-, medium-, and low-risk categories. High-risk sports include collision sports or those that carry a high incidence of catastrophic cervical spine injury and neuropraxia. This includes but is not limited to cheerleading, football, wrestling, ice hockey, skiing, snowboarding, and pole vaulting.[53,54] When functional cervical stenosis is present, many believe this represents an absolute contraindication for the return to contact sports.[45] However, this recommendation is based on low-quality evidence,[4] and therefore some advocate proper counseling on the increased risk of SCI in the athlete with asymptomatic spinal stenosis.[55] Medium-risk sports may include most other noncollision contact sports such as soccer, baseball, basketball, and equestrian sports. In this subgroup, epidemiologic data are not clear. Counseling should be provided, and a recommendation for cessation of play should be considered. Low-risk sports include most noncollision noncontact sports. In this subgroup, the risk for catastrophic injury is very low, and RTP can be recommended with appropriate counseling.

The athlete who has developed cervical myelopathy should be evaluated by a spine specialist. Athletes who have subsequently undergone an anterior cervical decompression and fusion present with a unique situation. A review of the literature by Daily suggests that "Surgical fixation with single-level ACDF to eliminate single level neurologic compression causing radiculopathy or myelopathy is a strong recommendation as a treatment option to return to full contact sports play." This recommendation is based primarily on one cohort study of 17 players who underwent ACDF in which an increased incidence of catastrophic injury after fusion was not seen. Further recommendations could not be made regarding multilevel fusions based on the lack of available studies. The practitioner should counsel patients on the lack of epidemiologic data in this subgroup and manage each on a case-by-case basis.

It is important to note that these recommendations are derived mostly from football injuries given the highest prevalence of catastrophic injuries in this subgroup. It is more difficult to apply these recommendations across different sports in which mechanisms of injury and predisposing body positions differ widely. A risk assessment may provide a framework for counseling patients given the lack of clear epidemiologic data. Each athlete and his or her position, the level of play, and personal preferences should be considered on a case-by-case basis.

SUMMARY

Each sport presents with unique risk factors and different mechanisms of injury, and therefore extrapolation of the data from one sport to another makes comparison difficult. The current evidence exploring the relationship of athletes and degenerative changes of the cervical spine leaves much to be debated, and future prospective longitudinal studies will be needed to clarify our understanding further. Such research will help structure clinical recommendations and improve sports safety and the care of athletes of all ages.

Currently, there is evidence to suggest that participation in collision sports is implicated in premature degeneration of the cervical spine. There is some evidence to suggest that the same is true with noncollision sports and activities that result in direct and indirect repetitive loads to the cervical spine over time. The risk factors have yet to be clearly identified. The natural history and sequelae of premature degeneration have yet to be elucidated.

Cervical spondylosis also appears to increase the severity, but not the frequency, of irreversible neurologic injury during collision sport participation. Prudence dictates that we not ignore the present evidence suggesting a link between neuropraxia and cervical stenosis. Proper screening for cervical stenosis in patients with transient neuropraxia with subsequent cessation of participation in collision sports if severe stenosis is present is suggested. There is no consensus for RTP guidelines in the setting of transient neurologic injuries in the athlete when severe degeneration is present, and each case must be considered individually with regard to the sport involved.

REFERENCES

1. Gillis H. High school sports participation increases for 20th consecutive year. Available at: http://www.nfhs.org/content.aspx?id=3505. Accessed September 15, 2009.
2. Golightly YM, Marshall SW, Callahan LF, et al. Early-onset arthritis in retired National Football League players. J Phys Act Health 2009;6(5):638–43.
3. Weir DR, Jackson JS, Sonnega A. University of Michigan Institute for social research, National Football League Player Care Foundation Study of Retired NFL Players. Available at: http://www.ns.umich.edu/Releases/2009/Sep09/FinalReport.pdf. Accessed September 10, 2009.
4. Dailey A, Harrop JS, France JC. High-energy contact sports and cervical spine neuropraxia injuries: what are the criteria for return to participation? Spine (Phila Pa 1976) 2010;35(21 Suppl):S200.
5. Cote P, Cassidy JD, Yong-Hing K, et al. Apophysial joint degeneration, disc degeneration, and sagittal curve of the cervical spine. Can they be measured reliably on radiographs? Spine (Phila Pa 1976) 1997;22(8):859–64.
6. Berge J, Marque B, Vital JM, et al. Age-related changes in the cervical spines of front-line rugby players. Am J Sports Med 1999;27(4):422–9.
7. Torg JS, Pavlov H, Genuario SE, et al. Neuropraxia of the cervical spinal cord with transient quadriplegia. J Bone Joint Surg [Am] 1986(68):1354–70.
8. Herzog RJ, Wiens JJ, Dillingham MF, et al. Normal cervical spine morphometry and cervical spinal stenosis in asymptomatic professional football players: plain film radiography, multiplanar computed tomography, and magnetic resonance imaging. Spine (Phila Pa 1976) 1991;16(6 Suppl):S178–86.
9. Odor JM, Watkins RG, Dillin WH, et al. Incidence of cervical spinal stenosis in professional and rookie football players. Am J Sports Med 1990;18(5):507–9.
10. Cantu RC. The cervical spinal stenosis controversy. Clin Sports Med 1998;17(1):121–6.
11. Cantu RC. Functional cervical spinal stenosis: a contraindication to participation in contact sports. Med Sci Sports Exerc 1993;25(3):316–7.
12. Hogan BA, Hogan NA, Vos PM, et al. The cervical spine of professional front-row rugby players: correlation between degenerative changes and symptoms. Ir J Med Sci 2010;179(2):259–63.
13. Boden SD, Davis DO, Wiesel SW, et al. Abnormal magnetic-resonance scans of the lumbar spine in asymptomatic subjects: a prospective investigation. J Bone Joint Surg [Am] 1990(72):403–8.
14. Gore DR, Sepic SB, Gardner GM. Roentgenographic findings of the cervical spine in asymptomatic people. Spine 1986(11):521–4.
15. Matsumoto M, Fujimura Y, Suzuki N, et al. MRI of cervical intervertebral discs in asymptomatic subjects. J Bone Joint Surg [Br] 1998;80(1):19–24.

16. Gerbino PG, D'Hemecourt PA. Does football cause an increase in degenerative disease of the lumbar spine? Curr Sports Med Rep 2002;1(1):47–51.
17. Micheli LJ. Overuse injuries in children's sports: the growth factor. Orthop Clin North Am 1983;14(2):337–60.
18. Gatt CJ Jr, Hosea TM, Palumbo RC, et al. Impact loading of the lumbar spine during football blocking. Am J Sports Med 1997;25(3):317–21.
19. Watson AW. Sports injuries in footballers related to defects of posture and body mechanics. J Sports Med Phys Fitness 1995;35(4):289–94.
20. Tall RL, DeVault W. Spinal injury in sport: epidemiologic considerations. Clin Sports Med 1993;12(3):441–8.
21. Ikata T, Miyake R, Katoh S, et al. Pathogenesis of sports-related spondylolisthesis in adolescents: radiographic and magnetic resonance imaging study. Am J Sports Med 1996;24(1):94–8.
22. Semon RL, Spengler D. Significance of lumbar spondylolysis in college football players. Spine (Phila Pa 1976) 1981;6(2):172–4.
23. Quarrie KL, Cantu RC, Chalmers DJ. Rugby union injuries to the cervical spine and spinal cord. Sports Med 2002;32(10):633–53.
24. Otis JS, Burnstein AH, Torg SJ. Mechanism and pathomechanics of athletic injuries to the cervical spine. In: Torg JS, editor. Athletic injuries to the head, neck, and face. 2nd edition. CRC Press; 1992. p. 438–56.
25. Milburn PD. The kinetics of rugby union scrummaging. J Sports Sci 1990;8(1):47–60.
26. O'Brien CP. "Rugby neck": cervical degeneration in two front row rugby union players. Clin J Sport Med 1996;6(1):56–9.
27. Thomas M, Haas TS, Doerer JJ, et al. Epidemiology of sudden death in young, competitive athletes due to blunt trauma. Pediatrics 2011;128(1):e1–8.
28. Scher AT. Rugby injuries to the cervical spine and spinal cord: a 10-year review. Clin Sports Med 1998;17(1):195–206.
29. Scher AT. Premature onset of degenerative disease of the cervical spine in rugby players. S Afr Med J 1990;77(11):557–8.
30. Albright JP, Moses JM, Feldick HG, et al. Nonfatal cervical spine injuries in interscholastic football. JAMA 1976;236(11):1243–5.
31. Lark SD, McCarthy PW. Cervical range of motion and proprioception in rugby players versus non-rugby players. J Sports Sci 2007;25(8):887–94.
32. Schneider RC, Papo M, Soto Alvarez C. The effects of chronic recurrent spinal trauma in high-diving: a study of Acapulco's divers. J Bone Joint Surg 1962;44A(4):648–56.
33. Sortland O, Tysvaer AT, Storli OV. Changes in the cervical spine in association football players. Br J Sports Med 1982;16(2):80–4.
34. Kartal A, Yildiran I, Senkoylu A, et al. Soccer causes degenerative changes in the cervical spine. Eur Spine J 2004;13(1):76–82.
35. Tsirikos A, Papagelopoulos PJ, Giannakopoulos PN, et al. Degenerative spondyloarthropathy of the cervical and lumbar spine in jockeys. Orthopedics 2001;24(6):561–4.
36. Scher AT. Injuries to the cervical spine sustained while carrying loads on the head. Paraplegia 1978;16(1):94–101.
37. Bono CM, Ghiselli G, Gilbert TJ, et al. An evidence-based clinical guideline for the diagnosis and treatment of cervical radiculopathy from degenerative disorders. Spine J 2011;11(1):64–72.
38. Bednarik J, Kadanka Z, Dusek L, et al. Presymptomatic spondylotic cervical cord compression. Spine (Phila Pa 1976) 2004;29(20):2260–9.
39. Nikolaidis I, Fouyas IP, Sandercock PA, et al. Surgery for cervical radiculopathy or myelopathy. Cochrane Database Syst Rev 2010;1:CD001466.

40. Powell JW, Barber-Foss KD. Injury patterns in selected high school sports: a review of the 1995–1997 seasons. J Athl Train 1999;34(3):277–84.
41. Thomas BE, McCullen GM, Yuan HA. Cervical spine injuries in football players. J Am Acad Orthop Surg 1999;7(5):338–47.
42. Eismont FJ, Clifford S, Goldberg M, et al. Cervical sagittal spinal canal size in spine injury. Spine (Phila Pa 1976) 1984;9(7):663–6.
43. Matsuura P, Waters RL, Adkins RH, et al. Comparison of computerized tomography parameters of the cervical spine in normal control subjects and spinal cord-injured patients. J Bone Joint Surg [Am] 1989;71(2):183–8.
44. Kang JD, Figgie MP, Bohlman HH. Sagittal measurements of the cervical spine in subaxial fractures and dislocations: an analysis of two hundred and eighty-eight patients with and without neurological deficits. J Bone Joint Surg [Am] 1994;76(11): 1617–28.
45. Cantu RC. Stingers, transient quadriplegia, and cervical spinal stenosis: return to play criteria. Med Sci Sports Exerc 1997;29(7 Suppl):S233–5.
46. Penning L. Some aspects of plain radiography of the cervical spine in chronic myelopathy. Neurology 1962;12:513–9.
47. Torg JS, Guille JT, Jaffe S. Injuries to the cervical spine in American football players. J Bone Joint Surg [Am] 2002;84-A(1):112–22.
48. Scher AT. Spinal cord concussion in rugby players. Am J Sports Med 1991;19(5): 485–8.
49. Torg JS, Naranja RJ, Stine RA. The relationship of developmental narrowing of the cervical spinal canal to reversible and irreversible injury of the cervical spinal cord in football players. J Bone Joint Surg [Am] 1996;78A:1308–14.
50. Brigham CD, Adamson TE. Permanent partial cervical spinal cord injury in a professional football player who had only congenital stenosis: a case report. J Bone Joint Surg [Am] 2003;85–A(8):1553–6.
51. Kelly JD 4th, Aliquo D, Sitler MR, et al. Association of burners with cervical canal and foraminal stenosis. Am J Sports Med 2000;28(2):214–7.
52. Torg JS, Glasgow SG. Criteria for return to contact activities following cervical spine injury. Clin J Sports Med 1991;1(1):12–26.
53. Gottschalk AW, Andrish JT. Epidemiology of sports injury in pediatric athletes. Sports Med Arthrosc 2011;19(1):2–6.
54. Cooper MT, McGee KM, Anderson DG. Epidemiology of athletic head and neck injuries. Clin Sports Med 2003;22(3):427,43, vii.
55. Davis G, Ugokwe K, Roger EP, et al. Clinics in neurology and neurosurgery of sport: asymptomatic cervical canal stenosis and transient quadriparesis. Br J Sports Med 2009;43(14):1154–8.

Spinal Cord Abnormalities in Sports

Mark R. Proctor, MD*, R. Michael Scott, MD

KEYWORDS

- Chiari malformation • Syringomyelia • Spinal cysts • Tethered spinal cord
- Spinal cord injury • Spinal cord tumors

KEY POINTS

- There are many anomalies of the spinal cord that may be detected in the evaluation of an athlete, several of which are incidental and not likely to affect his or her ability to participate in sports.
- Minor Chiari malformation (<5 mm cerebellar tonsillar descent) and small dilatations of the central canal of the spinal cord are often normal variants that require no further evaluation.
- Patients with significant Chiari malformations, spinal syringomyelia, and spinal cord tumors, cysts, or tethering should be evaluated by a neurosurgeon.
- Data to support return-to-play criteria for spinal cord anomalies are relatively sparse, and many of the recommendations in this article are based on consensus and experience.

Congenital and acquired brain stem and spinal cord anomalies, such as Chiari malformation, cysts within and around the spinal cord, tethered spinal cord, prior spinal cord injury, and spinal cord tumors may be present in competitive athletes. There is a paucity of information on the management of these conditions in athletes, however, and whether they represent a contraindication to play. This article attempts to clarify this confusing area by reviewing the literature and the consensus of experts in the field in hopes of providing readers with a practical common sense approach to the management of these issues.

CHIARI MALFORMATION
Background

Chiari malformation is generally defined as descent of the cerebellar tonsils 5 mm or more below the foramen magnum, the opening at the skull base where the spinal cord joins the brain. It is one of the more common incidental findings seen in neurosurgical

The authors have nothing to disclose.
Department of Neurosurgery, Children's Hospital Boston, Harvard Medical School, 300 Longwood Avenue, Boston, MA 02115, USA
* Corresponding author.
E-mail address: mark.proctor@childrens.harvard.edu

Clin Sports Med 31 (2012) 521–533
doi:10.1016/j.csm.2012.03.008
0278-5919/12/$ – see front matter © 2012 Elsevier Inc. All rights reserved.

practice, being detected in roughly 1% of individuals undergoing magnetic resonance imaging (MRI).[1] Additional patients may have what is called "tonsillar ectopia," another normal variant in which the cerebellar tonsils are between 1 and 5 mm beyond the foramen magnum. The Chiari malformation is so common that some authors have recently suggested it should be called the Chiari anomaly.[2]

Evaluation

The symptoms of a Chiari malformation may relate to either the brain or the spinal cord. When the cerebellar tonsils are descended beyond the level of the foramen magnum, they can crowd the structures located there, causing symptoms due to compression of the cerebellum, brain stem, and spinal cord.[2,3] The most common symptom of this crowding is headache, which is typically exacerbated by transient increases in intracranial pressure (called "tussive" headache, occurring when the patient coughs, laughs, or has some other transient spike in intracranial pressure related to physical exertion). These headaches are usually located in the occiput at the craniocervical junction, and the patient may describe them as either occipital headaches or neck pain. When the compression at the level of the foramen magnum makes it difficult for cerebrospinal fluid (CSF) to circulate normally out of the fourth ventricle, the Chiari malformation can lead to the development of syringomyelia, dilated cystic spaces within the spinal cord[4] (see "Syringomyelia"). Patients may rarely have cranial nerve findings from brain stem compression, including snoring, difficulty swallowing, double vision, or sleep apnea. Findings on MRI that might indicate a more severe Chiari malformation include altered CSF flow studies and pointed cerebellar tonsils,[5] as well as signal changes on MRI within the spinal cord (**Fig. 1A, B**).

Treatment

One difficulty with Chiari malformation is that many of its associated symptoms can be multifactorial, and the presence of the Chiari does not always imply that it is the cause of the symptoms. For instance, many patients suffering a concussion undergo imaging of the brain, and a coincidental Chiari malformation may be discovered because of its high prevalence in the population. Genuinely symptomatic patients can benefit from surgery, and most neurosurgeons would agree that asymptomatic Chiari malformation does not require surgery.[2,3,6,7] What are the reasons to consider operating on an athlete with asymptomatic Chiari malformation? One concern is that the Chiari malformation can become symptomatic over time, and therefore the surgery should be performed prophylactically.[8,9] The more concerning issue is that a patients with a significant Chiari malformation could present with a catastrophic central nervous system (CNS) injury after trauma owing to preexisting spinal cord or brain stem compression from the malformation; there are several anecdotal reports of this phenomenon occurring.[10,11] However, the true incidence of this event is probably quite low, as several studies that have looked prospectively at patients with Chiari malformation have failed to show any significant incidence of brain stem or spinal cord injury and suggest that the natural history is benign.[2,3,7] The surgery to decompress a Chiari does carry some risks, and the very low risk of spinal cord injury in the asymptomatic patient who suffers neck trauma needs to be weighed against the risks and potential complications of surgery. Although the literature has yet to define the exact degree of concern that a sport medicine clinician should have in this situation, most neurosurgeons do not advocate prophylactic surgery for asymptomatic Chiari malformations in competitive athletes.[6,12]

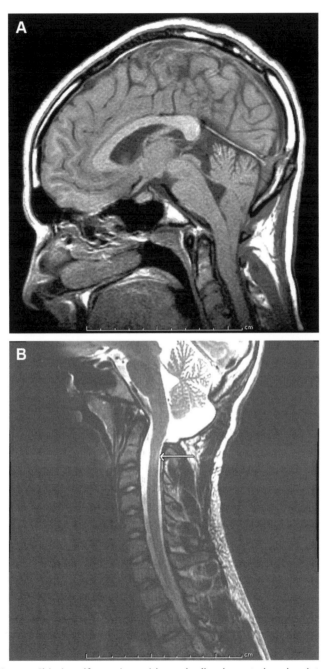

Fig. 1. (*A*) Severe Chiari malformation with markedly elongated and pointed cerebellar tonsils extending to the inferior level of C2. (*B*) On postoperative imaging, the Chiari is well decompressed but there is gliosis in the spinal cord, which precludes return to football (*arrow*).

Return to Play

Assuming a patient with Chiari malformation is asymptomatic and there are no radiographic findings to suggest a severe malformation as defined previously, there is no significant contraindication to return to play. In general it is our practice to allow these athletes to participate, but to also inform the athletes and their families of the potential concerns that the Chiari malformation may become symptomatic, or, as rarely reported, be implicated in the causation of severe neurologic injury. In general, evaluating such cases is complex enough that the decisions to play should be made in conjunction with a neurosurgeon. We believe that a severe Chiari malformation in an asymptomatic patient might be considered a relative contraindication to play in certain patients, but that the vast majority of athletes will not experience adverse effects from participating in sports with this condition. We do not limit patients who have required surgical decompression but are now neurologically intact from future participation in any sport.

SYRINGOMYELIA
Background

Syringomyelia is a condition in which fluid accumulates within the spinal cord and enlarges and distends it. The normal spinal cord has a central canal that runs its length and that in the developing fetus is an extension of the fluid-filled ventricular system of the brain. The central canal is generally not visible on routine MRI imaging studies because it is typically collapsed after birth. However, in the current era when many patients are undergoing high-quality MRI imaging, it is far more common to see the central canal on the MRI scan than it had been previously (**Fig. 2**). This has

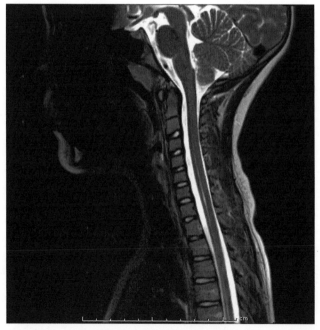

Fig. 2. Benign dilatation of the central canal. There is a long, thin streak of fluid, with no expansion of the spinal cord.

prompted many specialists to think of a small dilatation of the central canal as a normal variant that requires no treatment.[13] On the opposite end of the spectrum is the large syringomyelia cavity, which may be associated with conditions such as Chiari malformation, tethered spinal cord, spinal cord tumor, prior spinal cord injury, or prior infection around the spinal cord.[4] In general these are easily distinguishable on imaging. Between these two extremes are occasional patients with central canal expansion of unclear significance and prognosis.[14]

Evaluation

Imaging characteristics of the benign dilated central canal should include the absence of any other CNS pathology, a normal caliber of the spinal cord, and if contrast is administered, no enhancement. It is generally not recommended to give contrast in such patients, however, as the appearance of these dilated central canals on standard MRI is fairly characteristic. When the syrinx is widely dilated, the inferior and superior extents of the spinal cord, which are areas that may not have been visualized on the initial MRI, should be imaged by repeat spinal MRI to rule out a Chiari malformation or spinal cord tethering, and contrast administration may occasionally need to be considered.

A careful history will rule out preexisting conditions, such as Chiari-type symptoms as defined previously, prior meningitis, or prior spinal cord injury. A patient with a significant syringomyelia may have a cape-like "suspended" sensory loss to pain and temperature or a pain syndrome marked by unusual burning or dysesthetic pain. Back pain is a common finding in athletes, and is relatively unusual in patients with syringomyelia unless there is concomitant scoliosis. Physical exam findings can include reflex changes, including loss of an abdominal reflex, or hyperreflexia in the legs as compared to the reflexes in the arms.

Treatment

In neurosurgical practice it is now quite common to see athletes referred for syringomyelia, especially after imaging for back pain. The vast majority of these syrinxes are benign dilatations of the central canal.[13,14] In the absence of concerning findings on the physical exam, or concerning details in the history, no treatment or additional investigation is required for these findings. In general we do not repeat the MRI.[13] When a true syringomyelia is present, the treatment must be designed to treat the clinical and imaging findings.[15] For instance, if the syrinx is the result of CSF circulation alterations caused by a significant Chiari malformation, the neurosurgeon will recommend decompression of the Chiari malformation, which will secondarily cause the syrinx to regress[6,12] (**Fig. 3A, B**; see "Chiari Malformation"). In general, any syrinx-associated conditions including tumor, tethered cord, or postinfectious or traumatic spinal cord injury or Chiari malformation require referral to a neurosurgeon, and we would not recommend that the sports medicine physician manage these patients independently.

Return to Play

Athletes should not be restricted from play because of a benign dilatation of the central canal. The athlete should be reassured that this is a normal anatomic variant, and as long as there are no associated findings on imaging, no further workup is required.[13,14] There are no data to indicate that such athletes are at increased risk for spinal cord injury. Sports medicine physicians should refer an athlete with a large syrinx to a neurosurgeon for a confirmatory opinion.

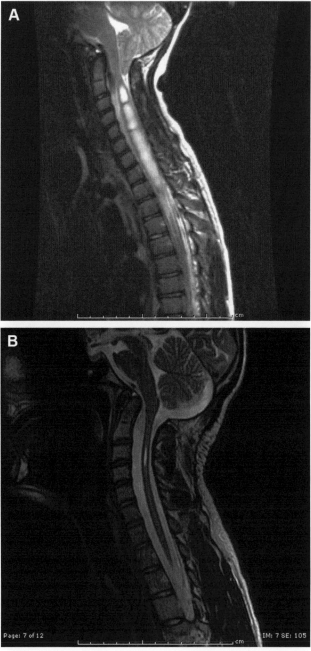

Fig. 3. (*A*) Chiari malformation with large syrinx expanding the spinal cord. (*B*) After surgery, the brain stem is decompressed and the syrinx has markedly reduced in size.

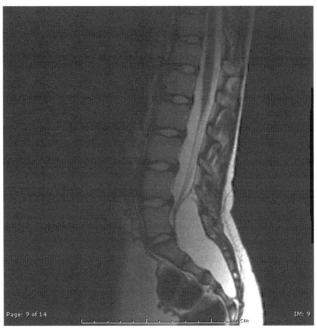

Fig. 4. Large meningocele at the base of the spine. Child presented with back pain and urinary incontinence that improved with surgery.

SPINAL CYSTS
Background

There are a variety of locations in which cysts may occur around the spinal cord, separate from syringomyelia, in which the fluid is within the spinal cord. They are relatively rare, and generalizations about management are difficult. Many of these cysts may be beneath the dura, the majority of which will be arachnoid cysts. When associated with an expansion of the dural sac along the nerve root, these cysts are called perineural cysts (or "Tarlov cysts").[16] Some of the cysts will occur extradurally or caudal to the end of the dural sac, and are referred to as meningoceles.[17,18] A relatively common location for these meningoceles is in the sacrum. Patients may present with deep tailbone pain, but also occasionally with bowel and bladder dysfunction (**Fig. 4**).

Evaluation, Treatment, and Return to Play

Patients with such cysts discovered on imaging should be referred to a neurosurgeon. Most patients will not require surgical intervention, and will be allowed to return to play. However, the lesions are unique enough that, as noted, neurosurgical referral is indicated.

TETHERED SPINAL CORD
Background

Tethered spinal cord refers to any condition in which the spinal cord is pathologically attached to the bones or soft tissues of the back. Many tethered spinal cords are discovered because of lumbar or sacral cutaneous stigmata, such as a dimple, hairy patch, fatty mass, discoloration of the skin, or other unusual findings such as a skin appendage. Most of these conditions will have been discovered in infancy or early childhood, and are therefore not likely to fall into the purview of the sports medicine physician. Others may present later in childhood or in teenage years with symptoms due to tension on the lower spinal cord, including back pain, bowel and bladder control difficulties, limb asymmetry or scoliosis, or neurologic dysfunction in a limb.[19,20]

Evaluation

Tethered spinal cord may not cause overt symptoms for the first several years of life, at a time when it is difficult to detect bowel or bladder dysfunction or for the child to express pain. Symptoms usually present during growth spurts (4–6 years and 8–13 years of age are common times for symptoms to present). Pain in the back or lower extremities, limb asymmetry, and scoliosis are potential reasons that athletes with this condition may present to a sports medicine physician. In general, objective findings on the neurologic examination that are not easily explained, or pain that persists despite routine treatments aimed at core and lower extremity strengthening, should prompt imaging to look for tethered spinal cord. Although the presence of a cutaneous lesion as noted previously will aid in the clinical diagnosis, such lesions in children or teenagers may be expected to be more subtle and difficult to detect.

Imaging findings for tethered spinal cord can vary significantly. Imaging may show thickening and fatty infiltration of the filum terminale (**Fig. 5**), which can occur with a lower-than-normal termination of the spinal cord or at the normal L1–2 level.[21] Some tethering lesions are extremely complex and may include large masses of fat,

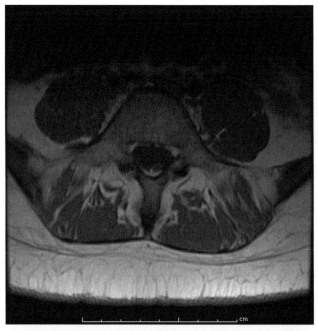

Fig. 5. Appearance of filum terminal thickened and infiltrated with fat on axial T1 MRI image.

congenital tumors, and other congenital abnormalities. Because tethering is most likely to affect the base of the spinal cord, the lower sacral nerves are most vulnerable. Urodynamic studies are often considered as an objective test to look for neuropathic bladder changes, especially if urinary incontinence or unexplained symptoms of urinary urgency or frequency exist.

Treatment

Certain patients with tethered spinal cord lesions may not develop symptoms, and we generally do not recommend treatment for an asymptomatic skeletally mature patient. Pain by itself may be incidental, so careful analysis by a neurosurgeon is important because surgery may be indicated if the patient has abnormalities on the neurologic exam or on other objective tests such as urodynamic evaluations of the nerve supply to the urogenital system.

Return to Play

In general, if spinal tethering is present on imaging, the patient should be referred to a neurosurgeon. If the patient is asymptomatic despite radiographic findings of tethered spinal cord, this should not be a contraindication to participation in sports. It has been our experience that such patients rarely present with rapid or catastrophic neurologic deterioration because of participation in activity, although we have seen patients become symptomatic after the initiation of activities that put additional stretch on the spinal cord or nerves emanating from it, such as the sciatic. When a tethered spinal cord is detected in asymptomatic athletes, we have recommended periodic clinical follow-up until full axial growth of the patient has occurred. The patients and families should also be counseled regarding the potential for the development of symptoms over time, and the risks and benefits of prophylactic surgery reviewed. After surgery, the course is generally benign and the athlete would have no limitations.[21]

PRIOR SPINAL CORD INJURY
Background

Spinal injury can generally be classified into one of three categories: (1) spinal column injury alone without any injury to the spinal cord, covered in another section of this article; (2) a spinal cord trauma causing permanent neurologic and/or radiographic abnormalities; (3) temporary neurologic abnormality followed by complete recovery, with no evidence clinically or radiographically of spinal cord injury.[22] This latter injury, often called spinal cord concussion or transient neuropraxia, seems to be a functional injury similar to a concussion.[23,24]

Evaluation

MRI is the study of choice to evaluate the spinal cord after spinal cord injury. Although radiographs and computed tomography (CT) scans may be normal, MRI can reveal an injury to the spinal cord itself (see **Fig. 1B**), or another lesion such as herniated disk or congenital stenosis that places the athlete at risk. The concept of "functional stenosis" is used to describe relative spinal cord compression in the setting of normal plain radiographic or CT findings. It reflects the fact that plain radiographs or CT scan may be inadequate to diagnose spinal compression, as the bony canal may be normal in the setting of soft tissue abnormalities such as disk herniation or ligamentous hypertrophy, or intrinsic spinal pathology such as syrinx or tumor.[25] Athletes who have suffered a transient neuropraxia but have normal MRI imaging do not appear to be at any increased risk for catastrophic spinal cord injury.[23,24] However, if there is an underlying anatomic lesion such as herniated cervical disk or spinal canal stenosis, the athlete's risk of spinal cord injury with subsequent trauma is increased.

Treatment and Return to Play

Any permanent neurologic injury or radiographic findings of structural changes in the spinal cord preclude participation in high-risk sports. The reserve capacity of the spinal cord is unknown, and the risk of second injury is increased. If the spinal cord and neurologic exam are normal but spinal canal stenosis exists, the abnormality may be amenable to correction by surgical measures. Once the anatomic abnormality has been corrected, the athlete may be able to return to play. In certain cases the athlete can return to some activities, but not other higher risk activities that involve the likelihood of severe flexion or extension movements of the neck.[22] We believe that most athletes with a transient neurologic deficit with normal imaging and clinical examination can return to play without increased risk of subsequent injury.[24]

SPINAL CORD TUMORS
Background

Intrinsic tumors of the spinal cord or tumors within the dura that compress the spinal cord are relatively rare, but we have seen several such patients present to our Sports Medicine department.[26] It is more common for tumors to occur in the bones and soft tissues, a topic discussed elsewhere in this article. Patients with intraspinal tumors often present with back and leg pain, and as expected, frequently have neurologic abnormalities when examined.

Evaluation

Symptoms that should prompt imaging include pain that is worse at night due to tumor swelling when recumbent, radiating pain that is worse with activity, as well as any unexplained abnormalities in the neurologic examination.

Treatment and Return to Play

When a spinal cord tumor is diagnosed, the patient should be referred promptly to a neurosurgeon. Return to play after surgery depends on the extent and success of surgery for the tumor, the length of bony exposure required, the subsequent stability of the spine, and the neurologic status of the patient, and must be individualized (**Fig. 6A, B**).

SUMMARY

Many types of spinal abnormalities can have an impact on an athlete's ability to participate in sports. One of the challenges in the current era is distinguishing the clinically relevant lesions from the incidental. Almost without exception, a Chiari malformation, significant syringomyelia or other cyst compressing the spinal cord or nerve roots, tethered spinal cord, or spinal tumor should prompt referral to a neurosurgeon. However, tonsillar ectopia (descent of the cerebellum less than 5 mm beyond the foramen magnum) and small dilatations of the central canal, are very commonly seen and appear to represent normal anatomic variants that place athletes at no increased risk of spinal injury, and should not be considered a contraindication to play. The recommendations made in this article are largely based on consensus and experience, but as we gain more clinical experience to correlate with the

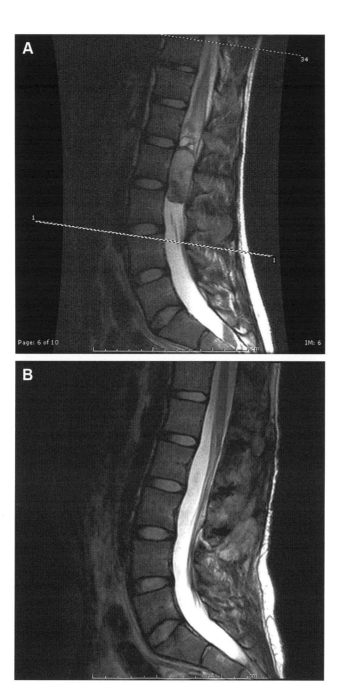

Fig. 6. (*A*) Large tumor at base of spinal cord in a 16-year-old athlete with severe back pain. (*B*) After surgery, she has returned to full activity. The pathology was myxopapillary ependymoma.

increasingly sophisticated imaging findings, we hope that these recommendations can be refined further.

REFERENCES

1. Meadows J, Kraut M, Guarnieri M, et al. Asymptomatic Chiari type I malformations identified on magnetic resonance imaging. J Neurosurg 2000; 92(6): 920–6.
2. Novegno F, Caldarelli M, Massa A, et al. The natural history of the Chiari type I anomaly. J Neurosurg Pediatr 2008;2(3):179–87.
3. Strahle J, Muraszko KM, Kapurch J, et al. Natural history of Chiari malformation type I following decision for conservative treatment. J Neurosurg Pediatr 2011; 8(2):214–21.
4. Strahle J, Muraszko KM, Kapurch J, et al. Chiari malformation type I and syrinx in children undergoing magnetic resonance imaging. J Neurosurg Pediatr 2011;8(2): 205–13.
5. Mauer UM, Gottschalk A, Mueller C, et al. Standard and cardiac-gated phase-contrast magnetic resonance imaging in the clinical course of patients with Chiari malformation type I. Neurosurg Focus 2011;31(3):E5.
6. Rocque BG, George TM, Kestle J, et al. Treatment practices for Chiari malformation type I with syringomyelia: results of a survey of the American Society of Pediatric Neurosurgeons. J Neurosurg Pediatr 2011;8(5):430–7.
7. Benglis D Jr, Covington D, Bhatia R, et al. Outcomes in pediatric patients with Chiari malformation type I followed up without surgery. J Neurosurg Pediatr 2011;7(4): 375–9.
8. Wan MJ, Nomura H, Tator CH. Conversion to symptomatic Chiari I malformation after minor head or neck trauma. Neurosurgery 2008;63(4):748–53 [discussion: 753].
9. Yarbrough CK, Powers AK, Park TS, et al. Patients with Chiari malformation type I presenting with acute neurological deficits: case series. J Neurosurg Pediatr 2011; 7(3): 244–7.
10. Callaway GH, O'Brien SJ, Tehrany AM. Chiari I malformation and spinal cord injury: cause for concern in contact athletes? Med Sci Sports Exerc 1996;28(10):1218–20.
11. Makela JP. Arnold-Chiari malformation type I in military conscripts: symptoms and effects on service fitness. Mil Med 2006;171(2):174–6.
12. Schijman E, Steinbok P. International survey on the management of Chiari I malformation and syringomyelia. Childs Nerv Syst ChNS 2004;20(5):341–8.
13. Magge SN, Smyth MD, Governale LS, et al. Idiopathic syrinx in the pediatric population: a combined center experience. J Neurosurg Pediatr 2011;7(1): 30–6.
14. Singhal A, Bowen-Roberts T, Steinbok P, et al. Natural history of untreated syringomyelia in pediatric patients. Neurosurg Focus 2011;31(6):1–5.
15. Roy AK, Slimack NP, Ganju A. Idiopathic syringomyelia: retrospective case series, comprehensive review, and update on management. Neurosurg Focus 2011; 31(6):1–9.
16. Lucantoni C, Than KD, Wang AC, et al. Tarlov cysts: a controversial lesion of the sacral spine. Neurosurg Focus 2011; 31(6):1–6.
17. Feigenbaum F, Hale S. Association between symptomatic giant sacral meningeal diverticulum and spinal cord tethering with thickened lipomatous filum. Spine 2011; 36(18):E1230–2.
18. Netra R, Min L, Shao Hui M, et al. Spinal extradural meningeal cysts: an MRI evaluation of a case series and literature review. J Spinal Disord Tech 2011;24(2): 132–6.

19. Hertzler DA 2nd, DePowell JJ, Stevenson CB, et al. Tethered cord syndrome: a review of the literature from embryology to adult presentation. Neurosurg Focus 2010;29(1):E1.
20. Filippidis AS, Kalani MY, Theodore N, et al. Spinal cord traction, vascular compromise, hypoxia, and metabolic derangements in the pathophysiology of tethered cord syndrome. Neurosurg Focus 2010;29(1):E9.
21. Kim AH, Kasliwal MK, McNeigh B, et al. Features of the lumbar spine on magnetic resonance images following sectioning of filum terminale. J Neurosurg Pediatr 2011; 8(4):384–9.
22. Bailes JE, Hadley MN, Quigley MR, et al. Management of athletic injuries of the cervical spine and spinal cord. Neurosurgery 1991;29(4):491–7.
23. Bailes JE. Experience with cervical stenosis and temporary paralysis in athletes. J Neurosurg Spine 2005;2(1):11–6.
24. Dailey A, Harrop JS, France JC. High-energy contact sports and cervical spine neuropraxia injuries: what are the criteria for return to participation? Spine 2010;35(21 Suppl):S193–201.
25. Proctor MR, Cantu RC. Head and neck injuries in young athletes. Clin Sports Med 2000;19(4):693–715.
26. O'Brien M, Curtis C, D'Hemecourt P, et al. Case report: a case of persistent back pain and constipation in a 5-year-old boy. Phys Sportsmed 2009;37(1):133–7.

Infectious, Inflammatory, and Metabolic Diseases Affecting the Athlete's Spine

Lionel N. Metz, MD[a], Rosanna Wustrack, MD[a],
Alberto F. Lovell, BS[b], Aenor J. Sawyer, MD, MSc[c],*

KEYWORDS

- Back pain • Spine infection • Orthopaedist • Spine inflammation
- Metabolic bone disease

KEY POINTS

- Spines of athletes compromised by infection, autoimmune disease, genetic factors, or malnutrition are at increased risk of injury.
- Genetically or metabolically weakened bones are at increased risk for fatigue fractures from the high-impact activities of athletes.
- Spinal deformity and weakness associated with autoimmune disease is challenging to athletic performance and also increases the risk of injury.
- It is paramount for any physician caring for athletes to have a working understanding of risk factors, presentation, and initial management of infectious, inflammatory, and metabolic diseases of the spine.

INTRODUCTION

The health and normal biomechanical function of the spine is vital for optimal athletic performance. The spine is vulnerable to a variety of insults that can be localized or systemic, acute or chronic, and that may preferentially affect patients of a certain age.

Disclosures: Aenor J. Sawyer, MD, MSc is a recipient of an SD Bechtel Jr Foundation Grant for Pediatric Bone Health Consortium and Chief Editor of the textbook *Bone Densitometry in the Growing Patient*, published by Springer.
Alberto F. Lovell, BS, wrote a portion of this article done while a research assistant at University of California, San Francisco, and is currently employed by Genentech Inc.
Lionel N. Metz and Rosanna Wustrack have nothing to disclose.
[a] Department of Orthopaedic Surgery, University of California, San Francisco, 500 Parnassus Avenue, MU320W, Box 0728, San Francisco, CA 94143-0728, USA; [b] Department of Orthopaedic Surgery, University of California, San Francisco, 533 Parnassus Avenue, HSE-641, Box 0514, San Francisco, CA 94143-051, USA; [c] Department of Orthopaedic Surgery, University of California, San Francisco, 500 Parnassus Avenue, Room MU311W, Box 0728, San Francisco, CA 94143-0728, USA
* Corresponding author.
E-mail address: SawyerA@orthosurg.ucsf.edu

Sports medicine specialists and orthopaedists must be familiar with spinal pathologies that may affect individuals with an active lifestyle. This ensures the recognition of spinal complaints and associated systemic symptoms, while expediting appropriate workup, initial management, and prompt referral of affected patients. This article is not as an exhaustive or systematic review of the literature, but a tool to empower physicians caring for athletes with the framework and knowledge to recognize, counsel, and begin to manage athletes with infectious, inflammatory, or metabolic spinal disorders.

SPINE INFECTIONS AND IMPLICATIONS FOR ATHLETES

Spine infections comprise bacterial, fungal, mycobacterial, and parasitic infections that occupy the vertebral body, disc, bony posterior elements, the paravertebral soft tissues, and/or the epidural space of the spinal axis and can occur by direct insult, extension from a nearby infection, or hematogenous seeding of spinal tissue through arterial or venous routes. Spine infections affect different demographics of patients as demonstrated in **Table 1**. In addition, infectious diseases of the spine can occur at an increased frequency in athletes with risk factors for infection due to immunocompromised health or a specific high-risk exposure. In the United States the most common spinal infection is pyogenic vertebral osteomyelitis, but in other regions of the world brucellosis and tuberculosis are more common etiologies.[1] When physicians care for athletes involved in international competitions, a variety of organisms must be included in the differential diagnosis for spine infection.

Pyogenic Vertebral Osteomyelitis

Acute pyogenic vertebral osteomyelitis (PVO) affects approximately 2.4 per 100,000 people per year in the United States, with a predilection for older patients.[2] The incidence increases with increasing age from 0.3 in 100,000 in patients younger than 20 years to 6.5 in 100,000 in patients older than 70 years.[2] The most common infectious organism is *Staphylococcus aureus*, followed by *Escherichia coli*.[2] Other organisms include coagulase-negative *Staphylococcus* species and gram-negative rods such as *Pseudomonas* and *Salmonella*. Strong risk factors for bacterial vertebral osteomyelitis are intravenous drug use, immunocompromised states such as human immunodeficiency virus (HIV) infection, diabetes mellitus, obesity, malnutrition, and congenital immunodeficiencies. Pharmacologically immunocompromised patients are also at risk for this complication. Consideration should be given to athletes using performance-enhancing steroids with possibly compromised immunity and increased susceptibility to infection. Wheelchair-dependent athletes deserve special consideration because they may develop spinal infections as a result of seeding from sacrococcygeal decubiti or recurrent urinary tract infections.

Vertebral osteomyelitis is an infection of the vertebral body and intervertebral disc, associated with epidural abscess in 17% (**Fig. 1A, B**) of cases and paravertebral abscess in 26% of cases. Most cases result from hematogenous seeding from distant infection or transient bacteremia found in intravenous drug abusers or immunocompromised hosts. Direct inoculation can result from penetrating trauma[3] and open fractures, or from prior operative or percutaneous procedures.[4] Direct extension from a retroperitoneal or retropharyngeal infection can also lead to vertebral osteomyelitis.[5] PVO secondary to intrapelvic infections due to seeding of the spine along Batson's plexus has been reported.[5] When hematogenous seeding of the vertebra is suspected, the primary site of infection is found in only 50% of cases; thus multifocal disease must also be ruled out.[2]

Table 1
Demographics of spinal infections

Type of Infection	Age Distribution	Association with Immunocompromise	Risk Factors	Frequency of Surgical Treatment	Risk of Late Deformity	Frequency of Neurologic Deficit
PVO	Older	Somewhat	IVDU, HIV, immunocompromise	Moderate	Moderate	Moderate to frequent
Pott	Children, any age	Yes, but not always	Endemic exposure	Moderate	Frequent	Moderate
Brucella	Men >40 years of age	No	Animal exposure	Low	Low	Low
Fungal	All	Yes, except coccidiomycosis and histoplasmosis	Immunocompromise, endemic areas	Low	Rare	Low

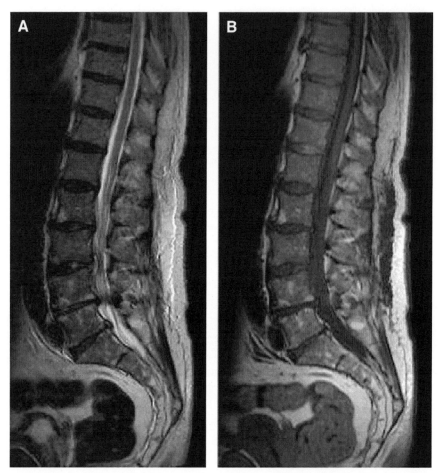

Fig. 1. MRI images demonstrate early PVO that was initially interpreted as L3–L4 disc extrusion of high water content on (*A*) Sagittal T2-weighted and (*B*) T1-weighted and images. The same patient had a repeat (*C*) Sagittal, T2-weighted; (*D*) T1-weighted MRI 18 days later which now demonstrates changes more typical of PVO at L3–L4 with enhancement of the posterior aspects of the endplates and an epidural abscess extending from L1 to L4. (*From* Dunbar JA, Sandoe JA, Rao AS, et al. The MRI appearances of early vertebral osteomyelitis and discitis. Clin Radiol 2010;65(12):974–81; with permission.)

Patients present with pain along the spinal axis in 86% to 92% of cases.[1,6] Back pain is commonplace in athletes; however, pain located in the midline rather than paraspinal pain, severe pain waking patients from sleep, pain not proceeded by training or trauma, and pain accompanied by history of fever are worrisome symptoms that should not be dismissed as routine. Although a history of fever, night sweats, and anorexia is common at presentation for PVO, initial clinical evaluation may reveal fever in fewer than 50% of cases.[2] Neurologic compromise occurs in about one third of patients.[6]

Uncontrolled PVO can lead to systemic infection and sepsis, spinal instability, or neurologic compromise resulting from either instability or epidural abscess.[7] When PVO is suspected, workup includes vital signs, a full extremity neurologic examination

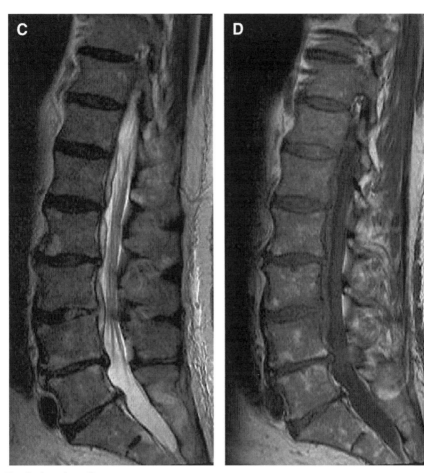

Fig. 1. (continued)

with documentation of rectal tone and perianal sensation, and laboratory analysis including complete blood count with differential (CBC), erythrocyte sedimentation rate (ESR), C-reactive protein level (CRP), and peripheral blood cultures. Elevated ESR and CRP have been reported in 98% and 100% of PVO cases, respectively.[2] CRP is also a sensitive marker of the clinical response to treatment and can indicate resolution or treatment failure when followed longitudinally. At least two peripheral blood cultures should be drawn before antibiotic administration and sent for routine culture as well as specialized culture for acid-fast bacilli and *Brucella* species in patients suspicious for those exposures.[2] Mylona and colleagues found 58% of blood cultures positive in their meta-analysis of clinical variables in PVO.[6] Imaging of suspected PVO includes full standing anterior–posterior (AP) and lateral radiographs of the spine as well as dedicated views of the suspected region. Magnetic resonance imaging (MRI) with gadolinium of the entire spine will show the extent of disease and detect epidural abscess, but cannot reliably predict structural stability of the spine. Computed tomography (CT) scan is more sensitive for determining the structural damage to the spine and augments preoperative planning. Treatment involves intravenous antibiotics, medical and nutritional optimization, and evaluation by an infectious diseases expert and spinal surgeon to determine whether operative débridement is required. Mylona and colleagues reported a relapse rate of 8% and a mortality rate of 6%.[6]

Spinal Brucellosis

Brucellosis is a systemic zoonotic bacterial infection caused by various facultative intracellular bacteria of the genus *Brucella*. The infection occurs worldwide, with the highest frequency seen in the Mediterranean, the Middle East, and Central and South America. Brucellosis is rare in the United States, with only about 200 cases reported annually.[8] Humans contract the infection by contact with domesticated animals. Working-age and middle-aged men are at highest risk, while children and elderly people are at lower risk. Although spinal involvement may occur in only 6% to 58% of cases,[9] brucellosis remains a frequent cause of spine infection in endemic areas, evidenced by a recent study from Greece citing it as the infectious organism in one third of spinal infections.[10]

Musculoskeletal manifestations of infection include spondylitis, sacroiliitis, arthritis, osteomyelitis, tenosynovitis, and bursitis.[11] The knee and the sacroiliac joints are more frequent sites of infection in children and young adults; however, the spine is the most frequent location of musculoskeletal brucellosis in older adults. Brucellar spondylitis presents most commonly in the lumbar spine (60%), followed by the thoracic (19%) and cervical (12%) spine, respectively.[11] Infection of the spine can be localized or diffuse, with multilevel involvement at presentation in about 6% to 14% of cases.[9,11,12] In local disease the infection has a predilection for the anterior superior vertebral endplate (**Fig. 2**) and the adjacent intervertebral disc, and can be mistaken for degenerative disc disease or erosive osteochondrosis in light of its predominant lumbar distribution.

MRI and postcontrast CT imaging can demonstrate associated paravertebral, psoas, and epidural abscesses as well as early disc and endplate changes not evident on plain films.[11] Brucellar spondylitis also has similarities in presentation and radiographic appearance to tuberculous spondylitis, spawning the term pseudo-Pott disease, and pyogenic spondylitis, which can make diagnosis difficult in the absence of positive cultures. Treatment with an antibrucellar antibiotic regimen and supportive therapy is effective in the majority of cases. Unless tissue is needed to confirm the diagnosis, surgery is rarely indicated in the absence of neurologic deficit.[13] Complications of late spinal deformity and neurologic compromise are rare.[11,13]

Pediatric Discitis and Pyogenic Vertebral Osteomyelitis

Pediatric discitis and pyogenic vertebral osteomyelitis can affect young athletes. Experts generally conclude that discitis is an isolated bacterial infection of the intervertebral disc and adjacent endplates. It is a mild manifestation of infectious spondylitis, in contrast to vertebral osteomyelitis with epidural or paraspinal abscess at the other end of the continuum.[14] These entities differ strikingly in their presentation, epidemiology, and prognosis.[15]

The anatomy of the pediatric blood supply explains both the pathoetiology and self-limited nature of discitis. In the immature spine, the circulation to the avascular disc traverses arterial channels in the cartilaginous endplate. These channels, which persist from fetal life until the ring apophyses fuse in the third decade of life, allow direct inoculation of the relatively immunoisolated disc tissue during episodes of bacteremia. Meanwhile, until about age 15 the vertebral body enjoys a rich anastomotic vascular network, which suppresses growth of interosseous septic emboli and extension of disc infection in most cases. Thus, vertebral body involvement is somewhat rare in children. In

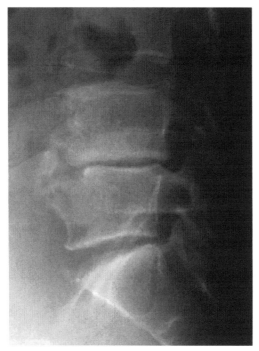

Fig. 2. Parrots' beak appearance on a lateral radiograph of the lumbar spine in a 54-year-old man with brucellar spondylitis. (*From* Chelli Bouaziz M, Ladeb MF, Chakroun M, et al. Spinal brucellosis: a review. Skeletal Radiol 2008;37(9):785–90; with permission.)

cases of pediatric discitis the infection may be self-limited, as the vertebral body's rich blood supply protects it from spread of the infection, and sustains a sufficient response to quell the neighboring disc infection even without antibiotics.[14,15]

Discitis classically has a bimodal pediatric age distribution with peaks in early childhood and adolescence.[16] Vertebral osteomyelitis is generally thought of as a disease affecting adults but there is also a peak in incidence among adolescents.[15,17] Fernandez and colleagues highlight the epidemiologic differences between patients presenting with discitis versus those presenting with vertebral osteomyelitis. They note that vertebral osteomyelitis was infrequently encountered in children younger than 3 years of age and discitis was rare in children older than 8 years of age, a finding that differs somewhat from that of Cushing.[15,16] Furthermore, discitis patients were far less likely to present with history of fever than PVO patients (28% vs 79%). Only three discitis patients had fevers exceeding 101°F, whereas all of those PVO patients with fever exceeded 102°F. Importantly, they note that radiographs were insensitive for PVO, and even in cases with strong clinical signs of spinal axis infection, discitis, and PVO were not radiographically distinguishable without MRI.

The incidence of discitis is estimated to be between 3 and 6 cases per 100,000, typically affecting children younger than 5 years of age.[1,16] Suspicion of pediatric spine infection is raised in patients with progressive refusal to sit, crawl, or walk without symptoms that localize to either lower extremity, whether fever is present or not. Symptoms will vary depending on age and may include abdominal pain, limp, or generalized irritability[14] and may have persisted for several weeks before presentation.

Although most patients with discitis are otherwise healthy, a history of antecedent infection such as otitis media or urinary tract infection is not uncommon.[14] The initial workup includes a full set of vital signs and physical examination of the spine and lower extremities including a spine-focused neurologic examination. **Evaluation of the limping child must include examination of the spine.**[14]

Laboratory workup includes CBC, ESR, CRP, and at least one peripheral blood culture. Imaging must include PA and lateral radiographs of the spine with dedicated views of the lumbar spine or other region of suspected infection (**Fig. 3A**). We advocate a low threshold for obtaining a spinal MRI containing T1-weighted axial and sagittal images and T2-weighted sagittal images (see **Fig. 3B**). MRI is helpful in cases of atypical clinical or radiographic presentation of discitis and in ill-appearing children where progression to PVO is a possibility. MRI is essential in cases with a neurologic abnormality, a poor clinical response to empiric discitis treatment, or when a presentation is worrisome for noninfectious spinal pathology. Technetium-99 bone scan is of limited utility in older children because it is nonspecific, but in a child too young to localize symptoms, it can help to distinguish spinal pathology from that of the sacroiliac joints, hips, and lower extremities.[14]

Workup of suspected discitis or osteomyelitis merits inpatient admission whether a firm diagnosis is made or not. Antibiotics are the mainstay of treatment and are empirically targeted at staphylococcal organisms in most cases. Obtaining blood

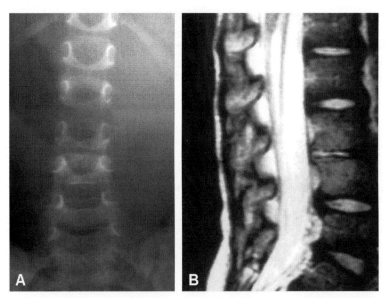

Fig. 3. (*A*) Pediatric discitis. Posteroanterior radiograph of a 3-year-old girl with a 2-week history of irritability and refusal to walk for 2 days. The disc space narrowing at L3/4 is consistent with discitis. (*From* Early SD, Kay RM, Tolo VT. Childhood diskitis. J Am Acad Orthop Surg 2003;11:414. © 2003 American Academy of Orthopaedic Surgeons. Reproduced with permission from the Journal of the American Academy of Orthopaedic Surgeons, Volume 11(6), pp. 413–20.) (*B*) T2 MRI pediatric discitis Sagittal T2-weighted MRI demonstrating loss of normal signal intensity and disc height at L3/4 and mild signal increase at adjacent vertebral bodies, consistent with discitis. (*From* Early SD, Kay RM, Tolo VT. Childhood diskitis. J Am Acad Orthop Surg 2003;11:417. © 2003 American Academy of Orthopaedic Surgeons. Reproduced with permission from the Journal of the American Academy of Orthopaedic Surgeons, 11(6):413–20.)

cultures before starting antibiotic therapy is preferable, but antibiotics should not be delayed for a toxic child. CRP should fall soon after initiation of treatment. An early increase in CRP indicates inadequate coverage and a late increase indicates inadequate duration of therapy or residual sequestrum. As with all pediatric musculoskeletal infections, immobilization is primarily a comfort measure; efficacy of bracing to prevent deformity is controversial. When an infection is unresponsive to treatment and blood cultures have not been useful, CT-guided percutaneous biopsy or even open biopsy may be required.[14,15] Follow-up radiographs at regular intervals for 12 to 18 months should be evaluated to rule out recurrence or late deformity.[14]

Tuberculosis and Pott Disease

Tuberculosis of the spine, known as Pott disease, is an infection of the spine and paraspinal soft tissues by *Mycobacterium tuberculosis* or a similar mycobacterial organism. The incidence of Pott disease varies widely and correlates both to the endemic incidence of tuberculosis (TB) and the endemic incidence of malnutrition and comorbid diseases such as HIV. In areas with a higher endemic burden of TB, there is a higher incidence of Pott disease in pediatric populations.[8] In the United States TB has an incidence of 3.8 cases per 100,000 persons, but has been reported up to 50 times higher in inner cities as recently as the 1990s. The proportion of spinal involvement varies; pediatric patients and HIV-positive patients are more likely to have extrapulmonary and spinal disease.[18] Some reports estimate greater than 60% extrapulmonary involvement in HIV-positive patients with TB.[19,20] Approximately 50% of musculoskeletal TB involves the spine.[21]

Outside the lungs, the spine is the second most common location of TB, following only lymph node involvement. The pathoetiology of spinal tuberculosis differs from that of pyogenic vertebral osteomyelitis in that nearly all cases of Pott disease result first from hematogenous spread from the lung, despite a substantial incidence of pulmonary involvement that remains subclinical. Hematogenous inoculation of the vertebral body is followed by extracorporeal spread along the path of the anterior longitudinal ligament, to adjacent as well as distant vertebral bodies. The posterior elements are often involved and are the sole area of involvement in 2% to 10% of lesions, a risk factor for paraplegia.[19] In serious cases spinal TB can lead to severe kyphotic deformity, as shown in **Fig. 4**, or neurologic compromise.[21]

The suspicion of Pott disease increases when back pain is accompanied by chronic malaise, weight loss, night sweats, or intermittent fevers in patients with a history of exposure to TB.[8] Pott disease can present with or without active pulmonary infection.[8] Laboratory workup includes white blood cell count (WBC), ESR, CPR, and imaging with full-length standing spinal radiographs and a full-spine MRI with gadolinium (**Fig. 5A, B**),[22] but also includes PA and lateral chest radiographs and a purified protein derivative (PPD) test. CT-guided biopsy of the lesion followed by polymerase chain reaction (PCR)-based rapid diagnosis and culture should be used to determine antimycobacterial sensitivities. If empiric therapy is used, multidrug-resistant (MDR) TB should be suspected if there is no significant improvement in 3 months. Tuberculous collections in the spine can be sterilized with current antitubercular drugs, which can penetrate infected granulation and caseous necrotic tissues, though levels in sclerotic bone typically remain subtherapeutic.[19] Treatment includes admission to the hospital for completion of workup, initiation of antimycobacterial chemotherapy, and airborne isolation precautions until cleared by a consulting infectious disease physician. These patients should still be regarded as potentially contagious through an airborne route, as positive sputum acid-fast bacillus (AFB) cultures in chest radiograph–negative patients with spinal TB have been reported.[23]

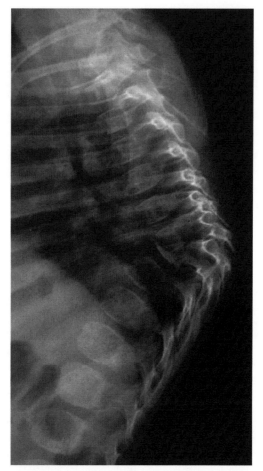

Fig. 4. Spinal TB kyphosis. A lateral radiograph of the thoracic spine of a 3-year-old child showing involvement of T7–T10 with severe kyphosis. (*From* Jain AK. Tuberculosis of the spine: a fresh look at an old disease. J Bone Joint Surg [Br] 2010;92:910.)

Although treatment is typically nonoperative in the absence of demonstrable instability, severe deformity, or neurologic compromise, surgical indications include (1) neurologic compromise; (2) unresponsiveness to antitubercular treatment or MDR TB; (3) kyphosis greater than 60° in an adult, less in a growing child (see **Fig. 4**); (4) panvertebral lesion; (5) intradural or intramedullary involvement; and (6) debilitating residual pain.[19] Débridement, stabilization, and corrective osteotomy have an important role in management of the progressive kyphosis typically associated with Pott disease. With ongoing antitubercular treatment, spinal hardware infection is unlikely.[19,24] Although "healed status" can be designated after 2 years without clinical or radiographic recurrence, late progression of kyphosis and associated neurologic deficit remain concerns.[19]

Fungal Infections of the Spine

Fungal infection of the spine is typically the result of systemic fungemia, which is rare in immunocompetent hosts. When patients presenting with fungemia or known

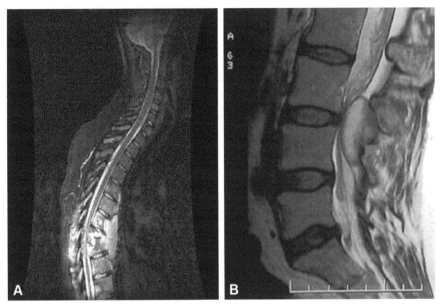

Fig. 5. (*A*) MRI showing spinal TB with destruction of vertebral bodies (*From* Ludwig B, Lazarus AA. Musculoskeletal tuberculosis. Dis Mon 2007;53(1):41; with permission.). (*B*) Isolated posterior element TB of L3 with epidural abscess (*red arrow*) causing neural compression. (*From* Nene AM, Pawar U. Tuberculosis of the spine 2011 update. ArgoSpine News & Journal 2011;23:105–9; with permission.)

localized fungal infections complain of back pain, suspicion of fungal spondylitis should be raised. These infections tend to be indolent, thus delay in diagnosis is common. Pain typically increases in proportion to local involvement as well as associated compression fractures and paravertebral abscesses.[8,25] Fungal organisms frequently reported to affect the spines of immunocompromised hosts include *Candida albicans* and other *Candida* species, *Nocardia asteroids*, and *Aspergillus fumigatus*.[26] Vinas and colleagues reviewed 39 published cases of spinal aspergillosis finding only monomicrobial infections that predominated in lumbar spine (54%), in a 78% male population with an average age of 40 years.[27]

Infections with disseminated *Coccidioides immitis,* and rarely *Histoplasma capsulatum* and related species, can affect the spine in immunocompetent hosts. Coccidiomycosis is a fungus endemic to California, Arizona, and the Southwestern United States as well as Northern Mexico that can cause systemic infection even in healthy patients; this includes infections of the axial and appendicular skeleton in 20% to 50% of disseminated cases.[28] There are an estimated 100,000 cases worldwide per annum.[29] Frazier and colleagues reviewed their experience in treating spinal fungal infections and found that 10 of 11 patients required surgical treatment in addition to antifungals,[26] though this retrospective study of surgical patients most likely overestimates the true proportion of cases that require surgical treatment.

Spinal Infections in Athletes

Postinfectious instability and deformity can result from any spinal infection and are a cause of late morbidity that may impair athletes. In addition to routine radiographic

---

Box 1
Forms of spondyloarthritis (SpA) recognized in adults

1. Ankylosing spondylitis
   a. Defined according to modified New York criteria: Definite disease requires radiographic sacroiliitis, either bilateral grade II–IV or unilateral grade III–IV, plus inflammatory back pain, limitation of lumbar motion, or decreased chest expansion.
   b. No lower age limit defined.
2. Undifferentiated SpA
   a. Defined by ESSG13 or Amor criteria, which factor in (but do not require) signs and symptoms of axial arthritis together with other features SpA, including gastrointestinal symptoms, psoriasis, and manifestations of psoriatic arthritis; MRI is not used in either classification system.
   b. ESSG and Amor criteria are usually used in adults, but no lower age limits have been defined and these criteria have been applied to children.
   c. "Axial spondyloarthritis" might now be considered a form of undifferentiated SpA.
3. Reactive arthritis
   a. Peripheral arthritis with onset typically within 6 weeks after certain infections of the gastrointestinal or genitourinary tracts.
   b. Classical extra-articular manifestations include rash (keratoderma blennorrhagicum and circinate balanitis), oral ulcers, conjunctivitis, enthesitis, and dactylitis.
4. Arthritis associated with IBD
   a. Coexisting arthritis and IBD, typically Crohn disease or ulcerative colitis; also referred to as enteropathic arthropathy.
   b. Arthritis is most commonly peripheral.
   c. Most frequently classified as SpA when sacroiliitis or spondylitis is present.
5. Psoriatic arthritis
   a. Coexisting arthritis and psoriasis, most often in the absence of rheumatoid factor.
   b. Frequently associated with nail pitting or onycholysis, dactylitis, and enthesis.
   c. Like IBD-related arthritis, most frequently considered a form of SpA when sacroiliitis or spondylitis is present.

Abbreviations: ESSG, European Spondyloarthropathy Study Group; IBD, inflammatory bowel disease; SpA, spondyloarthritis.

Data from Colbert RA. Classification of juvenile spondyloarthritis: enthesitis-related arthritis and beyond. Nat Rev Rheumatol 2010;6(8):477–85.

---

follow-up for up to 24 months, regular physical examination during the recovery period should include a spine examination with particular attention to progressive kyphosis and neurologic changes. Return to play after a spinal infection should be guided by a physical therapist after an orthopaedist or spine surgeon has determined participation to be safe. Any pain that is new, severe, or does not improve and any new neurologic symptoms are red flags, as are fevers and constitutional symptoms. If any question remains about the fitness of an athlete's spine, prompt referral back to a spine surgeon is indicated.

INFLAMMATORY AND AUTOIMMUNE DISEASES OF THE SPINE

Inflammatory disease is a well-established cause of spinal dysfunction. The various vertebroligamentous and capsular insertions and the discovertebral junction are targets of autoimmunity in seronegative spondyloarthropathies (SpA), whereas the synovial joints are targets primarily involved in rheumatoid arthritis and similar autoimmune processes. Among the inflammatory diseases that affect the adult spine are rheumatoid arthritis, ankylosing spondylitis, and the other SpA listed in **Box 1**.[30] Inflammatory diseases affecting the pediatric spine include enthesitis-related arthropathy,

Table 2
Modified New York diagnostic criteria for AS[a]

Clinical Criteria	Radiographic Criteria
Lower back pain and stiffness for >3 months that improves with exercise but is not relieved with rest	Bilateral sacroiliitis ≥ grade 2
Limited lumbar spine motion in frontal and sagittal planes	Unilateral sacroiliitis ≥ grade 3
Limitation of chest expansion	

[a] Definite AS; one clinical criterion plus one radiographic criterion. Probable AS; three clinical criteria and no radiologic criteria or one radiologic criterion and no clinical criteria.

Data from van der Linden S, Valkenburg HA, Cats A. Evaluation of diagnostic criteria for ankylosing spondylitis: a proposal for modification of the New York criteria. Arthritis Rheum 1984;27(4):361–8.

psoriatic arthritis, and undifferentiated arthritis. Both young and old athletes may suffer from autoimmune diseases affecting the spine. The most notable of these are ankylosing spondylitis and rheumatoid arthritis, which receive special attention in this section.

Ankylosing Spondylitis

Ankylosing spondylitis (AS) is the prototype of a group of autoimmune diseases called the SpA and can cause significant functional disability through its effects on the sacroiliac joints and axial skeleton.[31] AS is defined by the constellation of symptoms, signs, and radiographic findings that meet the modified New York criteria[32] as demonstrated in **Table 2**. Definite disease involves sacroiliitis of grade II–IV bilaterally or grade III–IV unilaterally in the presence of inflammatory back pain (**Box 2**) as well as either limitation of lumbar motion or decreased chest expansion. Harper and colleagues offer a diagnostic approach to the evaluation of inflammatory back pain in **Fig. 6**. The biological hallmarks of AS are its non-association with rheumatoid factor (an antibody to the F_c portion of one's own circulating immunoglobulin G [IgG] antibodies) and its association with human leukocyte antigen HLA B27. HLA B27 is a major histocompatibility complex (MHC) class I molecule involved in antigen presentation, expressed by more than 90% of affected patients,[33] far more prevalent than the 8% of nonaffected persons carrying the gene.[31]

Despite its strong association with HLA B27, fewer than 5% of patients with this gene will develop symptomatic AS. Incidence differs among the various subtypes of the *B27* allele.[33] It is unclear what events might trigger autoimmunity in AS; however, theories about a traumatic unveiling of previously immunoisolated antigens and

Box 2
Characteristics of inflammatory back pain

Age at onset <35 years

Insidious onset

Morning stiffness lasting >30 minutes

Improvement with exercise but not with rest

Alternating buttock pain

Awakens in second half of night

Data from Harper BE, Reveille JD. Spondyloarthritis: clinical suspicion, diagnosis, and sports. Curr Sports Med Rep 2009;8(1):29–34.

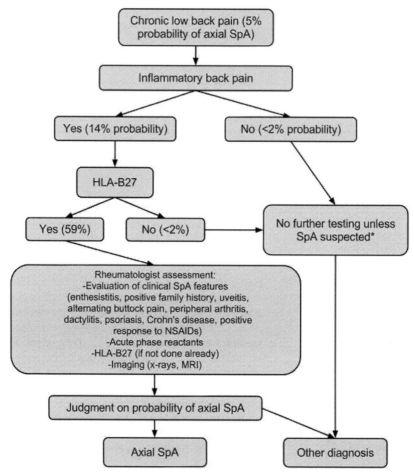

Fig. 6. Axial spondyloarthritis determination. A diagnostic approach to the patient with low back pain. (*From* Harper BE, Reveille JD. Spondyloarthritis: clinical suspicion, diagnosis, and sports. Curr Sports Med Rep 2009;8:29; with permission.)

various types of infectious triggers, including *Klebsiella*, have surfaced.[34] After the inciting event, inflammatory lesions appear at entheses throughout the axial skeleton followed by new bone formation at sites of prior inflammatory lesions,[35] thus the characteristic autofusion of sacroiliac joints and the spinal motion segments.

Although the exact prevalence of AS is not known owing to misdiagnoses and its often milder course in women, it is thought to affect approximately 1% of Caucasians, with a 3:1 male-to-female distribution.[31] At presentation, 90% to 95% of patients have intermittent inflammatory pain in the lumbar spine, described in **Box 2**. Physical examination reveals pain with percussion of the sacroiliac joints and a positive Flexion, ABduction, and External Rotation of the hip (FABER) or Gaenslen test. Spinal sagittal alignment shows varying degrees of lumbar hypolordosis, thoracic kyphosis, and cervical hypolordosis. Reduced motion in the lumbar spine is demonstrated on the Schober test with limited separation of lumbar surface landmarks with forward flexion. As the disease also affects the costovertebral joints of the thoracic spine,

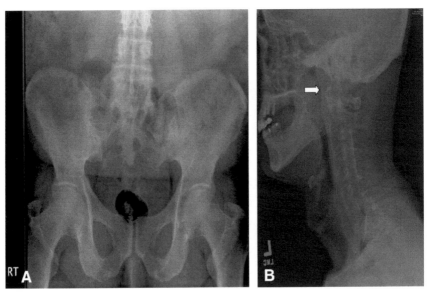

Fig. 7. (*A*) Bilateral grade III sacroiliitis with sclerosis, erosions, and joint space narrowing of bilateral sacroiliac joints. (*From* Harper BE, Reveille JD. Spondyloarthritis: clinical suspicion, diagnosis, and sports. Curr Sports Medicine Rep 2009;8:29; with permission.) (*B*) Cervical ankylosis. Fusion of C2–C7 with fracture of dens (*arrow*). (*From* Harper BE, Reveille JD. Spondyloarthritis: clinical suspicion, diagnosis, and sports. Curr Sports Med Rep 2009;8:29; with permission.)

reduced chest expansion with inspiration is a common finding. Laboratory tests reveal elevated ESR in 80% of AS patients, and CRP elevation is frequent, with a median highly sensitive CRP level of 4.8 mg/L in one cross-sectional study.[36] Rheumatoid factor and antinuclear antibody are typically negative.

Radiographic changes in AS include symmetric sclerotic sacroiliitis (**Fig. 7A**) in more than 85% of patients, and predominantly lumbar involvement in the first 20 years of the disease course, after which lumbar and cervical involvement are equal (see **Fig. 7B**).[37] Complete spine involvement is seen in 28% of patients with between 30 and 40 years of disease and in 43% of patients after their 40th year with AS.[37] Ossification begins at the vertebral rim and extends across the annulus fibrosus in line with and perpendicular to the spinal axis. So-called vertebral corner inflammatory lesions (CILs) are hyperintensities seen at the anterosuperior and anteroinferior corners of vertebral bodies on sagittal T2 and short T1 inversion recovery (STIR) MRI sequences as demonstrated in **Fig. 8**A, B. CILs signify active disease, as there is a four- to fivefold increased probability of new syndesmophyte formation at the site of these lesions within 24 months of their appearance on MRI.[35] The term bamboo spine describes the appearance of the vertically oriented syndesmophytes, calcified annulus fibrosus, and ossified anterior and posterior longitudinal ligaments on lateral radiographs.

AS causes progressive autofusion of the spine, which begins in the sacroiliac joints and lumbar spine and typically progresses proximally. The costovertebral joints are also affected, as shown in the MRI in **Fig. 8**B, leading to a progressive extrinsic restrictive lung disorder in some patients. A rigid thoracic kyphosis in conjunction with

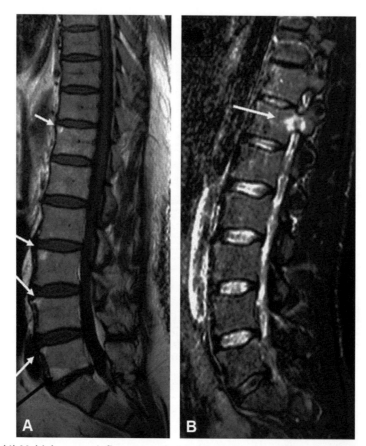

Fig. 8. (*A*) Multiple corner inflammatory lesions. Example of multiple corner inflammatory lesions (*white arrows*) with one endplate lesion (*black arrow*). (*B*) Axial spondyloarthropathy, posterior element T12 lesion. Inflammatory posterior element lesions on sagittal STIR MRI sequence, depicting posterior element/costovertebral inflammatory lesion at T12. (*From* Bennett AN, Marzo-Ortega H, Rehman A, Emery P, et al. The evidence for whole-spine MRI in the assessment of axial spondyloarthropathy. Rheumatology (Oxford, England) 2010; 49; 426–32; with permission.)

lumbar and cervical hypolordosis leads to the characteristic chin-in-chest deformity, which is painful, functionally limiting, and only partially compensated by obligate knee flexion and hip hyperextension.

Surgical management of AS is required in cases of fracture, fracture-associated epidural hematoma, neurologic compromise, and most commonly painful or function limiting deformity. Spinal fracture from minor trauma and low-energy falls can occur secondary to the long inflexible lever-arm of fused spinal segments. Additional vertebral fracture risk may be attributable to fragility that results from chronic inflammation, abnormal biomechanics, and drug-related osteopenia. Trauma in the athlete with AS and acute or delayed neck or back pain deserves close observation because the dreaded complication of neurologically devastating epidural hematoma associated with even radiographically subtle fractures can be delayed by days or weeks. MRI evaluation of the spine is imperative in all

Table 3	
Extra-Articular features of ankylosing spondylitis	
Organ System	**Manifestations**
Ophthalmic	Acute anterior uveitis
Cardiovascular	Aortitis
	Aortic valve insufficiency
	Thickening of aortic valve leaflets
	Subaortic fibrosis
	Conduction abnormalities
	Mitral valve insufficiency
	Left ventricular dysfunction
Gastrointestinal	Inflammatory bowel disease
Neurologic	Myelopathy and radiculopathy
	Cauda equina syndrome
	Vertebrobasiar insufficiency
	Peripheral neuropathy
Pulmonary	Interstitial fibrosis
	Restrictive thoracopathy
Renal	Amyloidosis
	Immunoglobulin A nephropathy

Data from Shamji MF, Bafaquh M, Tsai E. The pathogenesis of ankylosing spondylitis. Neurosurg Focus 2008;24(1):E3.

suspected spinal fractures in patients with AS, as radiographs are notoriously insensitive for subtle fractures, particularly in the lower cervical spine, the most frequently involved region. There is high in-hospital morbidity and mortality in AS patients with cervical spine injuries likely owing to preexisting restrictive pulmonary disease and AS-associated cardiopulmonary disease, as listed in **Table 3**.[31] Compared to patients with rheumatoid arthritis, few AS patients experience atlanto-axial subluxation (21% in a recent large series, and of these patients, just 23% required surgical stabilization[38]).

The mainstays of nonoperative treatment of AS include medications to target pain and inflammation in addition to physical therapy to combat impending deformity during autofusion. Medications are categorized into nonsteroidal anti-inflammatory drugs (NSAIDs), disease-modifying anti-rheumatic drugs (DMARDs), and biological immune-modulating drugs designed to block specific targets in the immune cascade (**Table 4**).[31] Physical therapy and ergonomics include extension directed spine exercises, as listed in **Table 5**,[39] deep-breathing exercises, and avoidance of spine flexion with pillow positioning.[40] Swimming and water therapy are cost-effective adjuncts to medical treatment and standard physical therapy.[40,41] Corset-style braces should be avoided because their efficacy is unproven, and potential adverse effects on respiratory capacity may be detrimental.

Biological treatments for AS held hope for prolonged disease remission; however, early trials have somewhat tempered enthusiasm for these drugs. AS manifests in the appendicular skeleton as an asymmetric, large-joint, pauciarticular arthritis in 30% of patients. Biological therapies have been effective in halting the progression of peripheral arthritis but are ineffective in preventing spinal ankylosis.[31]

With regard to athletics and physical activity in patients with AS, the orthopaedist should be cognizant of the documented benefits of exercise therapy and aerobic

Table 4
Drug therapy for inflammatory spinal disorders

Drug (chemical class)	Trade Name	Pill Size (mg)	Maximum Dose (mg/day or week*)	Frequency (per day)
Salicylates				
Aspirin	Bayer	81, 325	5200	4–6
	Ecotrin	325	5200	
Substituted salicylates				
Diflunisal	Dolobid	250, 500	1500	2
Propionic acid				
Ibuprofen	Motrin	200, 400, 500, 800	4500	4–6
Naproxen	Naprosyn	220, 375, 500	1500	2–3
Flurbiprofen	Ansaid	50, 100	300	2–3
Ketoprofen	Orudis	25, 50, 75, 200	300	1–4
Pyrole acetic acid				
Sulindac	Clinoril	150, 200	450	2–3
Indomethacin	Indocin	25, 50, 75SR	225	2–3
Benzeneacetic acid				
Diclofenac	Voltaren	25, 50, 75, 100SR	225	2–3
Diclofenac/ misoprostil	Arthrotec	50, 75, 200	225	2–3
Oxicam				
Piroxicam	Feldene	10, 20	20	1
Pyranocarboxylic acid				
Etodolac	Lodine	200, 300, 400XL, 500XL	1600	2–4
Naphthylalkanone				
Nabumetone	Relafen	500, 750	2000	2
COX-2 inhibitors				
Celecoxib	Celebrex	100, 200	400	2
Meloxicam	Mobic	7.5, 15	15	1–2
Disease-modifying antirheumatic drugs				
Hydroxychloroquine	Plaquenil	200	400	1–2
Sulfazalazine	Azulfidine	500	3000	1–3
Penicillamine	Cupramine	125, 250	125–750	1–2
Leflunomide	Arava	10, 20, 100	20	1
Methotrexate	Rheumatrex	2.5, 5, 7.5	25*	1/week
Azathioprine	Imuran	50	50–300	1
Etanercept	Enbril	25, 50	*	1/week
Adalimumab	Humira	40		2 weeks
Infliximab	Remicaide	3 mg–10 mg/kg		8 weeks

Data from Borenstein D. Inflammatory arthritides of the spine: surgical versus nonsurgical treatment. Clin Orthop Relat Res 2006;443:208–21.

Table 5 Exercises for spondyloarthritis		
Chest expansion	Single knee to chest	Leg slides out
Chin tuck	Double knee to Chest	Leg rotation
Neck rotation	Trunk rotation	Back extension
Neck side bending	Shoulder stretch	Trunk side bending
Hamstring stretch	Shoulder blade stretch	"Cat & camel"
Pelvic tilt	Bridging	Kneeling stretch
Hip flexor stretch	Trunk side bending	Trunk rotation
Calf stretch	Wall calf stretch	Corner stretch

Data from Harper BE, Reveille JD. Spondyloarthritis: clinical suspicion, diagnosis, and sports. Curr Sports Med Rep 2009;8(1):29–34.

exercise, the increased risk of low-energy spinal fracture, and possible cardiac disease associated with AS, as listed in **Table 3**.[33] Special attention to the stabilization and transport of an AS patient with a cervical spine injury should focus on maintaining the individual's native neck alignment, which may be more flexed than that of a healthy counterpart[42]; acknowledging this factor has been shown to reverse an acutely progressing neurologic deficit.

Rheumatoid Arthritis of the Cervical Spine

Rheumatoid arthritis (RA) is a T-cell–mediated autoimmune disease that manifests as a symmetric polyarthropathy affecting the joints of the axial and appendicular skeleton at the hands, wrists, feet, ankles, elbows, shoulders, hips, knees, and spine. One percent of persons in the United States have RA, with females affected approximately three times as often as males. Spinal involvement is less frequent than is seen in AS, and primarily involves the cervical spine, with clinically symptomatic disease affecting 40% to 80% of patients.[31] Cervical spine disease ranges in severity from referred pain and radiculopathy to frank nonambulatory myelopathy, brain stem compression, and even sudden death.

Despite extensive study, the pathogenesis of RA is incompletely understood. RA-mediated inflammation is manifested primarily in synovial joints. Clinically important serologic markers of disease include rheumatoid factor (RF) and anticyclic citrullinated peptide (anti-CPP) antibodies. RF-positive serology is 69% sensitive and 85% specific for RA, making it a key part of the diagnostic workup. Anti-CCP–positive serology is 67% sensitive and 95% specific for RA. In RA, cytokines such as tumor necrosis factor-alpha (TNF-α) and interleukin-1, which sustain the inflammatory cascade, have surfaced as the targets of most biological immune-modulating drugs as shown in **Table 4**. Inflammation leads to the synovial cell production of metalloproteinases, which destroy articular cartilage. Synovial cell and lymphocyte-driven differentiation of osteoclast precursor cells leads to bony erosion by active osteoclasts.[43] The long-term effect of inflammation is widespread osteoarticular damage.

Among the most serious musculoskeletal sequellae of RA is cervical spine instability, particularly of the exclusively synovial articulation of C1–C2. RA-associated inflammation leads to articular cartilage destruction, capsular and ligamentous laxity, and bony erosion. The C1–C2 articulation is stabilized primarily by capsular and ligamentous structures, as the facet surfaces lie in the axial plain and lend minimal anteroposterior stability from their bony articulation. For the same reason, the

Table 6
Ranawat classification of neurologic deficit

Classification	Clinical Criteria
Class I	Pain without neurologic deficit
Class II	Subjective weakness, hyperreflexia, dysesthesias
Class III	Objective weakness, long tract signs
Class IIIA	Class III, ambulatory
Class IIIB	Class III, nonambulatory

Data from Monsey RD. Rheumatoid arthritis of the cervical spine. J Am Acad Orthop Surg 1997;5(5):240–8.

atlanto-occipital articulation is subject to instability. Furthermore, subluxation can be seen in the subaxial cervical spine, which is a source of pain and neurologic compromise. The resulting deformities in the cervical spine are (1) subluxation of C1 on C2, usually anteriorly; (2) pseudobasilar invagination, which involves encroachment of the dens into the foramen magnum with impingement on the brain stem caused by erosion at the atlanto-occipital and/or atlanto-axial articulations; and (3) subaxial subluxation caused by facet erosion and capsuloligamentous laxity, which can involve multiple levels.[44]

Symptoms of cervical instability are occipital headache; sensation of movement of the head on the neck with changing head position; and neurologic symptoms such as syncope, myelopathy, Lhermite sign, weakness, vertigo, dysphagia, and cranial nerve involvement.[31] Neurologic abnormalities are present in one tenth to one third of patients with RA.[31,44] The Ranawat classification, shown in **Table 6**,[44] is frequently used to describe the severity of cervical myelopathy in RA and is used to measure improvement after surgical intervention.

Radiographic evaluation is indicated in any patient with RA and neck pain or neurologic symptoms. Radiographic abnormalities are present in 34% to 86% of patients with RA; this rate differs between reported cohorts secondary to differing study populations and radiographic techniques and criteria used. Radiographs should be adequate to evaluate the standardized radiographic criteria shown in **Box 3**,[45] and should include a PA view, a lateral series with flexion and extension views, and an open-mouth odontoid view of the cervical spine.[44] Standard radiographic measurements include the anterior atlanto-dens interval (AADI), posterior atlanto-dens interval (PADI; **Fig. 9A**), the McGregor line, and the Ranawat (see **Fig. 9B**) and Redlund–Johnell (see **Fig. 9C**) measurements.

An AADI of up to 2.5 mm in women and 3.0 mm in men is considered normal. As pseudobasilar invagination and anterior subluxation are of chief concern with increasing atlanto-axial instability, the PADI, which is the distance from the posterior aspect of the odontoid process to the anteriormost aspect of the posterior arch of the axis, should also be measured. A study by Boden and colleagues demonstrated that a PADI less than 14 mm had a sensitivity of 97% in predicting neurologic deficit, and that 94% of patients with a PADI greater than 14 mm were neurologically intact.[46]

Addition of MRI is indicated in the presence of new or progressive neurologic compromise, as radiographs do not appreciate synovial pannus, which can exert additional mass effect on the brain stem and spinal cord. An MRI of the cervical spine should be obtained for patients presenting with myelopathy, pseudobasilar invagination, or instability. MRI can also evaluate for myelomalacia and better characterize

Box 3
Roentgenologic criteria for rheumatoid arthritis of the cervical spine

1. Atlanto-axial subluxation of 2.5 mm or more.
2. Multiple subluxations of C2–C3, C3–C4, C4–C5, C5–C6
3. Narrow disc spaces with little or no osteophytosis
    a. Pathognomonic at C2–C3 and C3–C4
    b. Probable at C4–C5 and C5–C6
4. Erosions of vertebrae, especially vertebral plates
5. Odontoid, small, pointed; eroded loss of cortex
6. Basilar impression (odontoid above McGregor's line)
7. Apophyseal joint erosion; blurred facets; narrow spaces
8. Osteoporosis, generalized

From Bland JH, Van Buskirk FW, Tampas JP, et al. A study of roentgenologic criteria for rheumatoid arthritis of the cervical spine. Am J Roentgenol Radium Ther Nucl Med 1965;95(4):949–54.

active lesions. The midsagittal cervical MRI slice can be used to measure the cervicomedullary angle, which is normally 135° to 175°, but can be less than 135° in cases of instability or pseudobasilar invagination. The presence of hand deformity correlates closely with cervical involvement in RA. In cases in which instability is suspected, radiographic evaluation should be completed with CT of the cervical spine, which is much more sensitive in characterizing bony erosions and quantifying subluxation at the atlanto-axial junctions. Although CT scan is more sensitive and specific for determining the AADI, it is not able to demonstrate dynamic, reducible instability and is not routinely indicated when high-quality radiographs are within normal limits in a neurointact patient.

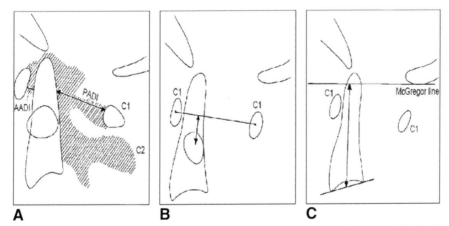

Fig. 9. Measurements for atlanto-axial instability. (*A*) Measurement of AADI and PADI. (*B*) The Ranawat method for measuring vertical settling. (*C*) The Redlund–Johnell method for measuring vertical settling. (*From* Monsey RD. Rheumatoid arthritis of the cervical spine. J Am Acad Orthop Surg 1997;5(5):240–8. © 1997 American Academy of Orthopaedic Surgeons. Reproduced with permission.)

The goals of management when RA affects the cervical spine are to avoid the development of an irreversible neurologic deficit or sudden death from undermanaged or unrecognized cervical instability.[44] Nonsurgical management of RA is targeted to interrupt the inflammatory cascade driving joint destruction and bony erosions with the goal of permanent disease remission. **Table 4** includes the medications commonly used to treat RA in the United States. Providers should be cognizant of bone fragility in RA patients, which results both from the disease process and its treatments.[47] Various treatments including calcium and vitamin D supplementation and bisphosphonate therapy are efficacious in reducing bone loss in RA.[47,48] Resistance training for patients with RA improves muscle strength and physical function; however, improvements in bone density have not been as evident.[49]

Surgical indications for cervical spine disease in RA are controversial, especially with asymptomatic instability. Strong indications are progressive myelopathy, severe pain refractory to nonoperative management, and symptomatic instability at the upper or lower cervical spine. Wolfs and colleagues found that deterioration rarely occurred in patients presenting with Ranawat I disease with or without surgery.[50] Ranawat II patients improved to Ranawat I 53% of the time after surgery, 40% remained unchanged, and 7% worsened. After surgical treatment, 56% and 21% of Ranawat IIIA and Ranawat IIIB patients, respectively, improved to Ranawat II and 38% of Ranawat IIIB patients improved to IIIA. Overall perioperative mortality is much higher and fusion rates are significantly lower than are reported for non-RA cases. Wolfs and colleagues also demonstrated 10-year mortality rates of 23%, 37%, 53%, and 70% for Ranawat I through IIIB, respectively.[50] Given instability and impaired fusion biology, instrumentation is imperative and stabilization of C1–2 can be performed posteriorly by Gallie or Brooks wiring, screw and rod constructs, and by various plating options when fusion is extended to the occiput. With significant proximal migration of the dens, fusion should always extend to the occiput.[44]

Many athletes of various skill levels are impaired by RA. The goals of care are to control the disease progression before cervical instability severely limits activities from pain and diminish the threat of neurologic injury. Athletics, in particular resistance training, may have benefits for maintaining strength and function and should be encouraged within safe limits. In patients with cervical spine instability, activities should be modified to minimize fall risk, and contact sports are contraindicated.[51] Activity limitations after surgical stabilization should be discussed with the operating spinal surgeon.

METABOLIC BONE DISEASE AND SPINE DISORDERS IN SPORTS

Metabolic bone disorders generally result in decreased bone strength from abnormal mineralization or structural deficits as seen in osteoporosis and osteomalacia. In adults, the manifestations of metabolic bone disorders of the spine are often associated with excessive bone loss resulting in skeletal insufficiency and subsequent micro or macro fractures. In the growing athlete, concerns also include abnormalities in acquisition of bone density and strength as well as bone loss. Despite the specific etiology, a condition that results in abnormal morphology, suboptimal mineralization, or inadequate microarchitecture of the vertebrae can ultimately lead to decreased mechanical properties and failure under loads, especially those experienced in athletic activities. This overview of the effects of metabolic bone disorders on the spine focuses on conditions most likely to be encountered in evaluating youth and adult sports participants.

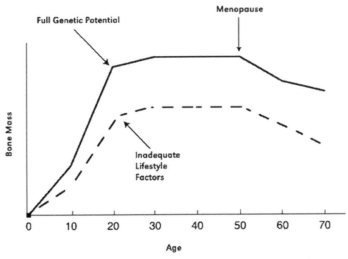

Fig. 10. Bone mass versus age across the lifespan. (*From* Heaney RP, Abrams S, Dawson-Hughes B, et al. Peak bone mass. Osteoporos Int 2000;11(12):985–1009; with permission.)

Bone Mass Acquisition and Maintenance

Adolescence is a critical time for bone acquisition; there is a 40% increase of bone mineral density during puberty.[52] Peak bone mass is achieved early in the third decade of life (**Fig. 10**) and is a significant predictor of postmenopausal osteoporosis[53] and fragility fractures in both men and women.[54] Genetic and lifestyle factors interact to determine actual bone mass accrual. Adequate nutrition and a balanced diet including calcium and vitamin D are important in both bone mass acquisition and maintenance. Weight-bearing sports have a highly positive effect on bone mineral content and density. Several studies have compared bone mineral density (BMD) among different sports. Among competitive athletes, volleyball players, gymnasts, and sprinters have the highest BMD whereas cyclists, cross-country skiers, and swimmers generally have the lowest.[52,55,56] Groudyte and colleagues studied 170 healthy adolescent girls who participated in competitive athletic programs and 33 controls who participated only in mandatory physical education classes. They found that BMD of the lumbar spine was most highly affected by low-impact versus high-impact sports and that rhythmic gymnasts had the highest BMD of the lumbar spine of out of all other athletes.[52] Nichols and colleagues tracked changes in BMD over a 7-year period in 19 competitive male cyclists and 18 controls. They found that the cyclists had a consistent pattern of lower BMD compared to controls at all bone sites at the initial and 7-year assessment.[57] As cyclists are at high risk for falls and accidents, the authors concluded that their coaches and health professionals should promote cross training with weight-bearing exercises to improve bone mass and minimize fracture risk.[57] Peer and Newsham published a report of a male collegiate track athlete who presented with bilateral L5 spondylolysis, L4 spondylolysis, and osteoporosis. This highlights the need to think of low BMD and stress fractures even in young men participating in high-level athletics.[58]

General Principles of Evaluation

All children and adolescents planning to participate in sports should undergo a pre-participation physical examination. In addition to the routine pre-participation data, the history should include any family background of metabolic bone disease and a history of fractures and nutritional intake, with specific questions concerning calcium and vitamin D intake as well as calorie restriction. In females, age at menarche and any periods of amenorrhea should be documented. The entire spine should be palpated for areas of tenderness. A focused physical examination of the spine should include posture and the Adam's forward bending test to screen for scoliosis or kyphosis. The provocative lumbar hyperextension test is helpful to screen for a stress fracture of the posterior elements. Positive findings warrant imaging studies as described below. If a stress reaction or stress fracture is noted, screening for an underlying metabolic bone disease is indicated.

Anterior-posterior (AP) and lateral radiographs of the entire spine should be obtained if the athlete has focal back pain or significant deformity on examination. Lateral and oblique radiographs focused on the lumbar spine are used to assess pars defects in the lumbar spine. Standard radiographs are less sensitive for early stress fractures compared to a CT scan or a single-photon emission CT scan (SPECT); therefore, advanced imaging may be indicated in the setting of a positive clinical picture with negative radiographs.[59] MRI can also detect stress fractures and has been shown to be as reliable as SPECT in diagnosing stress fractures in the spine.[60,11] Radiographs are not sensitive for detecting generalized bone loss; it has been estimated that once osteopenia is noted on radiography, there is already a 25% loss of bone mass.

BMD is clinically measured using dual-energy X-ray absorptiometry (DEXA). DEXA scanning has been the gold standard to evaluate BMD in adult osteoporosis and now through pediatric software algorithms, it can be used to measure BMD in children and adolescents. The International Society for Clinical Densitometry recommends using the z-score, the number of standard deviations away from the mean for age, sex, and ethnically matched peers, to assist in the diagnosis of osteoporosis in the pediatric population, but it cannot be used alone to diagnose osteoporosis.[53,61]

A metabolic bone panel is essential to assess nutritional status and calcium and vitamin D levels and to screen for secondary causes of poor skeletal health. A screening panel consists of a CBC with differential, a comprehensive metabolic panel (including calcium, phosphate, magnesium, aspartate aminotransferase [AST], alanine aminotransferase [ALT], alkaline phosphatase, and albumin), parathyroid hormone (PTH), thyroid-stimulating hormone (TSH), free thyroxine (T4) and 25(OH) vitamin D levels. Bone specific alkaline phosphatase, serum osteocalcin, serum type 1 procollagen (C-terminal or N-terminal), urinary collagen type 1 cross-linked N-telopeptide (NTX), and urinary collagen type 1 cross-linked C-telopeptide (CTX) are bone turnover markers sensitive to changes in bone formation and resorption.[62] Abnormalities in the metabolic bone panel should alert the physician if an underlying endocrinopathy or poor nutrition is contributing to the poor bone health and guide further evaluation.

Fractures of the Spine

Stress fractures

Stress fractures can be due to supraphysiologic loads or repetitive loads on normal bone and are considered fatigue fractures. **Fig. 11** depicts the stress–strain curve of biomaterials such as bone. Failure will occur once the load exceeds the intrinsic strength of the material. Insufficiency fractures are similar in appearance to fatigue fractures, but are the result of physiologic loads on structurally compromised bone.[63] Both conditions can and do occur simultaneously in some athletes, in other words overloading of abnormal bone. Among athletes, fractures of the spine can be due to

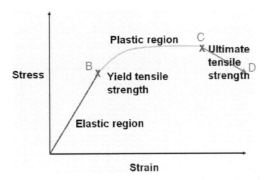

Fig. 11. Stress–strain curve. Point *B* is the yield point. Force beneath point *B* is in the elastic range and the bone will return to its original shape. Beyond point *B*, plastic deformation occurs. Point *C* is ultimate stress point and *D* is the fracture point.

a variety of mechanisms. Athletes are susceptible to trauma and high physical demands causing stress fractures. Several studies have found the tibia to be the most frequent bone affected by a stress fractures.[64,65] Stress fractures of the spine are less common and represent 0.4% to 0.6% of all stress fractures.[64,65] An increase in training volume and intensity, endurance running, low body mass index (BMI), and low BMD all increase the risk for a stress fracture among athletes.

Vertebral body fractures
The vertebral body has a high trabecular bone content and is more sensitive to estrogen withdrawal[66]; therefore, vertebral compression fractures are common in postmenopausal osteoporosis. Approximately 600,000 vertebral compression fractures occur annually in the United States, but only one third comes to clinical attention (www.nof.org). Although the majority occur in women, it is important to note that 20% occur in men. These fractures can also occur in young athletes and should be in the differential diagnosis when an athlete complains of thoracic or lumbar pain. McHugh and colleagues published a case of a T12 compression fracture in an 18-year-old male basketball player after a rebound.[67] Vertebral compression fractures can cause back pain, decreased mobility and a decrease in health-related quality of life (HRQL).[68] Stable fractures can be treated reliably with a thoracolumbar orthosis. Painful or unstable compression fractures can be treated with vertebral augmentation with reliable results.[69]

Pars fractures
Spondylolysis is a disruption of the pars interarticularis, often due to a fatigue or stress fracture.[70] The pars interarticularis is thin and susceptible to shear stresses across the lordotic lumbar spine (**Fig. 12**). The incidence of spondylolysis is 5% in the general population and has been reported to be 11% in gymnasts.[70,71] Fatigue fractures of the pars in athletes may result from repetitive forceful lumbar hyperextension as seen in gymnasts and football linebackers. Relative rest, activity modification, and bracing are the first lines of treatment. Fixation and bone grafting across the pars may be necessary to treat symptomatic recalcitrant spondylolysis. Bilateral pars fractures can result in gradual displacement of the vertebral body and may require posterior spinal fusion.

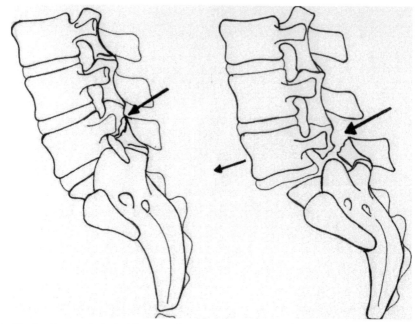

Fig. 12. Pars interarticularis: Diagram of the pars interarticularis demonstrating spondylolysis (*left*), and associated spondylolisthesis (*right*) with anterior subluxation of the L5 body to S1. The L5 pars is most susceptible to fatigue and fracturing.

Pedicle and lamina fractures

Several cases of pedicle stress fractures, "pediculolysis," have been reported in the literature.[72,73] Any part of the posterior neural arch can be susceptible to a stress fracture. Abel hypothesized that most normal activities concentrate stress through the pars interarticularis, causing the more common pars fracture. However, a more posterior-directed force, observed in joggers, can result in a stress fracture of the lamina. Conversely, ballet dancers experience anterior directed axial force and are more likely to fracture the pedicle.[74] Bilateral pediculolysis has been reported, but more commonly a stress fracture of the pedicle occurs in association with a contralateral spondylolysis.[75] Both pedicle and lamina fractures can also be due to high-energy trauma such as a fall from height or can be an iatrogenic injury.

Facet fractures

Facet fractures are more commonly due to high-energy trauma; however, facet fractures can occur as stress fractures in ballerinas as reported by Fehlandt and Micheli.[76,77] In contrast to stress fractures of the facet, those from trauma are typically unstable injuries and require surgical stabilization.

Eating Disorders and High-Intensity Sports

Poor nutrition retards skeletal development, causing low bone mass and an increase in fragility fractures. Overweight and obese children sustain more fractures compared to normal weight children, suggesting a negative effect of adiposity and sedentary behaviors on skeletal development.[53,78,79] Moderate exercise is recommended in adolescence to promote bone acquisition and in postmenopausal women to decrease the rate of bone loss.[80] However, high training volumes with high intensity may have the opposite effect on bone in men and women.[56,80] Athletes in sports that emphasize a low body weight such as wrestling, crew, ballet, and gymnastics have a higher incidence of stress fractures and lower BMD.[81] It is also important to recognize eating disorders or calorie restriction in athletes trying to "make weight." These athletes are at a higher risk for abnormal bone acquisition and insufficiency fractures.

Female athlete triad

The interrelationship among disordered eating, amenorrhea, and altered BMD in female athletes is termed the female athlete triad. It is a spectrum ranging from optimal energy availability, eumenorrhea, and optimal bone health to a pathologic state encompassing low energy availability, functional hypothalamic amenorrhea, and osteoporosis.[82] The true prevalence of female athlete triad is unknown. Two recent studies found a higher prevalence of eating disorders in female elite athletes compared to controls; 31% in "thin build sports," 5.5% in endurance athletes, and 25% in aesthetic and weight-class athletes compared to 9% in the general population.[83] Hoch found among club triathletes a 60% rate of calorie deficit and that 40% of female triathletes studied reported a history of amenorrhea.[84] Smaller studies have reported a high prevalence, 67%, of secondary amenorrhea in female runners and a rate of 22% of primary amenorrhea among cheerleaders, gymnasts and divers compared to 1% in the general population.[76] The critical energy needed for normal physiologic function after exercise is 30 kcal/kg.[82] Normal hormonal balance is disrupted within 5 days if the energy availability is reduced to less than 30 kcal/kg.[85] Gonadotropin-releasing hormone (GnRH) and luteinizing hormone (LH) are both decreased, disrupting the normal cycle of circulating estrogen and progesterone and causing amenorrhea. The exact mechanism, however, is unknown.

According to the AAP and Endocrine Society Task Force, a z-score of less than –2.0 plus additional risk factors for a future fracture (malnutrition, hypogonadism, eating disorders, and amenorrhea) define osteoporosis in the young athlete. Multiple mechanisms cause low BMD in the female athlete triad. Estrogen deficiency causes premature bone loss and inadequate bone formation. Estrogen deficiency is typically accompanied by chronic undernutrition, which also has a direct negative impact on bone health.

The American College of Sports Medicine recommends screening for the female athlete triad at all pre-participation physicals. A DEXA scan to measure BMD should be obtained in an athlete with a stress fracture or a low-impact fracture, after 6 months of amenorrhea or oligomenorrhea, and when an athlete exhibits disordered eating or an eating disorder.[82] All athletes with disordered eating should be referred to a mental health specialist for further evaluation.

The most important treatment component is to increase energy availability. Successful treatment requires a team approach including a physician; a team trainer; a dietitian; and in cases of eating disorders, a mental health specialist. Some athletes may need to be restricted from competition until they comply with a nutrition program. Although oral contraceptives are often used to address amenorrhea, increases in BMD among females with the female athlete triad are highly correlated to weight gain and less so with hormone replacement therapy or oral contraceptives.[82] Bisphosphonates stay in the body for a very long time and are rarely indicated for use in adolescent girls because of their unknown effect on fetal development.

Table 7
Rare metabolic bone diseases in adults

Disease	Description	Treatment
Paget's disease of bone	Weak, brittle bone prone to fracture and deformation; most common in the spine, pelvis, long bones and the skull.	Bisphosphonates, calcitonin, 1000–1500 mg of calcium and 400–800 IU of vitamin D daily.
Osteomalacia	A vitamin D deficiency leading to low available calcium and phosphate; result of insufficient nutritional quantities, renal tubular acidosis, malabsorption syndromes, chronic renal failure, hypophosphatemia, tumor-induced osteomalacia, and anticonvulsant therapy. The earliest symptoms are low back pain and thigh pain.	Weekly intravenous treatment with 10,000 IU of vitamin D for 4–6 weeks. For non-nutritional causes, treatment of the underlying condition can result in improved calcium and phosphorus homeostasis.
Osteitis fibrosa cystica	Overproduction of parathyroid hormone from hyperactive parathyroid glands causing stimulation of osteoclastic bone resorption: decreased bone mass, weakened bone, substitution of calcified matrix with fibrous tissue, and cyst-like brown tumors. Parathyroid adenoma, hereditary factors, parathyroid carcinoma, or renal osteodystrophy are all causes of osteitis fibrosa cystica.	Medical management consists of vitamin D treatment. Surgical treatment to remove the parathyroid glands is definitive.

Metabolic Diseases of the Spine in Older Adults

As athletes are continuing to participate in sports well into their 60s and 70s it is important to be aware of issues they face. Osteoporosis and osteopenia are the most common metabolic bone diseases affecting adults in the United States. In 2005, the National Osteoporosis Foundation (NOF) estimated 10 million people in the United States had osteoporosis and another 34 million were considered to have osteopenia. Additional less common metabolic bone diseases are listed in **Table 7**.

Metabolic bone disease in adults often manifests as vertebral compression fractures. Vertebral compression fractures due to osteoporosis occur with an annual estimate of 600,000 in the United States. In postmenopausal women the risk of sustaining future vertebral and extraspinal fractures is increased two- to ninefold in the first 2 years after sustaining a vertebral compression fracture.[57,86,87]

Fractures in adults, regardless of mechanism, should trigger the physician to ask about risk factors for metabolic bone disorders and when indicated, to obtain a metabolic bone laboratory panel and DEXA study. A lateral view should be included in the DEXA study to screen for vertebral compression fractures. The possibility of vertebral fracture should be considered in all athletes older than the age of 50 who present with acute back pain. Adequate intakes of vitamin D and calcium as well as regular weight-bearing exercises are the cornerstone of bone mass maintenance and fracture prevention. The NOF recommends that adults take 1000 to 1200 mg of calcium daily. Vitamin D recommendations currently range from 600 to 800 IU daily for adults.[88] Several studies have highlighted the prevalence of vitamin D deficiency in North America[89] and the need to screen for vitamin D deficiency.

Several classes of drugs have been approved by the US Food and Drug Administration (FDA) to treat osteoporosis in the adult including bisphosphonates, calcitonin, estrogens, hormone therapy, raloxifene, and PTH. The first line of treatment for adult osteoporosis is usually a bisphosphonate, which increases BMD by preventing osteoclastic resorption of bone. Both oral and intravenous forms of bisphosphonates reduce the risk of vertebral compression fractures and hip fractures.[90,91] Long-term use of bisphosphonate treatment has been associated with atypical femoral fractures. Larger studies need to be performed to better understand the relationship, but there may be a role for a drug holiday after 5 years of treatment if there is an improvement in BMD.[92]

Causes of Secondary Osteoporosis

Several disorders can affect BMD and bone quality such as juvenile inflammatory arthritis, diabetes, osteogenesis imperfecta, hyperthyroidism, hyperparathyroidism, Cushing syndrome, malabsorption syndromes, anorexia nervosa, and kidney disease. Common medications known to deleteriously affect bone are anticonvulsants, corticosteroids, and immunosuppressant agents.

SUMMARY

Sports and weight-bearing activities can have a positive effect on bone health in the growing, mature, or aging athlete. However, certain athletic activities and training regimens may place the athlete at increased risk for stress fractures in the spine. In addition, some athletes have an underlying susceptibility to fracture due to either systemic or focal abnormalities. It is important to identify and treat these athletes in order to prevent stress fractures and reduce the risk of osteoporosis in late adulthood. Therefore, the pre-participation physical examination offers a unique opportunity to screen athletes for metabolic bone disease through the history and physical examination. Positive findings warrant a thorough workup including a metabolic bone laboratory panel, and possibly a DEXA scan, which includes a lateral spine view.

REFERENCES

1. Quinones-Hinojosa A, Jun P, Jacobs R, et al. General principles in the medical and surgical management of spinal infections: a multidisciplinary approach. Neurosurg Focus 2004;17(6)E1.
2. Zimmerli W. Clinical practice. Vertebral osteomyelitis. N Engl J Med 2010;362(11): 1022–9.
3. Maier RV, Carrico CJ, Heimbach DM. Pyogenic osteomyelitis of axial bones following civilian gunshot wounds. Am J Surg 1979;137(3):378–80.
4. Fang A, Hu SS, Endres N, et al. Risk factors for infection after spinal surgery. Spine (Phila Pa 1976) 2005;30(12):1460–5.
5. Hopton B, Barron D, Ambrose S, et al. The flatulent spine: lumbar spinal infection secondary to colonic diverticular abscess: a case report and review of the literature. J Spinal Disord Tech 2008;21(7):527–30.
6. Mylona E, Samarkos M, Kakalou E, et al. Pyogenic vertebral osteomyelitis: a systematic review of clinical characteristics. Semin Arthritis Rheum 2009;39(1):10–7.
7. Carragee EJ. Instrumentation of the infected and unstable spine: a review of 17 cases from the thoracic and lumbar spine with pyogenic infections. J Spinal Disord 1997; 10(4):317–24.
8. Skaf GS, Kanafani ZA, Araj GF, et al. Non-pyogenic infections of the spine. Int J Antimicrob Agents 2010;36(2):99–105.

9. Zormpala A, Skopelitis E, Thanos L, et al. An unusual case of brucellar spondylitis involving both the cervical and lumbar spine. Clin Imaging 2000;24(5):273–5.

10. Sakkas LI, Davas EM, Kapsalaki E, et al. Hematogenous spinal infection in central Greece. Spine (Phila Pa 1976) 2009;34(15):E513–8.

11. Chelli Bouaziz M, Ladeb MF, Chakroun M, et al. Spinal brucellosis: a review. Skeletal Radiol 2008;37(9):785–90.

12. al-Shahed MS, Sharif HS, Haddad MC, et al. Imaging features of musculoskeletal brucellosis. Radiographics 1994;14(2):333–48.

13. Solera J, Lozano E, Martinez-Alfaro E, et al. Brucellar spondylitis: review of 35 cases and literature survey. Clin Infect Dis 1999;29(6):1440–9.

14. Early SD, Kay RM, Tolo VT. Childhood diskitis. J Am Acad Orthop Surg 2003;11(6):413–20.

15. Fernandez M, Carrol CL, Baker CJ. Discitis and vertebral osteomyelitis in children: an 18-year review. Pediatrics 2000;105(6):1299–304.

16. Cushing AH. Diskitis in children. Clin Infect Dis 1993;17(1):1–6.

17. Sapico FL, Montgomerie JZ. Pyogenic vertebral osteomyelitis: report of nine cases and review of the literature. Rev Infect Dis 1979;1(5):754–76.

18. Golden MP, Vikram HR. Extrapulmonary tuberculosis: an overview. Am Fam Physician, 2005;72(9):1761–8.

19. Jain AK. Tuberculosis of the spine: a fresh look at an old disease. J Bone Joint Surg [Br] 2010;92(7):905–13.

20. Watters DA. Surgery for tuberculosis before and after human immunodeficiency virus infection: a tropical perspective. Br J Surg 1997;84(1):8–14.

21. Jain AK, Dhammi IK. Tuberculosis of the spine: a review. Clin Orthop Relat Res 2007;460:39–49.

22. Nene AM, Pawar U. Tuberculosis of the spine 2011 update. ASN&J 2011;23(3):105–9.

23. Schirmer P, Renault CA, Holodniy M. Is spinal tuberculosis contagious? Int J Infect Dis 2010;14(8):e659–66.

24. Oga M, Arizono T, Takasita M, et al. Evaluation of the risk of instrumentation as a foreign body in spinal tuberculosis: clinical and biologic study. Spine (Phila Pa 1976) 1993;18(13):1890–4.

25. Kim CW, Perry A, Currier B, et al. Fungal infections of the spine. Clin Orthop Relat Res 2006;444:92–9.

26. Frazier DD, Campbell DR, Garvey TA, et al. Fungal infections of the spine: report of eleven patients with long-term follow-up. J Bone Joint Surg [Am] 2001;83-A(4):560–5.

27. Vinas FC, King PK, Diaz FG. Spinal aspergillus osteomyelitis. Clin Infect Dis 1999;28(6):1223–9.

28. Kushwaha VP, Shaw B, Gerardi JA, et al. Musculoskeletal coccidioidomycosis: a review of 25 cases. Clin Orthop Relat Res 1996;332:190–9.

29. Crum NF, Lederman ER, Stafford CM, et al. Coccidioidomycosis: a descriptive survey of a reemerging disease. Clinical characteristics and current controversies. Medicine [Baltimore], 2004;83(3):149–75.

30. Colbert RA. Classification of juvenile spondyloarthritis: enthesitis-related arthritis and beyond. Nat Rev Rheumatol 2010;6(8):477–85.

31. Borenstein D. Inflammatory arthritides of the spine: surgical versus nonsurgical treatment. Clin Orthop Relat Res 2006;443:208–21.

32. van der Linden S, Valkenburg HA, Cats A. Evaluation of diagnostic criteria for ankylosing spondylitis: a proposal for modification of the New York criteria. Arthritis Rheum 1984;27(4):361–8.

33. Shamji MF, Bafaquh M, Tsai E. The pathogenesis of ankylosing spondylitis. Neurosurg Focus 2008;24(1):E3.

34. Ebringer A. The cross-tolerance hypothesis, HLA-B27 and ankylosing spondylitis. Br J Rheumatol 1983;22(4 Suppl 2):53–66.

35. Maksymowych WP, Chiowchanwisawakit P, Clare T, et al. Inflammatory lesions of the spine on magnetic resonance imaging predict the development of new syndesmophytes in ankylosing spondylitis: evidence of a relationship between inflammation and new bone formation. Arthritis Rheum 2009;60(1):93–102.

36. Poddubnyy DA, Rudwaleit M, Listing J, et al. Comparison of a high sensitivity and standard C reactive protein measurement in patients with ankylosing spondylitis and non-radiographic axial spondyloarthritis. Ann Rheum Dis 2010;69(7):1338–41.

37. Jang JH, Ward MM, Rucker AN, et al. Ankylosing spondylitis: patterns of radiographic involvement—a re-examination of accepted principles in a cohort of 769 patients. Radiology 2011;258(1):192–8.

38. Ramos-Remus C, Gomez-Vargas A, Guzman-Guzman JL, et al. Frequency of atlantoaxial subluxation and neurologic involvement in patients with ankylosing spondylitis. J Rheumatol 1995;22(11):2120–5.

39. Harper BE, Reveille JD. Spondyloarthritis: clinical suspicion, diagnosis, and sports. Curr Sports Med Rep 2009;8(1):29–34.

40. Elyan M, Khan MA. Does physical therapy still have a place in the treatment of ankylosing spondylitis? Curr Opin Rheumatol 2008;20(3):282–6.

41. van Tubergen A, Hidding A. Spa and exercise treatment in ankylosing spondylitis: fact or fancy? Best Pract Res Clin Rheumatol 2002;16(4):653–66.

42. Maskery NS, Burrows N. Cervical spine control; bending the rules. Emerg Med J 2002;19(6):592–3.

43. Gravallese EM, Manning C, Tsay A, et al. Synovial tissue in rheumatoid arthritis is a source of osteoclast differentiation factor. Arthritis Rheum 2000;43(2): 250–8.

44. Monsey RD. Rheumatoid arthritis of the cervical spine. J Am Acad Orthop Surg 1997;5(5):240–8.

45. Bland JH, Van Buskirk FW, Tampas JP, et al. A study of roentgenologic criteria for rheumatoid arthritis of the cervical spine. Am J Roentgenol Radium Ther Nucl Med 1965;95(4):949–54.

46. Boden SD, Dodge LD, Bohlman HH, et al. Rheumatoid arthritis of the cervical spine: a long-term analysis with predictors of paralysis and recovery. J Bone Joint Surg [Am] 1993;75(9):1282–97.

47. Mawatari T, Miura H, Hamai S, et al. Vertebral strength changes in rheumatoid arthritis patients treated with alendronate, as assessed by finite element analysis of clinical computed tomography scans: a prospective randomized clinical trial. Arthritis Rheum 2008;58(11):3340–9.

48. Thornton J, Ashcroft D, O'Neill T, et al. A systematic review of the effectiveness of strategies for reducing fracture risk in children with juvenile idiopathic arthritis with additional data on long-term risk of fracture and cost of disease management. Health Technol Assess 2008;12(3):iii–ix, xi–xiv, 1–208.

49. Hakkinen A, Sakka T, Kautiainen H, et al. Sustained maintenance of exercise induced muscle strength gains and normal bone mineral density in patients with early rheumatoid arthritis: a 5 year follow up. Ann Rheum Dis 2004;63(8):910–6.

50. Wolfs JF, Kloppenburg M, Fehlings MG, et al. Neurologic outcome of surgical and conservative treatment of rheumatoid cervical spine subluxation: a systematic review. Arthritis Rheum 2009;61(12):1743–52.

51. Tassone JC, Duey-Holtz A. Spine concerns in the Special Olympian with Down syndrome. Sports Med Arthrosc 2008;16(1):55–60.

52. Gruodyte R, Jürimäe J, Saar M, et al. The relationships among bone health, insulin-like growth factor-1 and sex hormones in adolescent female athletes. J Bone Miner Metab 2010;28(3):306–13.

53. Loud KJ, Gordon CM. Adolescent bone health. Arch Pediatr Adolesc Med 2006; 160(10):1026–32.

54. Nordström A, Karlsson C, Nyquist F, et al. Bone loss and fracture risk after reduced physical activity. J Bone Miner Res 2005;20(2):202–7.

55. Beshgetoor D, Nichols JF, Rego I. Effect of training mode and calcium intake on bone mineral density in female master cyclist, runners, and non-athletes. Int J Sport Nutr Exerc Metab 2000;10(3):290–301.

56. Nichols JF, Rauh MJ. Longitudinal changes in bone mineral density in male master cyclists and nonathletes. J Strength Cond Res 2011;25(3):727–34.

57. Black DM, Arden NK, Palermo L, et al. Prevalent vertebral deformities predict hip fractures and new vertebral deformities but not wrist fractures. Study of Osteoporotic Fractures Research Group. J Bone Miner Res 1999;14(5):821–8.

58. Peer KS, Newsham KR. A case study on osteoporosis in a male athlete: looking beyond the usual suspects. Orthop Nurs 2005;24(3):193–9 [quiz: 200–1].

59. Lusins JO, Elting JJ, Cicoria AD, et al. SPECT evaluation of lumbar spondylolysis and spondylolisthesis. Spine (Phila Pa 1976) 1994;19(5):608–12.

60. Campbell RS, Grainger AJ, Hide IG, et al. Juvenile spondylolysis: a comparative analysis of CT, SPECT and MRI. Skeletal Radiol 2005;34(2):63–73.

61. Ellis KJ, Shypailo RJ, Hardin DS, et al. Z score prediction model for assessment of bone mineral content in pediatric diseases. J Bone Miner Res 2001;16(9):1658–64.

62. Brown JP, Albert C, Nassar BA, et al. Bone turnover markers in the management of postmenopausal osteoporosis. Clin Biochem 2009;42(10-11):929–42.

63. Daffner RH, Pavlov H. Stress fractures: current concepts. AJR Am J Roentgenol 1992;159(2):245–52.

64. Knapp TP, Garrett WE Jr. Stress fractures: general concepts. Clin Sports Med 1997;16(2):339–56.

65. Matheson GO, Clement DB, McKenzie DC, et al. Stress fractures in athletes: a study of 320 cases. Am J Sports Med 1987;15(1):46–58.

66. Rutherford OM. Spine and total body bone mineral density in amenorrheic endurance athletes. J Appl Physiol 1993;74(6):2904–8.

67. McHugh-Pierzina VL, Zillmer DA, Giangarra CE. Thoracic compression fracture in a basketball player. J Athl Train 1995;30(2):163–4.

68. Fechtenbaum J, Cropet C, Kolta S, et al. The severity of vertebral fractures and health-related quality of life in osteoporotic postmenopausal women. Osteoporos Int 2005;16(12):2175–9.

69. Esses SI, McGuire R, Jenkins J, et al. The treatment of symptomatic osteoporotic spinal compression fractures. J Am Acad Orthop Surg 2011;19(3):176–82.

70. Hensinger RN. Spondylolysis and spondylolisthesis in children and adolescents. J Bone Joint Surg [Am] 1989;71(7):1098–107.

71. Jackson DW, Wiltse LL, Cirincoine RJ. Spondylolysis in the female gymnast. Clin Orthop Relat Res 1976;117:68–73.

72. Sairyo K, Katoh S, Sasa T, et al. Athletes with unilateral spondylolysis are at risk of stress fracture at the contralateral pedicle and pars interarticularis: a clinical and biomechanical study. Am J Sports Med 2005;33(4):583–90.

73. Weatherley CR, Mehdian H, Berghe LV. Low back pain with fracture of the pedicle and contralateral spondylolysis: a technique of surgical management. J Bone Joint Surg [Br] 1991;73(6):990–3.

74. Abel MS. Jogger's fracture and other stress fractures of the lumbo-sacral spine. Skeletal Radiol 1985;13(3):221–7.

75. Gunzburg R, Fraser RD. Stress fracture of the lumbar pedicle: case reports of "pediculolysis" and review of the literature. Spine (Phila Pa 1976) 1991;16(2):185–9.

76. Fehlandt AF, Micheli LJ. Lumbar facet stress fractures in a ballet dancer. Spine 1993;18(16):2537–9.

77. Beals KA, Manore MM. Disorders of the female athlete triad among collegiate athletes. Int J Sport Nutr Exerc Metab 2002;12(3):281–93.

78. Goulding A, Taylor RW, Jones IE, et al. Spinal overload: a concern for obese children and adolescents? Osteoporos Int 2002;13(10):835–40.

79. Goulding A, Grant AM, Williams SM. Bone and body composition of children and adolescents with repeated forearm fractures. J Bone Miner Res 2005;20(12): 2090–6.

80. Braam LA, Knapen MH, Geusens P, et al. Factors affecting bone loss in female endurance athletes: a two-year follow-up study. Am J Sports Med 2003;31(6):889–95.

81. Hinrichs T, Chae E-H, Lehmann R, et al. Bone mineral density in athletes of different disciplines: a cross-sectional study. Open Sports Sci J 2010;3:129–33.

82. Nattiv A, Loucks AB, Manore MM, et al. American College of Sports Medicine position stand: the female athlete triad. Med Sci Sports Exerc 2007;39(10):1867–82.

83. Sundgot-Borgen J, Torstveit MK. Prevalence of eating disorders in elite athletes is higher than in the general population. Clin J Sport Med 2004;14(1):25–32.

84. Hoch AZ, Stavrakos JE, Schimke JE. Prevalence of female athlete triad characteristics in a club triathlon team. Arch Phys Med Rehabil 2007;88(5):681–2.

85. Loucks AB, Thuma JR. Luteinizing hormone pulsatility is disrupted at a threshold of energy availability in regularly menstruating women. J Clin Endocrinol Metab 2003; 88(1):297–311.

86. Cauley JA, Hochberg MC, Lui LY, et al. Long-term risk of incident vertebral fractures. JAMA 2007;298(23):2761–7.

87. Lindsay R, Silverman SL, Cooper C, et al. Risk of new vertebral fracture in the year following a fracture. JAMA 2001;285(3):320–3.

88. Jackson RD, LaCroix AZ, Gass M, et al. Calcium plus vitamin D supplementation and the risk of fractures. N Engl J Med 2006;354(7):669–83.

89. Holick MF. Vitamin D deficiency. N Engl J Med 2007;357(3):266–81.

90. Black DM, Cummings SR, Karpf DB, et al. Randomised trial of effect of alendronate on risk of fracture in women with existing vertebral fractures. Fracture Intervention Trial Research Group. Lancet 1996;348(9041):1535–41.

91. Black DM, Delmas PD, Eastell R, et al. Once-yearly zoledronic acid for treatment of postmenopausal osteoporosis. N Engl J Med 2007;356(18):1809–22.

92. Sellmeyer DE. Atypical fractures as a potential complication of long-term bisphosphonate therapy. JAMA 2010;304(13):1480–4.

Spinal Tumors Found in the Athlete

Megan E. Anderson, MD[a,b,c,*]

KEYWORDS

- Spine • Tumor • Adolescent • Aneurysmal bone cyst • Osteoid osteoma
- Osteoblastoma • Giant cell tumor • Hemangioma

KEY POINTS

- Spine tumors in the adolescent athlete population are uncommon.
- A careful history and physical examination can offer clues about a spine tumor.
- Plain x-rays and magnetic resonance imaging are often the most helpful imaging modalities.
- A high index of suspicion is necessary to identify these lesions.

Spine tumors are infrequently encountered in the adolescent athlete population. However, when they are not identified in a timely manner, the consequences can be significant: spinal deformity, neurologic deficits, longstanding pain, and more. It is thus important for all clinicians caring for athletes to keep neoplasia in their differential when they are evaluating an athlete with a spine complaint.

In this article, clues in presenting symptoms and appropriate imaging are discussed. Specific tumor types that are most commonly encountered in this population and their treatment will also be included. This is not intended as an exhaustive review of spine tumors in general but truly focused to the adolescent athlete.

PRESENTATION

Most athletes with a spine tumor present similarly to those with overuse syndromes or traumatic injuries: with pain. Pain that persists beyond the normal timeframe for an injury or overuse problem or pain that is of a much more severe intensity should prompt further investigation. Pain associated with signs of nerve root compression,

The author has nothing to disclose.

[a] Children's Hospital Boston, Department of Orthopaedic Surgery, Hunnewell 2, 300 Longwood Avenue, Boston, MA 02115, USA; [b] Beth Israel Deaconess Medical Center, Boston, MA, USA; [c] Harvard Medical School, Boston, MA, USA

* Children's Hospital Boston, Department of Orthopaedic Surgery, Hunnewell 2, 300 Longwood Avenue, Boston, MA 02115.

E-mail address: megan.anderson@childrens.harvard.edu

myelopathy, or spinal deformity should trigger a more urgent evaluation. Pain that is worse at rest and when lying down at night can be a worrisome feature as well.

Athletes may also present with a tumor as an incidental finding when they are being evaluated after trauma or overuse. Many of these lesions are benign, but consultation with a clinical spine tumor specialist or radiologist should be the default so that the appropriate workup and biopsy, if necessary, can be performed.

Physical examination should be directed to the area of concern (eg, upper extremities for cervical spine), checking for radicular nerve root or cord compression findings. The athlete should be evaluated for spinal deformity as well. An acute curve toward the side of pain may be a spastic scoliosis caused by inflammation from a tumor such as an osteoid osteoma. An acute kyphosis may indicate vertebral body collapse secondary to involvement of the vertebral body with tumor or Langerhans cell histiocytosis. Any of these findings warrant further evaluation with imaging studies.

Section Summary

Keep spine tumor in the differential for an athlete with back pain

- Back pain that persists longer than normal
- Pain that is more severe than normal
- Spinal deformity with pain
- Nerve root compression and/or myelopathy.

IMAGING

Plain radiographs are rarely diagnostic in the evaluation of a patient with a spine tumor. They may indicate clues, however, that should prompt further evaluation. Spinal deformity would be evident on full spine x-rays. The absence of the bony landmark of the pedicle, the "winking owl sign," may indicate that a pedicle is involved with tumor. Either of these findings would then necessitate further 3-dimensional imaging studies.

Magnetic resonance imaging (MRI) is extremely helpful in evaluating a patient with a spine tumor. The normal anatomy of the neighboring cord, cauda equina, or exiting nerve roots is demonstrated, along with their relation and proximity to the tumor. Soft tissue tumors, both intra- and extradural, are best delineated with this modality. Bone tumors are also nicely assessed with MRI where internal characteristics of certain tumors can be identified (these will be discussed with specific tumor types below). Computed tomography (CT) is better at evaluating the intraosseous extent and thus fracture risk associated with a spine tumor with bony involvement. CT can also identify internal osteoid, bone, or cartilage matrix formation within a tumor.[1]

Bone scan is really only useful when multiple lesions are suspected or if the clinician cannot easily localize the site of origin of an athlete with concerning spine pain. Otherwise, bone scan typically does not add to what may be gleaned from MRI and CT. It is, however, part of the staging process for a malignant primary tumor of bone.

Section Summary

- MRI is the basis for imaging most spine tumors
- CT is helpful for bone tumors and to assess fracture risk
- Bone scan can be useful to pinpoint the area of concern.

SPECIFIC TUMORS AND TUMORLIKE CONDITIONS
Enostosis

Also know as a bone island, enostoses are almost always incidental findings. They are more of a developmental abnormality than a true neoplasm, a result of incomplete bone resorption during bone maturation. They appear as dense areas of lamellar compact bone within cancellous bone and typically have a slightly brushed or spiculated border on CT. They are universally low signal on all MRI sequence and can have uptake on bone scan. Treatment is observation. A suspected enostosis that enlarges more than 25% in 6 months should be evaluated further.[2]

Osteoid Osteoma

Osteoid osteomas are very small lesions (>1.5 cm) that incite a tremendous inflammatory response. They are located in the spine in only 10% of cases, where most are lumbar, followed by cervical, thoracic, then sacral, in location, typically in the posterior elements.[2] They classically cause pain that is worse at night, unrelated to activity, and better with nonsteroidal anti-inflammatory drugs (NSAIDs) or aspirin. Painful scoliosis is a frequent association as noted above (**Fig. 1A**).

They are so small that they usually cannot be identified on plain radiographs. CT is the modality of choice where the small radiolucent nidus is often surrounded by a significant amount of sclerotic reactive bone (see **Fig. 1B**). Bone scan can help focus the area of concern, and then a CT can be performed of that area in detail if osteoid osteoma is suspected, if there is difficulty localizing the lesion. These lesions typically have a significant amount of uptake on a bone scan (see **Fig. 1C**). On MRI, the lesion is often obscured by the tremendous surrounding edema but is usually low to intermediate in signal on T1 and variable on T2 (see **Fig. 1D**).

Treatment ranges from long-term treatment with NSAIDs to surgical resection. The symptoms do tend to "burn out" over time, but this may take several years and the side effects of chronic NSAID use leads many to seek surgical intervention. Observation is of course the best option for osteoid osteomas in locations that are difficult to access. The painful scoliosis often resolves as the pain does, but may persist if the symptoms go on for over 15 months.[3] Radiofrequency ablation is an appealing technique, as it is minimally invasive with little recovery time and good success. However, it must be used with caution in the spine because of the proximity of neural elements.[4] Surgical excision usually provides immediate pain relief but must be balanced against the risks of the surgical approach and the needed resection and reconstruction. Intraoperative bone scan can assist in localizing and thus performing a complete resection in these cases (see **Fig. 1E**).[5]

Osteoblastoma

Osteoblastomas are very similar to osteoid osteomas pathologically but often differ in their presentation. Patients frequently complain of a dull pain not relieved by NSAIDs. They are less often associated with scoliosis. Osteoblastomas involve the spine 30% to 40% of the time and they can be locally aggressive.[1,2] On imaging they are larger than 2 cm and can be purely radiolucent or demonstrate internal osteoid matrix. The CT shows a geographic lesion that may expand and thin the cortex significantly. Most are either in the posterior elements or in the posterior elements with extension into the body. MRI shows a lesion that is hypointense on T1 and hyperintense on T2 sequences other than the mineralization, which is hypointense universally. They enhance after injection of contrast

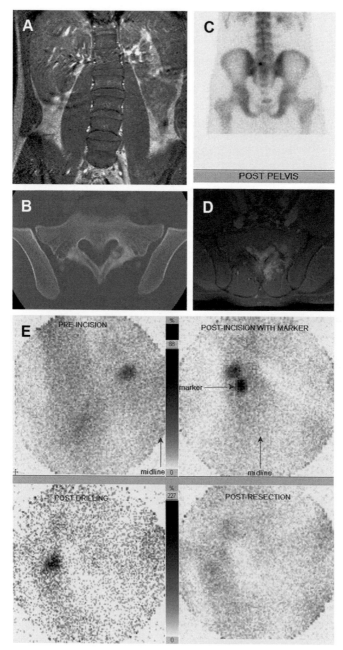

Fig. 1. Osteoid osteoma of the S1 lamina. (*A*) Inflammatory scoliosis noted on the coronal scout during the patient's MRI. (*B*) Axial CT image through the area of concern. Note the radiolucent nidus with central matrix mineralization surrounded by reactive sclerotic bone. (*C*) Bone scan shows significant uptake in the S1 lamina recorded from a posterior projection. (*D*) Axial MRI image T1 with fat saturation after contrast administration shows the significant inflammatory change around the lesion. (*E*) Bone scan images acquired during surgical resection of the S1 osteoid osteoma.

material. They often have a marked surrounding inflammatory response, termed the *flare phenomenon*, which may lead to overestimation of the size of the lesion.[1]

The preferred treatment is complete resection, but often curettage and bone grafting are the only possibility because of the risk of significant neurologic injury associated with the former. Recurrence rates are high, ranging from 10% to 20%.[3]

Aneurysmal Bone Cyst

Aneurysmal bone cysts involve the spine in 3% to 20% of cases, with the majority in the posterior elements, some expanding into the vertebral body.[1,2] These lesions are purely radiolucent on radiographs and CT and have a bubbly, expanded appearance with a very thin cortical shell (**Fig. 2A**). On MRI, fluid-fluid levels are common within large spaces within the lesion (see **Fig. 2B**). These are caused by the blood in these spaces separating into solid and fluid components.

Treatment depends on the location of the lesion. In areas that can be approached and removed surgically, excision is the treatment of choice and is associated with a lower recurrence rate. Curettage and bone grafting is associated with a higher recurrence rate and may be associated with significant blood loss intraoperatively, prompting many surgeons to advise preoperative embolization. A surgical approach is the treatment recommendation for an aneurysmal bone cyst associated with fracture or neurologic involvement.[3]

Recent series have pointed to success with multiple injection procedures for these lesions, especially in lesions that are difficult to approach. Selective embolization or sclerotherapy has been associated with good healing responses and low risks when performed by a subspecialized team (see **Fig. 2C**).[3]

Hemangioma

Hemangiomas are the most common benign bone tumor in the spine and are frequently found incidentally. They can be solitary or multiple, and most involve the vertebral body. When they are large or involve the pedicle, they can present a risk for fracture. This is particularly the case for transitional vertebral body levels.[6] On CT, the coarse striations of trabecular bone between the irregular vascular spaces are evident and give a honeycomb or polka dot appearance depending on whether they are imaged in line with the trabeculae or en face. On MRI, they have a high signal intensity on T1- and T2-weighted images because of the fatty tissue within them and fluid, respectively.[1]

If hemangiomas are an incidental finding and are reasonably small, no treatment is necessary. If they are large, growing in size, or present risk for pathologic fracture, they need to be treated surgically with excision and reconstruction.

Langerhans Cell Histiocytosis

Langerhans cell histiocytosis is the abnormal proliferation of histiocytes from the reticuloendothelial system and not a true neoplasia. Bone involvement is common, and spine location is notable in 10% to 15% of cases.[3] It tends to affect a younger athletic population, in the first and second decades most commonly. Although vertebral collapse into vertebra plana is common, symptoms are usually fairly mild and neurologic symptoms uncommon. If the classic appearance of vertebra plana with no soft tissue mass is identified, these lesions can be followed. Biopsy may injure the residual apophysis, which is necessary to restore height in these bodies.[3] In earlier stages when the lesions are radiolucent with local destruction, biopsy is necessary to rule out more aggressive and malignant lesions (**Fig. 3**). Often, this is the only

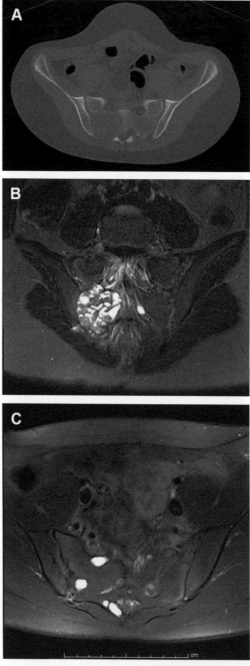

Fig. 2. Aneurysmal bone cyst of the right sacral ala. (*A*) Axial CT image shows thin cortices and expanded appearance of the bone. (*B*) Coronal T2 MRI image through the lesion shows multiple fluid-fluid levels. (*C*) Appearance of the same sacral aneurysmal bone cyst 2 years after 3 sclerotherapy injection procedures on an axial MRI image T2 sequence with fat saturation.

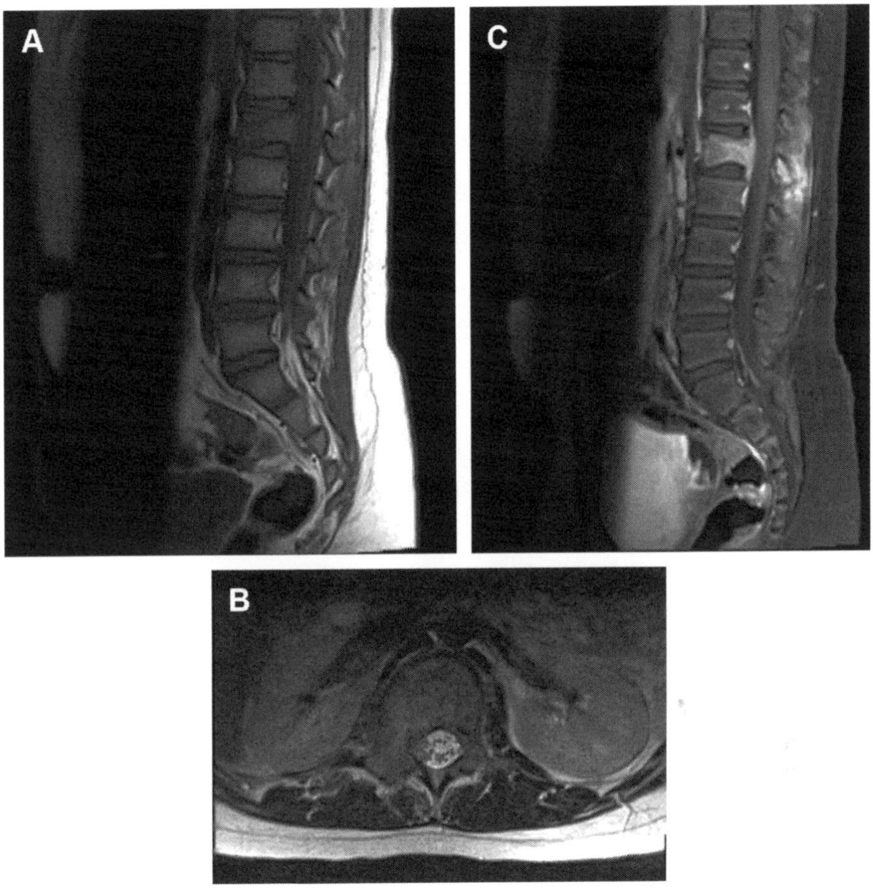

Fig. 3. MRI images of Langerhans cell histiocytosis involving the first lumbar vertebral body and pedicle. (*A*) There is subtle replacement of the fatty bone marrow signal and slight loss of height in the L1 vertebral body on this sagittal T1 sequence. (*B*) Involvement of the pedicle with permeative extension into the soft tissues and epidural space is evident on this axial T2 image. (*C*) The lesion is more apparent and appears aggressive on this sagittal T1 sequence with fat saturation after contrast.

treatment necessary, with or without cortisone injection, as the bone lesion can heal in after biopsy only. At first presentation, evaluation for the patient with Langerhans cell histiocytosis by an oncologist is helpful to evaluate the child for multisystem involvement, in which case systemic therapy would likely be indicated.

Giant Cell Tumor

Giant cell tumor of bone involves the spine in roughly 10% of cases, with the majority involving the sacrum.[2] Patients, mostly young adults, usually present with longstanding pain and occasional signs of nerve root impingement. Some tumors may reach a large size before diagnosis (**Fig. 4**). Imaging shows a radiolucent lesion with cortical thinning and expansion. They can cause enough local destruction to also cause pathologic fracture. MRI shows heterogeneous signal on all imaging sequences.

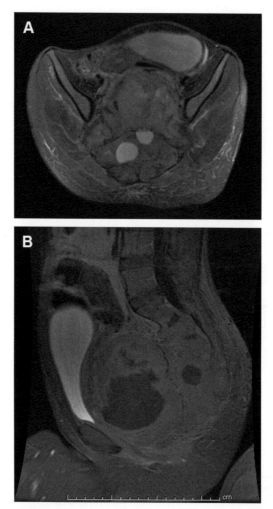

Fig. 4. MRI images of a very large giant cell tumor of the sacrum in a patient who presented with no pain but obstipation and urinary frequency. (*A*) Axial T2-weighted image. (*B*) Sagittal T1-weighted image with fat saturation after contrast administration.

Treatment is based on the size and location of the lesion. If it can be safely removed en bloc, that is usually preferred and can be curative. Often, however, these lesions are difficult to approach and remove entirely because of their location and significant vascularity. Denosumab, the RANK ligand inhibitor, is currently under investigation as an effective agent for unresectable and metastatic giant cell tumor of bone.[7] This may prove to be a monumental swing in the treatment of patients with giant cell tumors of the spine, but further investigation is necessary.

Malignant Tumors

Primary malignant tumors of the spine are rare but certainly can present in the athlete patient population. A high index of suspicion is necessary to diagnose these conditions, however, as most patients present with nonspecific pain. The pain, however, tends to be deep and unresponsive to medications, present independent of activity, worse at night (even waking the patient from sleep) or persistent for longer than traumatic or overuse syndromes. In the adolescent and young adult, the most common entities are osteosarcoma and Ewing sarcoma, but lymphoma and leukemia can also rarely present with spine involvement in this age group.

In addition to pain, many patients may have signs of neurologic compression caused by extension of tumor out of the bone or involvement of the epidural space. In these situations, spinal cord compression requires emergency management, ideally by a multidisciplinary team with experience in spine tumor treatment. Decompression most often requires surgery but can be achieved medically in tumors that are chemosensitive.[8] While steroids are frequently used in the acute setting of an athlete with suspected traumatic cord compression, they should not be used in the situation in which a malignancy is suspected before diagnosis, as some cases of leukemia or lymphoma may resolve entirely with steroids making diagnosis and staging impossible.

Osteosarcoma involves the spine in less than 5% of cases where it tends to arise in the vertebral body most commonly.[9] Imaging demonstrates an aggressive tumor with destruction of normal bone and matrix mineralization within the tumor of a variable extent (**Fig. 5**). In cases in which the tumor is very heavily mineralized, it may appear as an "ivory vertebra." Treatment involves chemotherapy and total spondylectomy or wide local excision, sometimes with the use of radiation as an adjuvant when total resection is not possible. Prognosis is poorer than nonspine osteosarcoma.[9]

Ewing sarcoma more commonly involves the spine in the setting of metastatic disease as opposed to presenting as a primary tumor (3%–6% of all Ewing sarcomas[2]). It most commonly involves the bone (**Fig. 6**) but can also arise in the soft tissues adjacent to the spine. Soft tissue masses from tumors that arise in bone primarily can be quite large (see **Fig. 6**), so neurologic impairment and cord compression are common. The tumors tend to be purely radiolucent and can cause enough bone destruction to cause vertebral body collapse and even vertebra plana. Treatment involves chemotherapy systemically and most commonly radiation therapy for local control. Surgical resection, especially in the rare case the tumor can be removed en bloc, however, may provide more durable local control.[10] Much like osteosarcoma of the spine, Ewing sarcoma on the spine carries a poorer prognosis.

Primary lymphoma of bone is rare and is most commonly a non-Hodgkin's diffuse large cell type. Occasionally, it involves in the spine, arising in the bone, epidural space, or retroperitoneal lymph nodes. Much like Ewing sarcoma, when it arises in bone, the soft tissue component can be very large and result in cord compression. Most lesions are radiolucent, but some can be mixed or sclerotic. Lymphoma can also be sclerotic enough to cause the "ivory vertebra" appearance, and these cases are more often Hodgkin's lymphoma. Treatment frequently involves laminectomy and biopsy for decompression and diagnosis then systemic chemotherapy. Radiation is used in some cases of spinal lymphoma to consolidate therapy, more so in adults than children.

When leukemia involves the spine, it tends to be acute lymphoblastic leukemia.[2] Often several vertebral bodies are involved, usually with radiolucent areas. Compression fractures can also be seen. The involved bone marrow has a lower signal on T1 and higher signal on T2 imaging by MRI. Patients may have systemic symptoms, such as fatigue, weight loss, fever, or lympadenopathy. Chemotherapy is the mainstay of treatment.

Soft tissue masses in the tissues adjacent to the bony spine or within or near the spinal cord itself may also rarely present in the athlete. These are so rare, however, they are beyond the scope of this paper.

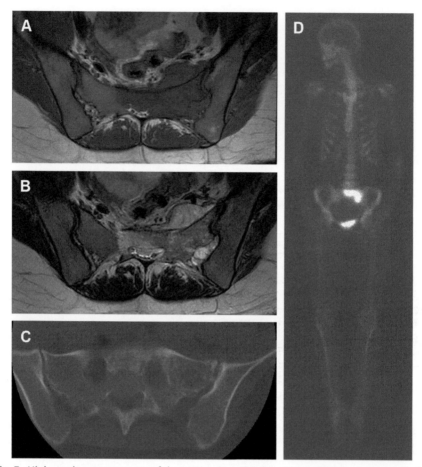

Fig. 5. High-grade osteosarcoma of the sacrum in a 25-year-old woman who presented with pain and radicular symptoms. The MR images show a marrow-replacing process with extension of the T1 hypointense (*A*) T2 hyperintense (*B*) tumor into the soft tissues. The lesion has a permeative appearance on CT (*C*) with areas of bone destruction mixed with subtle areas of matrix mineralization. There is intense activity in the lesion on bone scan (*D*) with no sites of bony metastasis.

Section Summary

- Malignant tumors of the spine are rare in adolescents
- Osteosarcoma and Ewing sarcoma are most common
- Lymphoma and leukemia can also be seen
- A high index of suspicion is necessary to diagnose these tumors.

SUMMARY

Spine tumors in the athlete are rare but should be included in the differential diagnosis of any patient in the adolescent or young adult age group with persistent

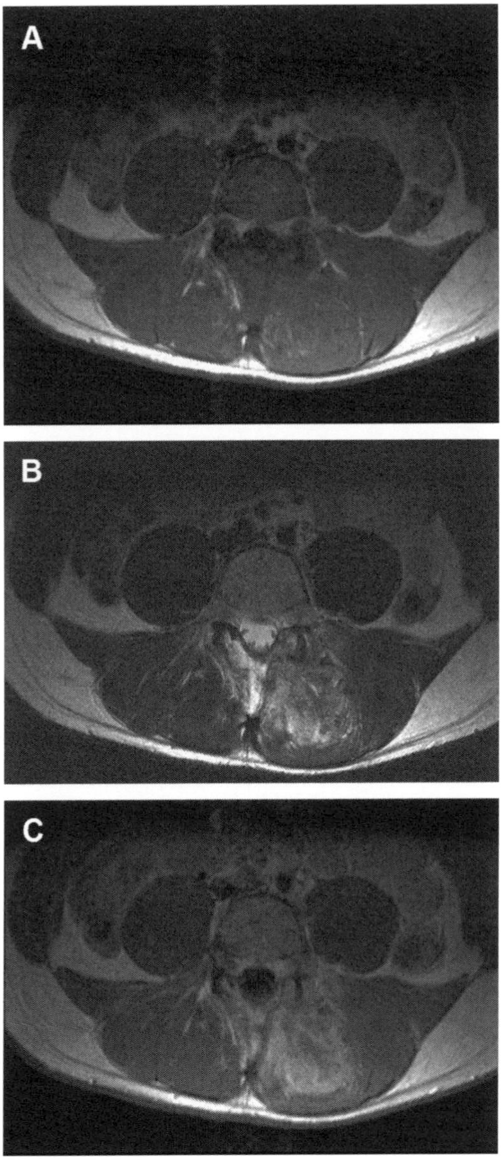

Fig. 6. Ewing sarcoma of the posterior elements of L4 in a 17-year-old boy who presented with pain in his lower back radiating down his left leg. The MRI showed a permeative and destructive mass of the posterior elements of L4 with extension into a large soft tissue mass: (A) axial T1-weighted image, (B) axial T2-weighted image, (C) axial T1-weighted image with fat saturation after the administration of gadolinium.

or severe pain. Presenting symptoms are often nonspecific, so a high index of suspicion is needed to diagnose these lesions in a timely fashion. Early recognition and referral to an appropriate multidisciplinary spine tumor center can greatly improve prognosis for these challenging cases.

REFERENCES

1. Rodallec MH, Feydy A, Larousserie F, et al. Diagnostic imaging of solitary tumors of the spine: what to do and say. Radiographics 2008;28(4):1019–41.
2. Abdel Razek AAK, Castillo M. Imaging appearance of primary bone tumors and pseudo-tumors of the spine. J Neuroradiol 2010;37(1):37–50.
3. Gasbarrini A, Cappuccio M, Donthineni R, et al. Management of benign tumors of the mobile spine. Orthop Clin North Am 2009;40(1):10–9.
4. Rybak LD, Gangi A, Buy X, et al. Thermal ablation of spinal osteoid osteomas close to neural elements: technical considerations. Am J Roentgenol 2010;195(4):w293–8.
5. Blaskiewicz DJ, Sure DR, Hedequist DJ, et al. Osteoid osteomas: intraoperative bone scan-assisted resection. J Neurosurg Pediatr 2009;4(3):237–44.
6. Vinay S, Khan SK, Braybrooke JR. Lumbar vertebral haemangioma causing pathologic fracture, epidural haemorrhage, and cord compression: a case report and review of the literature. J Spinal Cord Med 2011;34(3):335–9.
7. Thomas D, Henshaw R, Skubitz K, et al. Denosumab in patients with giant-cell tumor of bone: an open-label phase 2 study. Lancet Oncol 2010;11(3):275–80.
8. Wilne S, Walker D. Spine and spinal cord tumours in children: a diagnostic and therapeutic challenge to healthcare systems. Arch Dis Chil Educ Pract Ed 2010;95: 47–54.
9. Sundaresan N, Rosen G, Boriani S. Primary malignant tumors of the spine. Orthop Clin North Am 2009;40(1):21–36.
10. Boriani S, Amendola L, Corghi A, et al. Ewing's sarcoma of the mobile spine. Eur Rev Med Pharmacol Sci 2011;15(7):831–9.

Index

Note: Page numbers of article titles are in **boldface** type.

Clin Sports Med 31 (2012) 581–588
http://dx.doi.org/10.1016/S0278-5919(12)00039-7
0278-5919/12/$ – see front matter © 2012 Elsevier Inc. All rights reserved.

sportsmed.theclinics.com

Printed and bound by CPI Group (UK) Ltd, Croydon, CR0 4YY

14/10/2024

01773652-0001